EMERGENCY MEDICINE

PEARLS OF WISDOM

ORAL BOARD REVIEW
Third Edition

William Gossman, M.D.

Scott H. Plantz, M.D.

Jonathan Adler, M.D.

NOTE

The intent of Emergency Medicine Oral Board Review *Pearls of Wisdom,* Third Edition, is to serve as a study aid to improve performance on a standardized oral exam. It is not intended to be a source text of the knowledge base of emergency medicine, nor to serve as a reference in any way for the practice of clinical emergency medicine. The authors do not warrant that the information in this text is complete or accurate. The reader is encouraged to verify each answer in several references. All drug use indications and dosages must be verified by the reader before administration of any compound.

Printed in U.S.A.

The editors would like to extend thanks to Terri Lair for her excellent managing and editorial support.

Art Director/Cover Design: Cleiton Gonçalves

This book was produced using Times and Symbols fonts and computer based graphics with Macintosh® computers

ISBN: 1-58409-074-X

DEDICATION

For my wife, Sherry; daughters Casey and Taylor.

Bill

For my brother, Brad, for his love and support through all our trials and tribulations.

Scott

For my wife, Elise, for her love and support.

Jonathan

AUTHORS AND EDITORS

William Gossman, M.D.
Assistant Prof. of Emergency Medicine
Chicago Medical School
Research Director, Depart of Emergency Medicine
Mt. Sinai Medical Center
Chicago, IL

Scott H. Plantz, M.D.
Associate Prof. of Emergency Medicine
Chicago Medical School
Research Director
Mt. Sinai Medical Center
Chicago, IL

Jonathan Adler, M.D.
Massachusetts General Hospital
Instructor in Medicine
Harvard Medical School
Boston, MA

CONTRIBUTING AUTHORS AND EDITORS

Bobby Abrams, M.D., FAAEM
Attending Physician
Macomb Hospital
Macomb, MI

David F.M. Brown, M.D.
Assistant in Emergency Medicine,
Massachusetts General Hospital
Instructor in Medicine
Harvard Medical School
Boston, MA

Eduardo Castro, M.D.
Assistant in Emergency Medicine
Massachusetts General Hospital
Instructor in Medicine
Harvard Medical School
Boston, MA

James Corrall, M.D.
Clinical Instructor of Emergency Medicine
University of Illinois College of Medicine
St. Francis Medical Center
Peoria, IL

Bikram S. Dhillon, M.D.
Assistant Clinical Professor of Medicine
University of Illinois School of Medicine
Dept. of Emergency Medicine
Illinois Masonic Medical Center
Chicago, IL

Stephen Emond, M.D.
Assistant in Emergency Medicine
Massachusetts General Hospital
Instructor in Medicine
Harvard Medical School
Boston, MA

Craig Feied, M.D., FAAEM
Assoc. Prof. of Emergency Medicine
Director of Informatics
Dept. of Emergency Medicine
Washington Hospital Center
Washington, DC

Lindsey Harrell, M.D.
Holston Valley Group
Kingsport, TN

James Holmes, M.D.
Division of Emergency Medicine
U of C, Davis School of Medicine
Sacramento, CA

Eddie Hooker, M.D., FAAEM
Asst. Professor, Dept. of Emergency
University of Louisville
Louisville, KY

Lance W. Kreplick, M.D., FAAEM
Asst. Prof., University of Illinois
Director, Dept. of Emergency Medicine
Christ Hospital and Medical Center
Oak Lawn, IL

Joe Lex, MD, FAAEM
Attending Physician
Chestnut Hill Hospital
Philadelphia, PA

Bernard Lopez, M.D., FAAEM
Asst. Prof. of Surgery
Dept. of Emergency Medicine
Jefferson Medical College
Philadelphia, PA

Mary Nan Mallory, M.D., FAAEM
Asst. Prof. of Emergency Medicine
Dept. of Emergency Medicine
University of Louisville
Louisville, KY

David Morgan, M.D., FAAEM
Assistant in Emergency Medicine
Section of Emergency Medicine
Southwest Medical Center - Dallas, Texas

Edward Panacek, M.D., FAAEM
Associate Prof. of Medicine
Division of Emergency Medicine
U of California, Davis School of Medicine
Sacramento, CA

Carlo Rosen, M.D.
Assistant in Emergency Medicine
Massachusetts General Hospital
Instructor in Medicine
Harvard Medical School
Boston, MA

David C. Smith, D.O.
Chief of Emergency Services
Mike O'Callyhan Federal Hospital
Las Vegas, NV

Dana Stearns, M.D.
Assistant in Emergency Medicine
Massachusetts General Hospital
Instructor in Medicine
Harvard Medical School
Boston, MA

Jack "Lester" Stump, M.D., FAAEM
Attending Physician
Rogue Valley Medical Center
Medford, OR

Loice Swischer, M.D., FAAEM
Asst. Prof. of Emergency Medicine
Dept. of Emergency Medicine
Medical College of Philadelphia
Philadelphia, PA

Stephen H. Thomas, M.D.
Instructor of Internal Medicine
Harvard Medical School
Associate Director of Boston Medflight
Dept. of Emergency Medicine
Massachusetts General Hospital
Boston, MA

James Unger, M.D., FAAEM
Co-Director, Center for Emergency Medicine
Dept. of Emergency Medicine
Redding, CA

Thomas Widell, M.D.
Assistant Professor of Emergency Medicine
Chicago Medical School
Asst. Residency Director
Dept. of Emergency Medicine
Mt. Sinai Medical Center

Leslie Zun, M.D.
Associate Professor of Emergency Medicine
Chicago Medical School
Chairman of Emergency Medicine
Dept. of Emergency Medicine
Mt. Sinai Medical Center
Chicago, IL

John Wipfler, M.D.
Asst. Prof. of Emergency Medicine
University of Illinois College of Medicine
St. Francis Medical Center
Peoria, IL

WE APPRECIATE YOUR COMMENTS!

We appreciate your opinion and encourage you to send us any suggestions or recommendations. Please let us know if you discover any errors, or if there is any way we can make our *Pearls of Wisdom* Text more helpful to you. We are also interested in recruiting new authors and editors. Please call, write, fax, or e-mail. We look forward to hearing from you.

W.G., S.H.P. & J.N.A.

Send comments to:

Boston Medical Publishing Corporation
4780 Linden Street, Lincoln, NE 68516

Toll Free: 1-888-MBOARDS (626-2737)
Tel: 402-484-6118
FAX: 402-484-6552
E-MAIL: bmpcorp@inebraska.com

www.bmppearls.com

INTRODUCTION

Congratulations! Emergency Medicine Oral Boards *Pearls of Wisdom*, Third Edition, will help you learn some emergency medicine. Originally designed as a study aid to improve performance on the EM Oral Board Exam, "Pearls" is full of useful information. First intended for EM specialists, we have learned that *"Pearls"* unique format has also been useful to house officers and medical students rotating in the ED. A few words are appropriate discussing intent, format, limitations and use.

The primary intent of “Pearls” is to serve as a study aid to improve performance on the EM Oral Board Exam. To achieve this goal the text is written in three formats: a topic review, a rapid-fire question/answer format, and actual practice cases. Emphasis has been placed on distilling true trivia and key facts that are easily overlooked, are quickly forgotten, and that somehow seem to be needed on board exams.

The first third of the text is presented in a straightforward format with more basic facts. The second section of the book consists of random pathophysiology, procedure, and treatment pearls with some questions selected from the Emergency Medicine Written *Pearls of Wisdom, 6 Ed.* The questions are grouped into small clusters by topic presented in no particular order. The random Pearls section repeats much of the factual information contained in the Pearls Topics and builds on this foundation with greater emphasis on linking information and filling in gaps from the Pearls Topics. The final section of the text, Oral Boards Cases, is the most important, as it contains actual practice cases that should be used with your study partner to gain confidence and experience in attacking boards cases.

"Pearls" has limitations (directly proportional to those of the senior editor/authors!). We have found *many* conflicts between sources of information. Variation between the definition of “apneustic” breathing provided in Tintinalli vs. Stedman’s causes little consternation. Variations between half-life of paralyzing agents and of naloxone, or between rankings of stability of cervical spine fractures, provided in Tintinalli vs. Rosen are more concerning. We have tried to verify in other references the most accurate information. Some texts have internal discrepancies further confounding clarification of information.

"Pearls" risks accuracy by aggressively pruning complex concepts down to the simplest kernel - the dynamic knowledge base and clinical practice of emergency medicine is not like that! For the most part, the information taken as "correct" is that indicated in the texts, Emergency Medicine, A Comprehensive Study Guide, edited by Tintinalli, Krome and Ruiz and The Clinical Practice of Emergency Medicine, edited by Harwood-Nuss, Linden, Luten, Shepherd, and Wolfson.

New research and practice occasionally deviates from that which likely represents the "right" answer for test purposes. In such cases we have selected the information that we believe is most likely to be "correct" for test purposes. This text is designed to maximize your score on a test. Refer to your most current sources of information and mentors for direction for practice.

Most of *"Pearls"* is designed to be used, not just read. It is an *interactive* text. Use a 3x5 card and cover the answers; attempt all questions.

A study method we strongly recommend is oral, group study, preferably over an extended meal or pitchers. The mechanics of this method are simple and no one ever appears stupid.

One person holds *"Pearls"*, with answers covered, and reads the question. Each person, including the reader, says "Check!" when he or she has an answer in mind. After everyone has "checked" in, someone states their answer. If this answer is correct, on to the next one, if not, another person says their answer or the answer can be read. Usually the person who "checks" in first gets the first shot at stating the answer. If this person is being a smarty-pants answer-hog, then others can take turns. Try it, it's almost fun! Oral board cases can be reviewed in small groups as well, with one individual playing the examiner, one student, and the rest of the group providing comments.

"Pearls" is also designed to be re-used several times to allow, dare we use the word, memorization. One co-editor (Plantz), a pessimist, suggests putting a check mark in each box provided every time a question is missed. Thus, two boxes have been arbitrarily provided. If you fill all the boxes on two reviews of *"Pearls"*, forget this question! You will get it wrong on the exam!

Another suggestion is to place a check mark when the question is answered correctly once; skip all questions with check marks thereafter. Utilize whatever scheme of using the check boxes you prefer.

We welcome your comments, suggestions, and criticism. Great effort has been made to verify these topics, questions and answers, and cases. There will be information we have provided that is at variance with your knowledge. Most often this is attributable to the variance between original sources (previously discussed). Please make us aware of any errata you find. We hope to make continuous improvements and would greatly appreciate any input with regard to format, organization, content, presentation, or about specific questions. Please contact Terri Lair, our managing editor, at 1-888-MBOARDS (626-2737).

Study hard and good luck!

Bill, Scott, and Jon

TABLE OF CONTENTS

ORAL BOARD PREPARATION

"Learning to learn is to know how to
navigate in a forest of facts, ideas and theories,
a proliferation of constantly and changing items of knowledge.
Learning to learn is to know what
to ignore but at the same time not rejecting
innovation and research."

Raymond Queneau

GENERAL EXAM INFORMATION

1. Where:

The exam is located in Chicago and is administered twice a year. The earlier you register after the written exam, the greater the probability you will be admitted to the next test period.

2. Pass Rate:

Over eighty percent.

3. Expenses:

Exam fee plus cost of hotel and travel.

4. Duration of Exam:

About 4 hours with two 20 minute breaks.

5. Number of Cases Comprising the Exam:

Five single cases administered (each lasting 15 minutes of actual testing), and two triples (each lasting 30 minutes of actual testing). One single case will consist of a field-test case and will not be scored.

6. Time of the day:

Morning or afternoon. They will assign you a day and a time slot. You may request to change the time and the day of the exam. If submitted early, your request is usually granted.

7. Scoring:

7.1 The eight point scale contains the following sections.

A. **Data Acquisition**: The data acquisition evaluation will be based on how efficiently and completely you acquire important data based upon the patient's medical history, the physical exam, and the laboratory results. This involves a reasonable use of labs, X-rays, etc., as well as obtaining relevant information from family physicians and consultants. If paramedics, family members, or friends of the patient are present, consult with them liberally as **they have important information required for managing the case.**

B. **Problem Solving**: You will be rated on your ability to diagnose a problem in an organized and thoughtful manner. How well you anticipate potential problems and then prepare for these situations accordingly will also be examined. (For example: Maintain airway equipment near the bedside of a patient diagnosed with anaphylactic reaction.)

C. **Patient Management**: Your skills to formulate a correct and timely treatment program will be tested. You must be able to effectively communicate your management, administer correct drug doses, use appropriate ACLS and ATLS algorithms, and obtain suitable consultations in a timely fashion.

D. **Resource Utilization**: This section will ascertain your ability to utilize available resources to aid in caring for your patient. Such resources include the Poison Control Center, the pharmacy, textbooks, and consultants. If you are unsure of something **DON'T GUESS,** you may be labeled as dangerous.

E. **Health Care Provided**: The examiner will ask two questions: **1)** Did the patient receive timely and appropriate medical treatment, and **2)** Did the patient's condition improve by the care provided? The patient should improve due to the treatment you provided.
F. **Interpersonal Relations**: You will be evaluated on your ability to interact with patients and family members in a compassionate and informative manner. All procedures or painful examination techniques must be explained to the patient before they are conducted. In addition, always assume an unconscious patient can still hear and warn him/her of impending painful maneuvers and procedures.
G. **Clinical Competence (Overall)**: This is the single most important rating of the eight scoring criteria. Overall, how well did you do? The examiner will judge your level of proficiency by accessing your combined cognitive and procedural skills in providing emergency care in this setting.

7.2 The eight performance ratings are scored on an 8 point scale for each oral case.
A. **Very Acceptable (7,8)**: The examiner does not have significant criticisms of the candidate's ability to diagnose and manage the case.
B. **Acceptable (5,6)**: All critical actions were addressed and no dangerous actions were undertaken.
C. **Unacceptable (3,4)**: One or more critical actions were not taken and/or one or more dangerous actions were implemented.
D. **Very Unacceptable (1,2)**: Gross negligence and/or mismanagement was observed.

7.3 Pass/Fail Criteria: A candidate passes the exam by fulfilling one of the following two pass/fail criteria.
A. The average score calculated from all of the cases is 5.75 or higher.
B. The highest and lowest cases are averaged. If this score and the scores from the remaining four cases are all 5.00 or above, you pass.

8. Examination Procedures:

8.1 Obtain initial vital signs and a brief history. While discussing medical history, communicate with the examiner as you would talk to a real patient.
8.2 Perform a physical exam. Remember you will be in charge. Nothing will be done unless you ask for it.
8.3 Order labs, X-rays, etc., without "shot gunning".
8.4 Review labs, X-ray results, etc. Abnormal lab values will not be highlighted.
8.5 Based upon all the information gathered, make a diagnosis and take the appropriate actions. The patient will deteriorate or improve based upon your actions.
8.6 The examiner will end the case, ask one or more questions, and then excuse you.
8.7 Feedback will not be provided.

9. Strategies:

9.1 Take your time and approach the exam systematically.
9.2 Ask for general information. For example: "What do I see as I observe the patient?"
9.3 Develop a system for taking notes and practice it.
9.4 Be direct in verbalizing your actions.
9.5 Listen to the examiner's feedback and cues.
9.6 If certain information cannot be obtained, continue to manage the case.
9.7 Don't verbally interpret X-ray and ECG findings unless asked to do so.
9.8 Know the dosages for commonly used drugs.
9.9 Use consultants as needed.
9.10 Acknowledge that all the examiner's information is correct.
9.11 Normal lab values will be provided.
9.12 Look up information, if necessary.

SUGGESTED OUTLINE OF ATTACK

The following outline provides one method of consistently approaching and treating an exam patient. This system includes a "Primary Survey", which may be interrupted for acute interventions and ordering of tests, a "Secondary Survey", and provision of treatment and disposition. A brief outline is provided below; details of each phase are described in the following sections. It is usually important to cover all of these issues during each case. The editors strongly encourage you to develop your own individualized approach to the patient based on the current history, the physical, and on the treatment approach of your own practice.

PRIMARY SURVEY

Obtain a complete set of vital signs, which may include bilateral BPs and use of a rectal probe. Ask "When I walk in the room, what do I see?"

A. Airway - Includes a c-spine, check for rate and depth of respirations, pooled secretions, gag reflex, and tracheal deviation.

B. Breathing - Air management, effort, breath sounds bilaterally and chest movement.

C. Circulation - BP, capillary refill, skin color and temperature. Perform interventions as determined thus far, i.e., restrain, security, c-spine precautions, intubation, needle thoracostomy/chest tube, etc. Consider interrupting Primary Survey here to order other interventions or tests.

D. Disability - GCS (Motor 6, Verbal 5, Eye 4) and perform a brief neuro exam.

E. Expose - Undress, perform a swift abbreviated exam, roll patient, check skin and look for medical alert tags.

F. Finger and Rectal Exam - Check for gross bleed, occult blood, high riding or "boggy" prostate, and blood at urethral meatus. Pass Foley prn.

G. NG tube and check aspirate.

H. History - A complete history requires AMPLE FRIENDS.

A Allergies.
M Meds
P Past medical history.
L Last meal.
E Events/Environment and chief complaint.

F Family medical history, family, friends and family doctor as sources of information.
R Records, ROS.
I Immunizations.
E EMS personnel as sources of information.
N Narcotic and other drugs/substances of abuse.
D Doctor for admission and consultation.
S Social history (living environment, etc.).

Consider pausing here at the end of the Primary Survey to re-evaluate vital signs and to order additional tests and treatments.

SECONDARY SURVEY

General.
Skin.
HEENT.
Neck.
Lungs/Heart/Chest.
Back.
Abdomen.
Extremities.
Neuro.
Vascular.
Perineum/Rectum/Vagina/Pelvis.

Re-evaluate at the end of the secondary survey and consider ordering further treatment, tests, consultations, and a disposition.

THE PRIMARY SURVEY

Obtain a complete set of vital signs, may include bilateral BPs and use of a rectal probe. Ask "When I walk in the room, what do I see?"

1. Airway

1.1 Assessment: Along with the c-spine.

A. Immobilize c-spine if indicated.
B. Place patient in a Philadelphia or a hard collar.
C. Log-roll patient on to a backboard.
D. Position sandbags or foam blocks to both sides of his/her head.
E. Anchor chin and forehead straps to the board.

1.2 Ask patient if he/she can breath: If yes, move on to "breathing", if no, stop and correct the problem.

A. Perform the chin lift maneuver.
B. Clear the airway of foreign bodies asking if the patient is pooling secretions.
C. If above maneuvers do not work, a definitive airway is required (oropharyngeal, nasopharyngeal, orotracheal, or cricothyrotomy).
D. If intubation is required, pre-oxygenate with 100% O_2 by using a bag-valve-mask. Auscultate the chest and obtain a postintubation chest X-ray.
E. Continue to maintain the c-spine in a neutral position.

2. Breathing:

2.1 Assessment:

A. Expose the neck and chest.
B. Determine rate and depth of respirations.
C. Inspect and palpate the neck and chest for tracheal deviation, for unilateral and bilateral chest movements, and for any signs of injury, such as bruising, crepitance, and tenderness.
D. Auscultate the chest bilaterally.

2.2 Management:

A. Administer a high concentration of oxygen.
B. Treat a tension pneumothorax.
C. Seal an open pneumothorax.
D. Place the patient on a pulse oximeter.

3. Circulation:

3.1 Assessment:

A. Inspect color of skin and presence of rash and petechiae.
B. Ascertain pulse rate and regularity.
C. Determine capillary refill.
D. Obtain blood pressure, if time permits.
E. Find sources of external bleeding.

3.2 Management:

A. Initiate two large bore IVs (14-16 gauge) of warm LR or NS if indicated.
B. Simultaneously obtain appropriate labs.
C. Apply direct pressure to bleeding sites.

D. Place the patient on a cardiac monitor.

3.3 Order:

IV (Bilat Ant Cubital), O_2, monitor, ABG, ECG, X-ray (Csp, CXR, pelvis), labs and coma protocol.

3.4 Treatment:

D_{50}, Narcan, Thiamine, Td.

4. Disability-Brief Neurological Exam:

4.1 Assessment:

A. Determine the level of consciousness by using the Glasgow Coma Scale (GCS).
B. Assess the pupils for size, equality, and reaction.
C. Test the patient's ability to move all extremities.

4.2 Management:

Consider using the following coma protocol:

A. Thiamine, 100 mg IV (not indicated in children less than 10).
B. Narcan, 2 mg IV in adults or 0.01-0.1 mg/kg in pediatrics.
C. Glucose, 50-100 mL of $D_{50}W$ for adults patients, 2-4 mL/kg of $D_{25}W$ = 0.5-1.0 g/kg for pediatric patients ages 1 month to 8 years, and 0.5-1.0 g/kg of $D_{10}W$ for the neonate.

5. Exposure:

5.1 Completely undress the patient.
5.2 Look for a medic alert tag and check his/her wallet for potential medical information.
5.3 Prevent hypothermia.

6. Finger and Foley:

Finger in every orifice. Check for contraindications to placement of Foley, pass prn.

7. NG:

7.1 After assessment of the pelvic bones, genitalia, and rectum, insert all appropriate catheters.

8. History:

Acquisition of a detailed history will aid in determining a diagnosis as well as in obtaining points in the data acquisition, problem solving, interpersonal relations, and clinical competence sections of the performance criteria. Developing a systematic approach and practicing it will help you in collecting the pertinent information in an efficient, complete, and timely manner. The following mnemonic may be useful: **AMPLE FRIENDS.**

A = Allergies.
M = Medications.
P = Past medical history.
L = Last meal.
E = Events/environment related to the injury or illness (History of Present Illness or HPI).

F = Family history, friends, and family doctor (as historians).
R = Records.
I = Immunizations.
E = EMTs and paramedics.
N = Narcotic and other substances of abuse.
D = Doctor for admission including consultants.
S = Social history (alcohol, tobacco, living conditions).

THE SECONDARY SURVEY

1. General:

1.1 Take another look at the patient.
1.2 Recheck vital signs.

2. Skin:

2.1 Check for lacerations, bruising, abrasions, or any abnormal lesions.
2.2 Reassess turgor, color, and capillary refill.

3. Head and Maxillofacial:

3.1 Assessment:
- A. Inspect and palpate the entire head and face for lacerations, contusions, and fractures.
- B. Re-evaluate the pupils while examining the eyes for hemorrhage, penetrating injury, jaundice, visual acuity, and the presence of a contact lens.
- C. Recheck level of consciousness.
- D. Evaluate ears and nose for cerebrospinal fluid leakage and check for a septal hematoma.
- E. Inspect the mouth for evidence of trauma.

3.2 Management:
- A. Maintain an adequate airway.
- B. Control hemorrhage.
- C. Prevent secondary brain injury.

4. Neck:

4.1 Assessment:
- A. Remove the anterior part of the c-collar and inspect for JVD, tracheal deviation, scars, deformity, or masses.
- B. Palpate for tenderness, deformity, swelling, or subcutaneous emphysema.
- C. Auscultate for carotid bruits.

4.2 Management:
- A. Maintain adequate in-line immobilization and protection of the c-spine.
- B. Obtain a cross table lateral c-spine X-ray with the intent of obtaining a complete series in time.

5. Lungs / Heart / Chest:

5.1 Assessment:
- A. Inspect for symmetrical rise and fall, bruising, wounds, hemorrhage, flail segment, and use of accessory muscles. Palpate for tenderness and crepitation.
- B. Auscultate the anterior chest wall and posterior bases for bilateral breath sounds and any adventitious sounds.

5.2 Cardiac:

Listen for murmurs, rubs, gallops, or clicks and distant or muffled tones.

5.3 Management:

A. Obtain a chest X-ray if it hasn't already been ordered.
B. Place the patient on a cardiac monitor and ask for a rhythm strip. Perform an ECG if indicated.
C. Perform a tube thoracostomy if indicated.
D. Perform a pericardiocentesis if indicated.

6. Back:

6.1 Assessment:

A. Log roll the patient while maintaining alignment of the entire spinal column.
B. Palpate, from top to bottom, all areas of the occiput, neck, back and buttocks.
C. Inspect for deformity, wounds, abrasions, ecchymoses, or tenderness.
D. Auscultate the posterior aspect of the chest.

6.2 Management:

Order X-rays if indicated.

7. Abdomen:

7.1 Assessment:

A. Inspect the anterior abdomen for signs of blunt and penetrating injury, deformity, gross appearance (distended or flat), surgical scars, and pregnancy.
B. Auscultate for presence or absence of bowel sounds.
C. Percuss for dullness or subtle rebound tenderness.
D. Palpate for rebound tenderness, guarding, rigidity, pulsatile mass, or thrill.
E. Compress the pelvis while examining for tenderness, abnormal motion, deformity, or crepitance.
F. Request a fetal heart tone monitor prn.

7.2 Management:

A. Transfer the patient directly to the operating room if indicated.
B. Perform a peritoneal lavage if necessary. Consider a CT scan if the DPL is equivocal and the patient is stable.
C. Obtain a pelvic X-ray.
D. Apply pneumatic antishock garment, if indicated for stabilizing a significant pelvic fracture.

8. Extremities:

8.1 Assessment:

A. Inspect upper and lower extremities for the presence of deformities, an expanding hematoma, open wounds, or abrasions.
B. Palpate for sensation, tenderness, crepitation, abnormal movement, and the
C. presence/absence of pulses.
D. Monitor compartment pressure if indicated.

8.2 Management:

A. Apply appropriate splinting devices for fractures as indicated.
B. Relieve pain by prescribing a medication and/or reducing fractures and dislocations.
C. Administer tetanus immunization and antibiotics if indicated.
D. Treat compartment syndrome aggressively.
E. Perform an escharotomy with circumferential burns.
F. Order an angiogram if indicated.
G. Obtain X-rays of suspected fracture sites as indicated. If it hurts after a traumatic event, acquire an X-ray.

9. Neurologic:

9.1 Assessment:

A. Re-evaluate the pupils and level of consciousness.
B. Determine the GCS.
C. Evaluate the upper and lower extremities for motor and sensory responses.
D. Evaluate the DTRs and note the presence/absence of pathologic reflexes (Babinski and ankle clonus).
E. Check cerebellar function
F. Evaluate the gait if possible.
G. Evaluate cranial nerve function.
H. Perform mini-mental status exam prn.

9.2 Management:

A. Continue to ventilate and oxygenate. Hyperventilate if a head injury is present.
B. Ensure that the patient is adequately immobilized.

10. Vascular:

10.1 Assessment:

A. Evaluate symmetry and strength of pulses.
B. Re-evaluate for bleeding sites.

10.2 Management:

A. Apply pressure dressings to bleeding sites and tie bleeding vessels when appropriate.
B. Arrange for a surgical consultation as appropriate.

11. Perineum / Rectum / Vagina / Pelvis:

11.1 Perineal Assessment:

A. Inspect the perineum and genitalia for wounds, swelling, urethral bleeding, or for a scrotal hematoma.
B. Inspect the testicles for swelling, pain, nodules, or for the presence of a varicocele.

11.2 Rectal Assessment:

A. Check the anal sphincter tone.
B. Assess the bowel wall integrity examining for the presence of bone fragments, tenderness, or gross blood.
C. Palpate the prostate noting its position, size, and quality.

11.3 Vaginal Assessment:

A. Check for blood in the vaginal vault.
B. Examine for retained tampons, lacerations, or for the presence of bone fragments.
C. Note for any indications of cervical motion tenderness, abnormal discharge, an enlarged uterus, enlarged ovaries, or for an adnexal mass and/or tenderness.

11.4 Pelvis:

A. Check for pelvis deformity or laxity.
B. Pelvic rock is no longer encouraged.

11.5 Management:

A. Perform a perineum/rectum/vaginal exam at the end of the primary survey if a DPL and a Foley catheter are required.
B. Treat injuries and obtain appropriate consultations.

Complete procedures and order additional tests. Evaluate all results, complete history, notify family contacts, and consult with personal physicians and specialists.

PEARLS

***All problems exist until proven otherwise.**

***All patients with chest pain require a rectal.**

***All patients that need thrombolytics actually have a contraindication.**

***All children are abused.**

***All cardiac patients become hypotensive when given morphine or nitroglycerin.**

***All alcoholics have multiple problems.**

***All seizure patients dislocate something.**

***All pills are somewhere.**

***All patients have allergies.**

***All overdoses are real and need a psychiatric consult.**

***All joints are septic.**

***All patients with an altered level of consciousness have fallen and require a c-collar and backboard.**

***All patients with a soft collar need it replaced with a hard collar.**

***All patients with an abnormal temperature need a rectal probe.**

***All seizure patients are noncompliant with their medication.**

***All single encounter patients need to be admitted.**

***All burns have CO poisoning.**

***All pain that goes away will be replaced by something worse.**

***All patients that have an arrhythmia will eventually need to be shocked.**

***All patients with "the flu" have CO, or some other toxin ingestion, or a dangerous infection.**

***All children under 3 months will need a septic work-up.**

***All females are pregnant.**

***All patients that wake up with D_{50} will need admission.**

***All patients with a pneumothorax need to be quickly needled.**

***All trauma and burn patients are at risk for myoglobinuria.**

***All females of child-bearing age with abdominal pain have ectopics.**

***All children with a head injury have hemophilia.**

***All pearls have exceptions.**

PEDIATRIC PEARLS

1. **Parkland Formula:** Weight (kg) x Percent Burn x 4 = 24 hour total (give 1/2 over the first 8 hours followed by the other 1/2 over the next 16 hours).

2. **ETT Size:** (16 + age) / 4

3. **Pediatric Weight:** (Age x 3) + 6 = Wt in Kg

4. **Pediatric BP:**
   < 1 year of age < 90 Systolic BP
   > 1 year of age 80 + (2 x age) = Systolic BP
   Diastolic BP = 2/3 of the Systolic BP

5. **Pediatric Fluid Bolus:** 20 mL/kg

6. **Blood (PRBCs):** 10 mL/kg in children

7. **Fluid Maintenance:**

4 cc/kg/hour	1st 10 kgs of weight
2 cc/kg/hour	2nd 10 kgs of weight
1 cc/kg/hour	for each kg over 20

8. **Foley catheter and nasogastric tube sizes:**

age	0-5 y	8 y	10 y	12 y
size	5 F	8 F	10 F	12 F

9. **Chest tube sizes:**

age	0-6 y	6-10 y	10-12 y
size	10-20 F	20-30 F	30-38 F

PEARL TOPICS

"The ultimate measure of a man is not where he stands in moments of comfort and convenience, but where he stands at times of challenge and controversy."

Martin Luther King, Jr.

CARDIOVASCULAR

CARDIAC LIFE SUPPORT

1. Ventricular Fibrillation/Pulseless Ventricular Tachycardia Algorithm (VF/VT):*

1.1 Access ABCs.
1.2 Perform CPR until a defibrillator is attached.
1.3 FV/VT are present on monitor.
1.4 Defibrillate up to 3 times with 200 J, 300 J, and 360 J.
1.5 Persistent VF/VT.
1.6 Continue CPR.
1.7 Intubate.
1.8 IV Access.
1.9 Administer epinephrine, 1 mg IV push, repeat q 3-5 minutes or vasopressin 40 U IV, as a single dose, 1 time only.
1.10 Defibrillate with 360 J within 30-60 seconds.
1.11 Medication sequence includes:

- A. Lidocaine, 1.0-1.5 mg/kg IV push, repeat in 3-5 minutes to a maximum dose of 3 mg/kg, or amiodarone 300 mg IV push, repeat 150 mg IV x 1 (max 2.2 g/24 hr).
- B. Magnesium sulfate, 1-2 g IV in torsades de pointes, suspected hypomagnesemic state, or refractory VF.
- C. Procainamide, 30 mg/minute in refractory VF to a maximum total dose of 17 mg/kg.
- D. Sodium bicarbonate, 1 mEq/kg IV, should be used if the following conditions are present:
  - Pre-existing bicarbonate-responsive acidosis.
  - Tricyclic antidepressant overdose.
  - Long cardiac arrest.
  - Hypoxic lactic acidosis.
  - Spontaneous circulation after long cardiac arrest.
  - Suspicion of hyperkalemic state

1.12 Defibrillate 360 J, 30-60 seconds after each dose of medication. Pattern should be drug-shock, drug-shock.

2. Pulseless Electrical Activity Algorithm (PEA):*

Pulseless Electrical Activity includes electromechanical dissociation (EMD), pseudo dissociation (EMD), idioventrical rhythms, ventricular escape rhythms, ventricular escape rhythms, bradysystolic rhythms, and postdefibrillation idioventricular rhythms.

2.1 Continue CPR.
2.2 Intubate.
2.3 IV access.
2.4 Consider possible causes, including:

- A. Hypovolemia.
- B. Hypoxia.
- C. Cardiac tamponade (pericardiocentesis).
- D. Tension pneumothorax (needle decompression).
- E. Hypothermia.
- F. Pulmonary embolism.
- G. Drug overdoses.

H. Hyperkalemia.
I. Acidosis.
J. Acute myocardial infarction.

2.5 Administer epinephrine, 1 mg IV push, and repeat q 3-5 minutes.
2.6 If bradycardia is < 60 bpm, give atropine, 1 mg IV, and repeat q 3-5 minutes to a total dose of 0.03 to 0.04 mg/kg.

3. Tachycardia Algorithm:*

3.1 Access ABCs, IV, O_2, and monitor. Obtain an ECG and a CXR.
3.2 Unstable tachycardia includes chest pain, SOB, altered mental status (AMS), low BP, Shock, CHF, or AMI. When the ventricular rate is > 150 bpm, cardiovert or administer *medications* based on arrhythmia.
3.3 For stable atrial fibrillation and atrial flutter, consider diltiazem, β-blockers, verapamil, digoxin, procainamide, quinidine, and anticoagulants.
3.4 For stable PSVT, Wide-Complex tachycardia, and VT, consider the following.

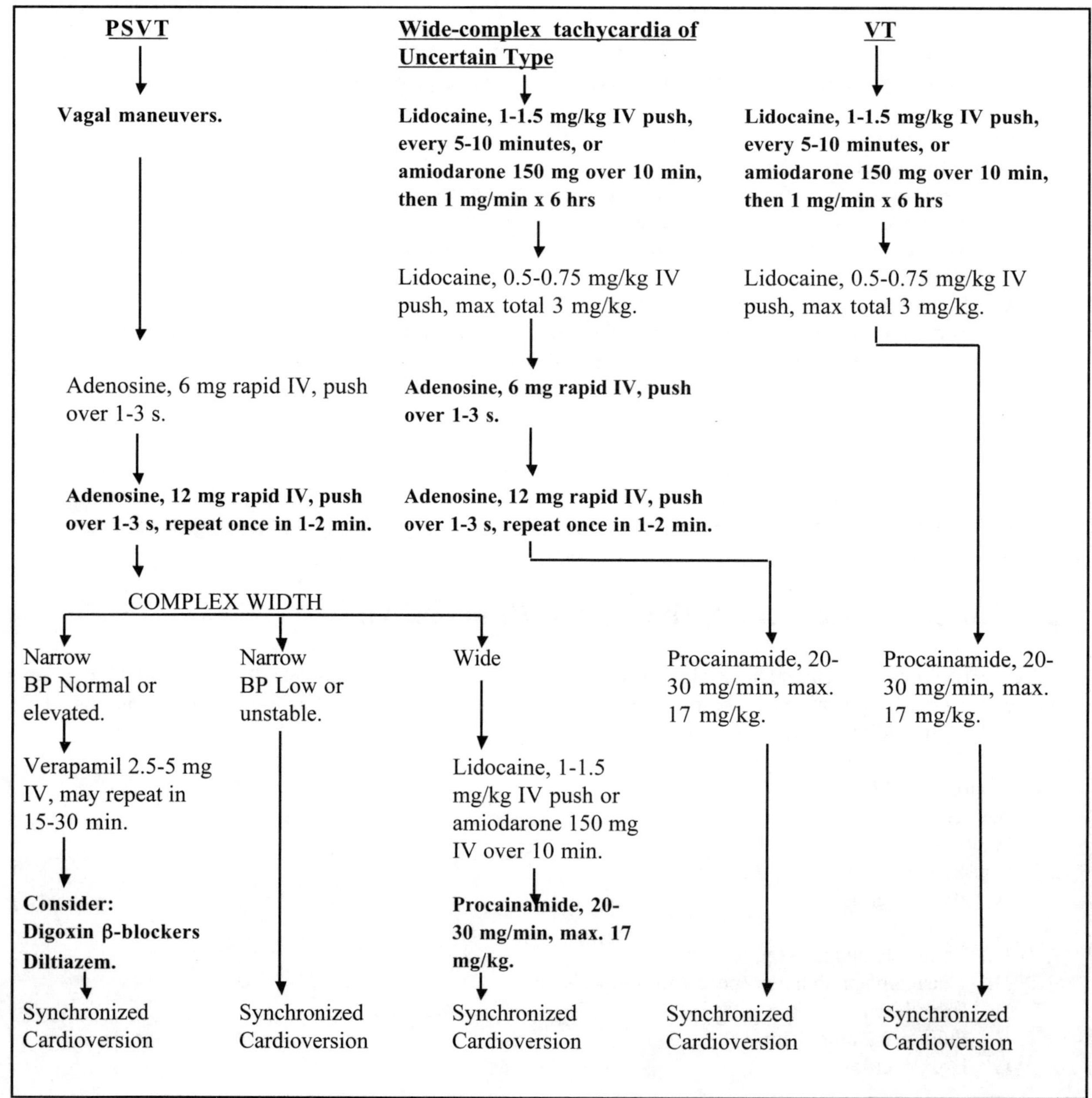

4. Asystole Algorithm:*

4.1 Continue CPR.
4.2 Intubate.
4.3 IV Access.
4.4 Confirm asystole in more than one lead.
4.5 Consider possible causes, including:
- A. Hypoxia.
- B. Hyperkalemia.
- C. Hypokalemia.
- D. Pre-existing acidosis.
- E. Drug overdose.
- F. Hypothermia.

4.6 Initiate immediate transcutaneous pacing.
4.7 Administer epinephrine, 1 mg IV push and repeat q 3-5 minutes.
4.8 Administer atropine, 1 mg IV push, and repeat q 3-5 minutes to a total of 0.03 -0.04 mg/kg.
4.9 Consider "termination of efforts".

5. Bradycardia Algorithm:*

5.1 Access ABCs.
5.2 Start IV, O_2, and monitor.
5.3 Check vital signs.
5.4 Obtain history, perform a physical exam, and order ECG, CXR, and electrolytes.
5.5 Bradycardia (< 60 bpm).
5.6 Consider serious signs or symptoms, including:
- A. Chest pain.
- B. SOB.
- C. AMS.
- D. Low BP.
- E. Shock.
- F. CHF.
- G. AMI.

5.7 If there are any serious signs/symptoms, perform the following intervention sequence.
- A. Administer atropine, 0.5-1.0 mg.
- B. Initiate transcutaneous pacing.
- C. Administer dopamine, 5-20 μg/kg per minute.
- D. Prescribe isoproterenol.

5.8 If no serious signs/symptoms exists, observe the patient in the ICU.

*Adapted from American Heart Association Emergency Cardiac Care Handbook.

CARDIOVASCULAR CASES

1. Advanced Cardiac Life Support:

1.1 Advanced Cardiac Life Support (ACLS) includes:
- A. **Airway:** Open airway with a modified jaw thrust maneuver and place an oropharyngeal airway. If this fails, secure airway by intubation or by cricothyrotomy.
- B. **Breathing**: Assess breathlessness and ventilate patient by using a bag-valve ventilation or a ET tube.
- C. **Circulation**: Confirm pulselessness and initiate closed-chest compressions. IV access and administer rhythm-appropriate drugs.
- D. **Defibrillate:** Or cardiovert as indicated.

2. Asystole:

Asystole is normally produced by a profound myocardial injury resulting in cardiac arrest. The outcome is usually fatal. Causes include myocardial infarction, hypoxia, hyperkalemia, hypokalemia, acidosis, drug overdose, hypothermia, and trauma.

2.1 Clinical Evaluation:

A. **Signs:** No heartbeat or pulse.
B. **Work-up:** No cardiac activity on monitor. Must be confirmed by two leads.

2.2 RX:

A. Support ABCs, CPR, IV, O_2, and monitor.
B. Initiate immediate transcutaneous pacing.
C. Treat with epinephrine, 1 mg IV push, and repeat q 3-5 minutes for adults. Use 0.01 mg/kg for the pediatric patient.
D. Administer atropine, 1 mg IV for the adult and 0.02 mg/kg for a child. Repeat q 3-5 minutes to total of 0.04 mg/kg, minimum dose 0.1 mg.
E. Consider transvenous pacing.
F. **Disposition:** Admit the patient to the ICU.

3. Atrial Fibrillation:

Atrial Fibrillation is the most common arrhythmia. In atrial fibrillation, multiple atrial ectopic foci stimulate irregular ventricular responses. The enlarged and poorly contracting left atrium induces the onset of thrombus formation, emboli, and stroke. Etiologies include coronary artery disease, congestive heart failure, cardiomyopathy, thyrotoxicosis, rheumatic heart disease, hypertension, alcohol ingestion, and pulmonary embolism.

3.1 Clinical Evaluation:

A. **Symptoms:** AF is often chronic in long-standing arteriosclerotic heart disease and maybe asymptomatic. In paroxysmal AF, palpitations and skipped beats may be accompanied by weakness and a feeling of faintness.
B. **Signs:** The rhythm is irregularly irregular with a rate of 80-180 bpm. The rate in chronic AF is usually 80-120 bpm. Some of the beats may not be transmitted to the peripheral circulation, resulting in a "Pulse deficit".
C. Multifocal atrial tachycardia, PSVT.
D. **Work-up:** ECG shows small irregular baseline undulations accompanied by irregular QRS-complexes and no clear p-waves.

3.2 RX:

A. Support ABCs, IV, O_2, and monitor.
B. If the rate is less than 120 bpm, usually no immediate treatment is required.
C. Anticoagulation therapy should be considered for AF > 48-72 hours duration prior to pharmacologic therapy or cardioversion.
D. For rate control, consider β-blockers, such as esmolol, metoprolol, propranolol, or calcium-channel-blockers, including diltiazem or verapamil. However, these two classes of drugs are negative inotropic agents and can cause hypotension. Begin digoxin or provide additional digoxin to patients already taking it.
E. Unstable patients with chest pain, dyspnea, hypotension, congestive heart failure, or cardiac ischemia, require immediate cardioversion after sedation. Start with 100 J of synchronized energy, and increase to 200, 300, and 360 J as needed.
F. **Disposition:** Admit to Telemetry or CCU.

4. Atrial Flutter:

Atrial flutter occurs when there is an ectopic focus originating from a small area in the atrium.

4.1 Clinical Evaluation:

A. **Symptoms:** Heart palpitations, with or without symptoms. Causes include coronary artery disease, COPD, and rheumatic heart disease.

B. **Signs:** Cardiac rate is typically about 150 bpm (2:1 block) and the rhythm is usually regular. Rates of 75 bpm occur with 4:1 block. Rate and rhythm may be irregular, alternating between a 2:1 and a 4:1 block.

C. **Work-up:** ECG shows characteristic "sawtooth" flutter waves with an atrial rate between 250 and 350 bpm. AV block is usually present, commonly 2:1, but 4:1 and alternating blocks are not uncommon.

4.2 RX:

A. Support ABCs, IV, O_2, and monitor.

B. β-blockers or calcium-channel blockers should be used to control the rate (refer to the "Atrial Fibrillation" section).

C. Unstable patients can usually be converted with 50 J of synchronized energy, increased as needed.

D. **Disposition:** Admit to Telemetry or to the CCU.

5. Bradyarrhythmias:

5.1 Clinical Evaluation:

A. **Symptoms:** A slow heart rate is < 60 bpm and the rate may be regular or irregular. Athletes and other individuals may have normal resting heart rates < 60 bpm. Remember, "Treat the patient, not the monitor".

B. **Signs:** Symptomatic bradycardias include sinus bradycardia, sinus arrest, 2° AV blocks (types I and II), and 3° AV block.

5.2 RX:

A. Support ABCs, IV, O_2, and monitor.

B. Administer atropine, 0.5-1.0 mg for adults and 0.01-0.02 mg/kg for peds, IV q 3-5 minutes to a total of 3 mg for the adult patient and 0.04 mg/kg for the pediatric.

C. Initiate transcutaneous pacing if available.

D. Administer dopamine, 5-20 μg/kg/minute for adults and for peds.

E. Administer epinephrine, 2-10 μg/minute and 0.05-2 μg/kg/minute for adults and peds, respectively.

F. Administer isoproterenol, 2-10 μg/minute for adults and 0.05-2 μg/kg/minute for the pediatric patient.

6. Paroxysmal Supraventricular Tachycardia (PSVT):

Paroxysmal Supraventricular Tachycardia is characterized by a sudden increase in heart rate, i.e., usually 140 to 200 bpm. This condition is induced by the impulse re-entering the AV node. PSVT arises in patients with accessory tracts that bypass part of the normal conducting system, such as in Wolff-Parkinson-White Syndrome. PSVT usually occurs in healthy individuals. Causes of PSVT include congenital (mitral valve prolapse), accessory conduction pathways, Wolff-Parkinson-White, hyperthyroidism, and arteriosclerotic heart disease.

6.1 Clinical Evaluation:

A. **Symptoms:** Heart palpitations, sometimes accompanied by weakness, dizziness, or faintness.

B. **Signs:** The heart rate is between 120-280 bpm, with an average rate of 160-200 bpm, and the rate is regular.

C. **DDX:** Digitalis toxicity, A-Flutter with 2:1 block, VT.

D. **Work-up:** An ECG shows narrow-complex QRS without P-waves.

6.2 RX:

A. Support ABCs, IV, O_2, and monitor. Attempt appropriate vagal maneuvers, such as carotid message, and then follow with the Tachycardia algorithm.

B. **Disposition:** Stable patients who do not present dangerous causes and who respond well to treatment can usually be discharged. Others require admission, often to telemetry.

7. Premature Ventricular Contractions (PVC):

Premature Ventricular Contractions are caused by one or more ectopic foci in the ventricle. PVCs are exacerbated by ischemia, electrolyte abnormalities, digoxin toxicity, and sympathomimetic drugs.

7.1 Clinical Evaluation:

A. **Symptoms:** PVCs are common in the normal patient but are significant in a patient with active cardiac ischemia

B. **Signs:** The Rhythm is irregularly irregular or regularly irregular if in bigeminy or trigeminy.

C.

D. **Work-up:** The cardiac monitor shows a wide QRS with no P-wave and a deflection opposite to the normal QRS.

7.2 RX:

A. Treatment is usually not necessary unless PVCs are frequent (approximately > 6/minute), multifocal, or in runs. In the setting of myocardial ischemia or infarction with these criteria, administer lidocaine, 1 mg/kg IV bolus, and start 2-3 mg per minute IV drip.

B. Consider magnesium sulfate in the setting of a myocardial infarction.

C. **Disposition:** Admit to Telemetry or the ICU if the patient is associated with concerning circumstances, i.e., ischemia, infarction, run of VT.

8. Pulseless Electrical Activity (PEA):

In Pulseless Electrical Activity, the electrical activity of the heart is not sufficient enough to stimulate a muscle contraction. The prognosis is poor unless a specific cause is known and then, if possible, quickly reversed. Reversible causes include hypovolemia, usually resulting from bleeding, hypoxia, cardiac tamponade, tension pneumothorax, hypothermia, massive pulmonary embolism, drug overdoses, hyperkalemia, and acidosis.

8.1 Clinical Evaluation:

A. **Symptoms:** Although observed in the setting of a cardiac arrest due to severe ischemic heart disease, reversible causes are important to recognize.

B. **Signs:** A pulse is not present but an impulse is displayed on the cardiac monitor.

C. **Work-up:** Ensure that a cardiac rhythm is displayed on the monitor. Order K^+, ABG STAT.

8.2 RX:

A. ABCs, CPR, IV, O_2, and monitor.

B. Administer epinephrine, 1 mg IV, repeat q 3-5 minutes for the adult and 0.01 mg/kg for the pediatric patient.

C. Consider an intermediate, 2-5 mg escalating, 1 mg, 3 mg, 5 mg, or a high dose, 0.1 mg/kg, of epinephrine.

D. Administer atropine, 1 mg IV, repeat q 3-5 minutes to a total dosage of 3 mg for the adult, and for peds, 0.02 mg/kg to a total of 0.04 mg/kg.
E. Consider HCO_3 if acidosis is suspected.
F. Treat hypovolemia with volume infusion of NS, followed by PRBCs if indicated.
G. Treat hypoxia by ventilating the patient.
H. For cardiac tamponade, perform pericardiocentesis.
I. Treat tension pneumothorax with needle decompression and insert a chest tube.
J. **Disposition:** Admit to ICU.

9. Ventricular Fibrillation (VF):

Ventricular Fibrillation is the most common cause of cardiac arrest. With this condition, the electrical activity of the heart is chaotic and no heart beat is present. The onset of VF is induced by severe ischemia, heart disease, and acute myocardial infarction.

9.1 Clinical Evaluation:

A. **Symptoms:** Commonly seen in severe ischemic heart disease with or without infarction.
B. **Signs:** No pulse.
C. **DDX:** Asystole.
D. **Work-up:** Cardiac monitor shows irregular waves in more than one lead.

9.2 RX:

A. Support ABCs, including CPR, IV, O_2, and monitor. (Refer to the “VF/VT” algorithm.)
B. **Disposition:** Admit the patient to ICU.

10. Ventricular Tachycardia (VT):

Ventricular Tachycardia is defined as three or more consecutive PVCs from an ectopic focus in the ventricle at a rate of over 100 bpm. There are two types of VT, "stable with a pulse”, and "pulseless." VT that results in symptomatic cardiac ischemia is considered unstable. Causes of VT include myocardial infarction, hypertrophic cardiomyopathy, drug toxicity, hypoxia, alkalosis, and electrolyte abnormalities.

10.1 Clinical Evaluation:

A. **Symptoms:** VT typically occurs in the setting of severe ischemic heart disease or myocardial infarction.
B. **Signs:** The rhythm is regular with a rate between 150 bpm and 200 bpm.
C. **Work-up:** Monitor indicates wide QRS complexes in sustained manner or in short bursts. The rate is greater than 100 bpm, the rhythm is usually regular, and the QRS axis is generally constant.

10.2 RX:

A. Support ABCs, CPR, IV, O_2, and monitor.
B. **Pulseless VT** is treated similarly to Ventricular Fibrillation (refer to “VF/VT” algorithm section).
C. An atypical VT (Torsade de Pointes) shows gradual alteration in the amplitude and the direction of electrical activity. Treat this condition with magnesium sulfate, 2 g IV over 2 minutes followed by 1 g/hour IV. Attempt transcutaneous "overdrive" pacing or isoproterenol to accelerate cardiac rhythm. Return to a slower sinus rhythm.
D. **Disposition:** Admit to CCU.

11. Abdominal Aortic Aneurysm (AAA):

Etiology: 90% atherosclerotic. Location: 98% infrarenal.

11.1 Clinical Evaluation:

A. **Symptoms:** Symptoms begin with a leaking or a rapidly expanding aneurysm. The typical patient is an older male with severe, constant, low abdominal and/or back pain which is not relieved by position. Pain may be present in the lower back, scrotum, or perineum.

B. **Signs:** Vitals may show hypotension which is an unstable condition characterized by a severe leak or impending rupture. Unequal extremity pulses, abdominal tenderness in the suprapubic region with radiation to the lumbar area, and pulsatile abdominal mass may be present and suggests AAA.

C. **DDX:**

Shock Present: Hemorrhagic pancreatitis, perforated viscous, and mesenteric infarction.

Shock Not Present: Renal colic, diverticulitis, lumbar disk disease/compression fracture, small bowel obstruction, appendicitis, and peritonitis.

D. **Work-up:** Start two or more large bore IVs. Order CBC, SMA-7, PT, PTT, T&C 10 U, and an ECG. Abdominal plain film is often useful and demonstrates a bulging calcified aorta on the lateral view. An ED ultrasound can detect an aneurysm but cannot identify if it is leaking. A CT is diagnostic but can only be used in the stable patient.

11.2 RX:

A. Support ABCs, IV, O_2, and monitor. Maintain SBP 90-100 with IVF, blood, and consider use of MAST.

B. Rush the unstable patient, i.e., hypotensive and/or in severe abdominal distress, to the OR for immediate surgery.

C. Admit the more "stable" patient to the ICU and continue evaluation for possible surgery. If the patient is symptomatic and AAA is not stable, something is changing.

12. Acute Aortic Dissection:

The main cause of Acute Aortic Dissection is necrosis of tunica media from atherosclerosis of the tunica intima eroding into the muscle layer. Dissection involves intimal tear, hematoma formation in the tunica media, and the creation of a false aneurysm.

A. Daily (Stanford) Type A (DeBakey I & II): Involves the ascending aorta and is usually best managed with surgery. The mortality rate of the untreated is approximately 75%. With treatment, the rate decreases to approximately 20%.

B. Daily (Stanford) Type B (DeBakey III): Involves the descending aorta only. No surgery was formally considered the best management of this condition. The mortality rate with treatment is approximately 10%. Type B dissections are associated with limb or organ ischemia. Patients with progressive conditions, despite medical treatment, should be considered for surgical management.

12.1 Clinical Evaluation:

A. **Symptoms:** A typical patient is an older hypertensive male with a sudden onset of severe chest pain, "tearing" quality, and radiation to the back.

B. **Signs:** Rales, diastolic murmur of aortic insufficiency, differences in left and right or upper and lower extremity blood pressures and pulses. Abdominal tenderness and/or pulsatile mass, and neurologic deficits are caused by compromised arterial supply. Signs of cerebrovascular accident are present if the carotid arteries are involved.

C. **DDX:** New onset angina, stable or unstable angina, variant (Prinzmetal's) angina, MI, pericarditis, pneumonia, pulmonary embolus, pneumothorax, chest wall pain, biliary disorders, and GI disorders, such as gastritis, pancreatitis, dyspepsia, peptic ulcer, esophagitis, and esophageal spasm.

D. **Work-up:** Obtain an ECG, CBC, SMA-7, PT, PTT, and T&C 6-8 U. CXR may show mediastinal widening, prominent ascending aorta, enlargement of the aortic knob, and/or pleural effusion. Order a CT or an aortography if the patient is stable. Consider transesophageal echocardiography if it is available in the ED.

12.2 RX:

A. Support ABCs, IV, O_2, and monitor.
B. Type A requires immediate surgery.
C. Type B requires medical or surgical management.
D. Other interventions:
   - To decrease the force of a contraction, prescribe β-blockers, including esmolol (Brevibloc), 500 μg/kg IV over 1 minute, then infuse at 50 μg/kg/minute, **or** propranolol, 1 mg/minute to total of 10 mg.
   - Start nitroprusside (Nipride), 0.5 μg/kg/minute IV, and lower systolic pressure to 100 to 120 mm Hg. Observe for organ perfusion and neurological status. Do not overshoot BP.
E. **Disposition:** Transfer the patient to the ICU or to surgery.

13. Acute Myocardial Infarction (AMI):

Acute Myocardial Infarction is necrosis of the heart muscle resulting from an acute coronary artery occlusion. The standard of therapy is rapid lysis or angioplasty as soon as possible for the appropriate individuals.

13.1 Clinical Evaluation:

A. **Symptoms:** When present, pain may be substernal, severe, steady, "squeezing", "heavy", "tight", or "pressure-like", often radiating to left jaw or shoulder. Nitrates do not relieve the pain. Associated symptoms include nausea, vomiting, dyspnea, diaphoresis, palpitations, and weakness.
B. **Signs:**
C. The patient may often be anxious, pale, or diaphoretic. An arrhythmia may be present.
D. Anterior MI is more common in younger patients. Hypertension and tachycardia are typical. Bradycardia may be present if 2° A-V block or complete heart block develops.
E. For inferior MI, bradycardia may occur.
F. Note precordial bulges, gallops, S3, S4, murmurs, and JVD if right sided failure. Rales if left sided failure.
G. **DDX:** onset of angina, stable or unstable angina, variant (Prinzmetal's) angina, aortic dissection, pericarditis, pneumonia, pulmonary embolus, pneumothorax, chest wall pain, biliary disorders, and GI disorders, such as gastritis, dyspepsia, peptic ulcer, esophagitis, and esophageal spasm.
H. **Work-up:** Obtain the following.
I. elevations in leads, II, III, and aVF (inferior wall); V1-3 (anteroseptal); I, aVL and V4-6 (lateral); and V1-6 (anterolateral). ST depression in leads, V1-3 (posterior). Nonspecific ST and T wave abnormalities in subendocardial myocardial infarction.
J. Cardiac enzymes: CK-MB fraction elevates in 4-8 hours, peaks in 24 hours. Check troponin level.
K. Pulse oximetry or ABG, CBC, SMA-7, LFTs prn, PT, PTT and CXR.

13.2 RX:

A. Support ABCs, IV, O_2, and monitor.
B. **Consider beginning thrombolytic therapy protocol within 30 minutes of arrival.**

   Precise indications: Choice of agent and dosing regimen for thrombolysis depends on local practice and current research. Thrombolytic therapy should be provided within 30 minutes of ED presentation to all patients diagnosed with an acute myocardial infarction exhibiting a ST segment elevation as long as there is no contraindication. Thrombolysis is a dangerous treatment because of the risk of inducing intracranial hemorrhage. This treatment should be initiated only under the supervision of the ED attending physician. Be prepared for hypotension and reperfusion arrhythmia. Consider adjunctive therapies, including, β-blockade, nitroglycerin, and magnesium sulfate.

   Contraindications: Active GI bleeding, prolonged CPR, intracranial aneurysm, AVM or tumor, history of hemorrhagic cerebrovascular accident, pregnancy, intracranial or spinal surgery, or trauma within 2 months.

   Relative contraindications: Recent surgery or trauma, history of cerebrovascular accident, and coagulopathy.

   Some Suggested Guidelines:

Front-Loaded t-PA (rt-PA, Alteplase, Activase): Gently reconstitute two 50 mg vials with 50 mL diluent each. Add contents of each of the vials to 100 mL of D_5W for a final concentration of 0.5 mg/mL. Start a dedicated IV line and use an infusion pump. Withdraw 15 mg bolus (30 mL) from bag. Inject bolus by MD. Start infusion, 50 mg (100 mL) over 30 minutes. Then infuse 35 mg (70 mL) over the next 60 minutes.
Dose patients < 65 kg with 1.25 mg/kg t-PA given over 90 minutes followed by 15% IV bolus by MD, 50% over 30 minutes, 35% over the next 60 minutes. Inject 20 mL of NS into an empty IV bag at the end of the dose and infuse to ensure all the t-PA is delivered. Administer heparin during the t-PA infusion at 100 units/kg IV bolus followed by an infusion of 1000-1200 units/hour.

Streptokinase: Reconstitute two 750,000 IU vials each with 5 mL of NS obtained from a 250 mL NS bag. Add contents from both vials, 1.5 MU, to the 250 mL bag for a final concentration of 6000 IU/mL. Start a dedicated IV with an infusion pump.
Infuse streptokinase over 60 minutes. Inject 20 mL of NS into an empty IV bag at the end of a dose and infuse to ensure that all the streptokinase is delivered. Heparin is no longer clearly indicated after the infusion but consider 12,500 units sq for 12 hours.

Anistreplase (APSAC, Eminase): Reconstitute with 5 mL of sterile water. Infuse 30 units IV over 5 minutes. Start an IV of D_5 1/2 NS. There is no need for heparin.

Reteplase (r-PA, Retavase, Reptilase): Derivative of rt-PA that is effective as rt-PA and may work more quickly. Infuse 10 units IV over 2 minutes followed by a repeat dose in 30 minutes. Heparin must be used to prevent reclosure.

C. Give aspirin, 160-325 mg po, pr, or chewed.
D. Administer NTG SL or spray x 3 q 5 minutes apart while starting IVs. Add NTG paste or initiate an IV drip at 10-50 μg/minute and titrate to pain and SBP.
E. Treat with β-blockade, especially for fast rates, such as metoprolol, 5 mg IV q 5 minutes x 3.
F. A heparin-thrombolytic therapy protocol may dictate timing of heparin. Common dosing is 5000 units IV load or 80 units/kg load and 18 units/kg/mdrip.
G. Consider providing additional analgesia, usually morphine.
H. Consult a cardiologist for consideration of cardiac catheterization. If angioplasty is to be performed start a GPIIb/IIIa inhibitor (abciximab, eptifibatide, or tirofiban).
I. **Disposition:** Admit to the CCU.

14. Hypertensive Emergencies:

Hypertension is defined as a sustained elevated blood pressure (S > 140 mm Hg or D > 90 mm Hg). Urgency exists with a diastolic blood pressure of about 120 mm Hg or greater, without evidence of end-organ damage is exhibited. A hypertensive emergency is characterized by an acute elevation in blood pressure resulting in a end-organ damage. This condition usually involves the cardiovascular, renal, and central nervous systems. Hypertensive emergencies require ED intervention and admissions, usually with a goal of lowering diastolic pressure about 25% in the first day. Hypertensive urgencies require ED intervention but often the patient may be safely discharged with a close follow-up. Incidental hypertension does not usually require ED intervention and out patient follow-up is appropriate.

14.1 Clinical Evaluation:

A. **Symptoms:** Headache, nausea, vomiting, visual disturbances, chest pain, shortness of breath, orthopnea, confusion, stupor, coma, and abdominal pain.
B. **Signs:** Neurological deficits, seizures, fundal abnormalities, rales, pulmonary edema, hemorrhage, thrombosis, embolus, acute renal failure, dyspnea, and murmurs.
C. **DDX:** Acute myocardial infarction, congestive heart failure, thoracic aortic dissection, coarctation of aorta, renovascular disease, and primary aldosteronism.
D. **Work-up:** Obtain an ECG, CBC, SMA-7, U/A, CXR, and a head CT.

14.2 RX:

A. Support ABCs, IV, O_2, and monitor.
B. Lower symptomatic BP or asymptomatic BP of 220/120 mm Hg by using labetalol, 20 mg IV, then 40-80 mg IV q 10 minutes until an adequate response or 300 mg is infused or a nitroprusside infusion, 0.5-10 μg/kg/minute (avoid in pregnancy), **or** hydralazine bolus, 5-15 mg (preferred in pregnancy), or nitroglycerin infusion, 50-100 μg/minute or nifedipine, 10-20 mg capsule q 20-30 minute, **or** phentolamine bolus, 5-10 mg q 5-15 minutes.
C. Specific Disease State Recommendations:
   For hypertensive encephalopathy, use nitroprusside or labetalol.
   For CNS events, use nitroprusside.
   For myocardial ischemia, use nitroglycerin infusion or labetalol or oral nifedipine.
   For CHF, use nitroprusside or nitroglycerin.
   For eclampsia/preeclampsia, use hydralazine.
   For interactions between MAO inhibitors and foods or drugs, use phentolamine or labetalol.
   For antihypertensive withdrawal, use labetalol or nitroprusside.
   For renal failure, use nitroprusside or labetalol.
   For cocaine toxicity use a benzodiazepine as the first agent.
D. **Disposition:** Send patient home if he/she has uncomplicated hypertension. Admit the patient if the BP is difficult to control and if complications arise, including altered mental status, cardiovascular disease, renal disease, or cerebrovascular disease.

15. Cerebrovascular Hypertensive Emergencies:

Main complications associated with Cerebrovascular Hypertensive Emergencies are intracerebral and subarachnoid hemorrhages. Hypertensive encephalopathy is a rare condition and occurs when the blood pressure exceeds the limits of auto-regulation by the blood-brain barrier. Blood enters the brain tissue which induces cerebral edema. (Refer also to "Intracranial Hemorrhage" in the Neurology section.)

15.1 Clinical Evaluation:

A. **Symptoms:** The onset of intracranial bleeding is usually rapid. It usually transpires in an awake patient experiencing a severe headache that is often accompanied by an alteration in the level of consciousness. Seizures may occur. Hypertensive encephalopathy develops over 24 to 48 hours.
B. **Signs:** Focal signs indicate location of bleed. Coma may be present. A stiff neck may be displayed with a subarachnoid hemorrhage. Retinal hemorrhages and papilledema may be exhibited in hypertensive encephalopathy.
C. **Work-up:** Order CBC, SMA-7, U/A, ECG, PT and PTT. A CT shows a bleed in most cases. A lumbar puncture is positive for blood with a subarachnoid hemorrhage if the CT is not conclusive.

15.2 RX:

A. Support ABCs, IV, O_2, and monitor.
B. Hypertension involving a hemorrhagic stroke often resolves without treatment.
C. For high pressures, > 220/130, the drug of choice is sodium nitroprusside (Nipride). Begin at 0.5 μg/kg/minute IV and titrate to diastolic of 80-100 mm Hg. Do not overshoot. Sodium nitroprusside is light sensitive; therefore, protect the drug by wrapping the delivery container in aluminum foil.
D. A second choice is an α-1 and a β-blocker. Administer labetalol (Normodyne, Trandate). Begin with 20 mg IV over 2 minutes with repeated boluses of 40 mg followed by 80 mg every 10 minutes to a total of 300 mg. Continue infusion at 2 mg/minute.
E. Consider rapid reversal of coagulopathy for patients on Coumadin.
F. **Disposition:** Transfer the patient to ICU/CCU or to surgery.

16. Chest Pain:

Chest Pain may arise from the musculoskeletal components of the chest wall or from the intrathoracic viscera, such as the heart, great vessels, esophagus, and pleura. Distinguish minor causes of chest pain from life-threatening causes. Generally, peripheral pain is clearly localized and visceral pain is poorly localized. Often the cause of chest pain cannot be determined.

16.1 Clinical Evaluation:

A. **Symptoms:** Obtain a description of the pain, such as character, location, radiation, duration, sudden or gradual onset, precipitating events, associated symptoms, aggravating/alleviating factors, and timing of previous episodes. Determine PMH, including previous coronary artery disease/myocardial infarction, medications, diabetes, smoking, elevated cholesterol, alcohol, and drugs, such as cocaine. Acquire an appropriate family history. Classic descriptions are rarely encountered, except during board exams.

Pulmonary embolism: Sudden pleuritic pain, accompanied by dyspnea. The patient has a history of risk factors, including immobilization and/or leg pain and swelling.

Myocardial infarction: Sudden substernal or precordial rushing, dull, tight, or pressure-like pain radiating to neck, jaw, or arms. The pain is not relieved by nitroglycerin and lasts more than 30 minutes. This condition is accompanied by nausea, vomiting, and diaphoresis.

Unstable angina: Chest pain that increases in severity or frequency or requires less exertion to precipitate. The first episode of squeezing pain occurs at rest and lasts less than 30 minutes. The pain is not relieved by nitroglycerin.

Acute aortic dissection: Sudden excruciating retrosternal pain radiating to back. Patient has history of hypertension.

Pneumonia: Gradual pleuritic pain with a productive cough and a fever.

Pneumothorax: Sudden onset of sharp pleuritic pain in young slender patients or in patients with COPD.

Acute pericarditis: Gradual pleuritic retrosternal pain, which is relieved by leaning forward, is accompanied by a fever.

Other causes of chest pain are valvular disease, pleurisy, esophagitis, hiatal hernia, peptic ulcer, costochondritis, and radiculitis.

B. **Signs:**

Pulmonary embolism: Tachypnea and tachycardia, edema and tenderness in thigh or calf.

Myocardial infarction: Shock, arrhythmia, paradoxical splitting of S2, gallops, and murmurs.

Dissecting aneurysm: Hypertension and differences in pulses in arms and legs, hemiparesis, pulsatile mass.

Pneumonia: Temperature elevation, rales, and consolidation.

Pneumothorax: Decreased breath sounds on one side.

Costochondritis: Chest wall tenderness.

C. **Work-up:** Order CBC, SMA-7, cardiac enzymes, pulse oximetry or ABG, and ECG. X-ray studies may reveal the following conditions.

Pneumothorax: Air in pleural space.

Pneumonia: Lung infiltrates.

Myocardial infarction: Pulmonary congestion or edema if accompanied by heart failure.

Dissecting aneurysm: Widened mediastinum.

Pulmonary embolism: Elevated hemidiaphragm, Hampton's hump, Westermark's sign, atelectasis

16.2 RX:

A. Support ABCs, IV, O_2, and monitor. (Refer to specific diseases.)
B. **Disposition:** Discharge patients with minor causes of chest pain, such as costochondritis and uncomplicated pneumonia in a healthy person. Individuals with all other conditions should be admitted to floor bed, ICU, CCU, or to surgery.

17. Congestive Heart Failure (CHF):

In Congestive Heart Failure, the heart cannot pump blood at a flow rate sufficient to meet the needs of the peripheral tissues. Possible causes of an acute presentation, such as acute left ventricular dysfunction, include tachyarrhythmia, bradyarrhythmia, and acute myocardial infarction. Chronic left ventricular dysfunction resulting from a chronic fluid overload, as displayed in valvular heart disease, must also be considered.

17.1 Clinical Evaluation:

A. **Symptoms:** Dyspnea, PND, orthopnea, nocturia, edema, chest pain, and previous cardiac disease.
B. **Signs:** Respiratory distress, tachycardia, tachypnea, hypotension, JVD, hepatojugular reflex, rales, murmurs, pulsatile liver, or cyanosis.
C. **DDX:** Constrictive pericarditis, cardiac tamponade, myocardial infarction, or pulmonary embolism.
D. **Work-up:** Order pulse oximetry, ABG, CXR, CBC, SMA-7, CPK with isoenzymes, sputum for Gram's stain and C&S, and ECG.

17.2 RX:

A. Support ABCs, IV, O_2, and monitor.
B. CPAP may be helpful in avoiding intubation.
C. Provide PEEP if patient requires intubation.
D. Keep patient in a sitting position if possible.
E. Insert a Foley for monitoring I/Os, IVs, and TKO.
F. Anticipate BP drop as patient's failure improves. (Refer also to "Acute Pulmonary Edema/Hypotension" algorithm.)
G. Consider administrating the following medications:
    Furosemide, 20-80 mg IV over 1-2 minutes q 30 minutes, may repeat several times. Double dose each time if there is no response. The first dose of Furosemide is double the patient usual dose.
    NTG spray or SL x 3 while monitoring BP. NTG paste or IV titrated to effect and BP.
    Morphine sulfate, 1-4 mg IV and repeat q 5-10 minutes for effect.
    For atrial fibrillation, consider digoxin, loading dose of 0.25-0.5 mg IV, followed by 0.25 mg IV q 6 hours to a total dose of 1.0 mg, **or** 8-12 μg/kg lean body weight, **or** 6-10 μg/kg in renal failure.
    Titrate for urine output and BP with dobutamine, 2.5-10 μg/kg/minute, **or** dopamine, 1-20 μg/kg/minute.
    Treat bronchospasms with albuterol, 2.5 mg in NaCl Nebs q 30-60 minutes.
    For hypertension, consider nitroprusside, 0.5-10 μg/kg/minute IV.
H. **Disposition:** Admit the patient to the ICU if there is evidence of pulmonary edema. The patient may be treated on a medical floor if he/she has improved and is stable after ED management with appropriate monitors. Patients with chronic congestive heart failure and mild worsening symptoms but who are responsive to IV diuretics may be discharged after adjustments in the chronic drug regimen have been made, a consultation with the patient's physician has been obtained, and a follow-up within 24-48 hours has been arranged. All patients with new onset congestive heart failure or pulmonary edema require admission.

18. Pulmonary Embolism:

Pulmonary Embolism most commonly occurs when the venous thrombi in the deep venous system dislodge and enter the pulmonary arterial circulation.

18.1 Clinical Evaluation:

A. **Symptoms:** Risk factors include prolonged bed rest, elderly, CHF, carcinoma, CVA, pregnancy, oral contraceptives, postoperative, leg trauma, and obesity. Patients often present with anxiety, chest pain, dyspnea, agitation, hemoptysis, and syncope.

B. **Signs:** Exam results may include tachycardia, tachypnea, low grade fever, hypotension, rales, rub, decreased breath sounds, and evidence of phlebitis or DVT.

C. **DDX:** Myocardial infarction, angina, pneumonia, pleural effusion, pneumothorax, musculoskeletal chest pain, pleurisy, and pericarditis.

D. **Work-up:** Obtain baseline labs, including a PT, PTT and D-Dimer.

CXR: Usually normal, may show non-specific abnormalities. Elevated hemidiaphragm, infiltrate or small pleural effusion may be present.

ECG: S1Q3T3 pattern or incomplete right BBB. Non-specific ST-T wave changes and tachycardia may be present.

ABG: Normal or decreased pO_2, decreased pCO_2, and alkalosis. Hypoxia is common. Ninety percent of patients exhibit $pO_2 < 80$ mm Hg. A normal A-a gradient is very uncommon in a pulmonary embolism.

V-Q scan: Positive if multiple segmental or lobar perfusion defects with normal ventilation. A normal scan excludes a pulmonary embolism. Normal ventilation with decreased perfusion is suggestive of a pulmonary embolism. Low and intermediate probability scans often require pulmonary arteriography for conformation. High probability requires immediate anticoagulation.

Doppler studies: If a diagnosis is suspected but not confirmed by a V-Q scan, many clinicians will order venous Doppler studies of the lower extremities. A low or intermediate V-Q scan result in the presence of a DVT is highly indicative of a PE.

Pulmonary angiogram: Intraluminal filling defects and/or arterial cutoffs suggest a PE.

CT scan of the chest: Good for detecting emboli in large pulmonary vessels but misses peripheral clots in small vessels.

Echocardiogram: Right ventricular dysfunction. Valuable in unstable patients who can not leave the ED.

18.2 RX:

A. Manage airway and maintain adequate oxygenation with supplemental O_2.

B. Manage pain as needed.

C. Treat with heparin, 80 units/kg bolus, followed by continuous IV infusion at 18 units/kg/hour.

D. Use Thrombolysis or Embolectomy on patients with hypotension requiring vasopressors and with angiographically documented PE. May be considered empirically for a patient in extremis.

t-PA, 100 mg over 2 hours **or** streptokinase, 250,000 IU load over 30 minutes, followed by 100,000 units/hour for 24 hours, **or** urokinase, 4,400 IU/kg load over 10 minutes, followed by 4,400 IU/kg/hour for 12-24 hours.

STAT thoracic surgery consult for consideration of embolectomy.

E. **Disposition:** Admit and treat patients with pulmonary embolism or individuals suspected of having a pulmonary embolism, i.e., the condition has not been eliminated.

19. Syncope:

Syncope is a sudden transient loss of consciousness characterized by unresponsiveness, loss of postural tone, and spontaneous recovery. Near-syncope or presyncope is the feeling of faintness. The etiologies are similar for both conditions. Life-threatening causes need to be excluded. Common origins are vasovagal (diagnosis of exclusion), hypoglycemia, arrhythmia, and drugs. Less common causes include oxygen deficit (COPD, anemia, pulmonary embolism, and CO poisoning), seizures (epilepsy and alcohol withdrawal), cardiac (valvular disease, arrhythmia, or ischemia), cerebrovascular accident/TIA (mostly vertebro-basilar), infection (CNS and sepsis), hyperventilation syndrome, and GI hemorrhage.

19.1 Clinical Evaluation:

A. **Symptoms:** Determine events immediately preceding the episode, including associated symptoms, i.e., chest pain, palpitations, prodrome, dyspnea, or headache. The patient usually has a history of cardiac, pulmonary, or endocrine disease and/or a prior history of syncope or seizure disorder.

B. **Signs:** Evaluate vital signs and check for orthostatic hypotension. Pinpoint or dilated pupils may suggest toxidrome. Carotid bruits suggest cerebral ischemia. Evaluate neurologic status, including mental status, sensory, motor, reflexes, and cerebellar signs. **Heme check stools**.

C. **DDX:** Drop attacks, seizure, black out from alcohol, and coma.

D. **Work-up:** Order finger stick glucose, CBC, SMA-7, T&C, PT, drug screen, and ECG. Determine pulse oximetry, ABG, and CXR. Obtain a CT if a neurologic cause is suspected.

19.2 RX:

A. Treat the patient as necessary depending on the findings/tests.

B. **Disposition:** Patients with syncope, resulting from seizure, vasovagal episode, corrected hypovolemia, and hypoglycemia, who improve in ED and who have no complications can usually be safely discharged. Admit patients, especially the elderly, with conditions due to an arrhythmia, valvular disease, cerebrovascular accident, subarachnoid hemorrhage, pulmonary embolism, aortic dissection, or myocardial infarction, as well as those individuals with undetermined causes to a monitored bed.

DERMATOLOGY

DERMATITIS

1. Toxicodendron Dermatitis:

Toxicodendron Dermatitis is caused by a poison sumac that has 7-13 leaflets per leaf. Poison ivy and oak have U or V shaped leaves with 3 leaflets. The blister fluid does not contain allergens.

1.1 Clinical Evaluation:

A. **Symptoms:** Rash occurs 1-10 days post exposure. It is spread by clothes, animals, and fingernails.
B. **Signs:** Erythema, pruritus, papulovesicles in linear pattern, vesicles, and bullae.
C. **DDX:** Herpes simplex, bullous pemphigoid, seborrheic dermatitis, atopic dermatitis, nummular eczema, lichen simplex chronicus, xerosis, and stasis dermatitis.

1.2 RX:

A. For mild cases, apply calamine or steroid creams, and use po antihistamines for pruritus.
B. For severe cases that involve larger surface areas, apply Domeboro compresses tid and treat with potassium permanganate baths and po antihistamines. Consider po prednisone administered in a long course, 40-60 mg initially tapered over 2-3 weeks.

PURPURIC LESIONS

1. Henoch-Schönlein Purpura (H-S-P):

Henoch-Schönlein Purpura is a vasculitis of the small vessels characterized by palpable purpura, arthritis, abdominal pain, and nephritis.

1.1 Clinical Evaluation:

A. **Symptoms:** The onset is gradual to abrupt. A low grade fever, malaise, and colic are common symptoms. Abdominal pain may also be present. This condition is most common in children aged 4-11 years. H-S-P tends to be contracted in the spring or after an infection.
B. **Signs:** Palpable purpura appears on the extremities, face, and ears. Diffuse abdominal pain and arthritis may be evident. Edema may be present on the face and ears.

1.2 RX:

A. Resolves in 1-4 months.
B. Anti-inflammatory agents may be used for fever and arthritis.
C. Treat with corticosteroids, such as prednisone 1-2 mg/kg/day, for angioedema and severe GI symptoms. Steroids do not help alleviate the lesions.
D. **Disposition:** Outpatient therapy is appropriate unless complications occur like renal failure, secondary infection of vasculitis lesions, or intestinal tract perforations.

2. Thrombotic Thrombocytopenic Purpura:

Thrombotic Thrombocytopenic Purpura is characterized by fever, a change in mental status, renal insufficiency, and microangiopathic hemolytic anemia. The mortality rate is 80%.

2.1 Clinical Evaluation:

A. **Symptoms:** Familial bleeding disorder, infection, which includes hemorrhagic *E. coli*, drug history, easy bruising, epistaxis, menorrhagia, or prolonged bleeding post surgery. Most cases occur in individuals ranging in ages between 10-40 years.

B. **Signs:** Flat, non-palpable purpura in areas of pressure, petechiae < 3 mm, and ecchymosis > 3 mm. Fluctuating neurological symptoms may occur, including stroke, seizures, and altered mental states. Hematuria, proteinuria, jaundice or pallor may be present. Purpura may involve the mucous membranes and optic fundi.

C. **Work-up:** Order CBC, PT, PTT, platelet count, type and cross, SMA-7, and U/A. A bone marrow biopsy may need to be performed as an inpatient..

2.2 RX:

A. Treatment includes corticosteroids, splenectomy, plasmapheresis, anticoagulation, aspirin, and dipyridamole. ED management is focused on diagnosis and treatment of acute complications.

B. Consult dermatology.

C. Maintain platelet counts above 20,000. One unit of platelets increases the count by 5-10,000.

D. **Disposition:** ICU admission is required for patients who are in septic shock and those with an intracranial hemorrhage.

3. Idiopathic Thrombocytopenic Purpura:

Idiopathic Thrombocytopenic Purpura is a decrease in the circulating number of platelets when there is no evidence of disease or toxic exposure. This condition is caused by the IgG antiplatelet antibody. The acute form occurs in children, 2-6 years old, usually following a viral prodrome. The chronic form of the disease is contracted by adults. The latter condition presents with no prodrome, easy bruising, prolonged menses, and mucosal bleeding.

3.1 Clinical Evaluation:

A. **Symptoms:** Tendency of bruising, gingival bleeding, menometrorrhagia, menorrhagia, recurrent epistaxis, and neurologic symptoms secondary to intracerebral bleeding.

B. **Signs:** Petechiae and purpura. Non-palpable spleen (absence of an enlarged spleen is an essential diagnostic criteria). Neurologic deficits secondary to intracerebral bleeding. Heme positive stools.

C. **DDX:** Lupus, urticaria, lymphoma, and telangiectasias.

D. **Work-up:** Obtain PT, PTT, CBC, and platelet count. Order a quantitative test for an antiplatelet antibody.

3.2 RX:

A. Treat acute ITP with prednisone, 1-2 mg/kg/day for 4 weeks, then taper. Patient should be considered for a splenectomy. Administer IV gamma globulin, 1-2 g/kg single dose.

B. For chronic ITP, use prednisone, 60 mg/day for 4-6 weeks, then taper. A high dose of IV gamma globulin may be used for some emergencies.

C. Aspirin is contraindicated.

D. Avoid gamma globulin if the patient has IgA deficiency.

E. Obtain a hematology consult.

F. Other therapies include vincristine, vinblastine, danazol, plasmapheresis, azathioprine, cyclophosphamide, and interferon.

G. **Disposition:** Consider outpatient management unless the individual has a platelet count

H. < 20,000. Admit patients with active bleeding.

LIFE THREATENING DERMATOSES

1. Staphylococcal Scalded Skin Syndrome (SSSS):

1.1 Clinical Evaluation:

A. **Symptoms:** Affects **primarily** children between 6 months to 6 years. SSSS is caused by an exotoxin that is produced by *Staphylococcus aureus.* Prodrome of fever, malaise, and skin tenderness are indicative of the approaching condition.

B. **Signs:** The mucous membranes are not involved but painful erythema and blistering of the skin are present. Nikolsky's sign is evident, i.e., the epidermis separates from the basal layer with pressure. Bullae and vesicles begin around mouth.

C. **DDX:** Toxic epidermal necrolysis, drug reactions, Kawasaki disease, Meningococcal or possibly gram negative sepsis, Rocky Mountain Spotted Fever, and Streptococcal scarlet fever.

D. **Work-up:** Biopsy blister and obtain *Staphylococcus aureus* culture from the nose or the oropharynx.

1.2 RX:

A. Administer, nafcillin, 50-100 mg/kg/day IV, **or** dicloxacillin, 50 mg/kg/day po.

B. Manage fluids and electrolytes.

C. **Disposition:** Admit.

2. Toxic Epidermal Necrosis (TEN):

This disease is contracted primarily by adults. A sign of this condition is the skin sloughing in large sheets. Toxic Epidermal Necrosis is believed to be a severe form of erythema multiform. The mortality rate is greater than 50%.

2.1 Clinical Evaluation:

A. **Symptoms:** Affects adults primarily. Flu-like prodrome that is precipitated by drugs or blood products. Skin is painful, hot, and red. Blisters and sloughing of skin develops.

B. **Signs:** Mucous membrane is involved. Entire thickness of the epidermis desquamates from the dermis. Nikolsky's sign is positive.

C. **DDX:** Staphylococcal Scaled Skin Syndrome, drug reactions, Kawasaki disease, Meningococcal or possibly gram negative sepsis, Rocky Mountain Spotted Fever, and streptococcal scarlet fever.

D. **Work-up:** Perform a biopsy.

2.2 RX:

A. Remove agent. Manage fluids and electrolytes similar to that used for burn treatments.

B. Consult a dermatologist and an ophthalmologist for eye involvement.

C. Corticosteroids are controversial.

3. Toxic Shock Syndrome:

Toxic Shock Syndrome is an acute multisystem illness associated with *Staphylococcus aureus* infections.

3.1 Clinical Evaluation:

A. **Symptoms:** The exotoxin of *Staphylococcus aureus* induces the toxic shock syndrome. The symptoms are fever > 38.9 °C, hypotension, rash, and the involvement of 3 organ systems. The condition is linked to tampons and nasal packing. Headache, arthralgia, vomiting, and diarrhea are exhibited.

B. **Signs:** Diffuse, blanching, macular erythroderma rash, pharyngitis, conjunctivitis, vaginitis, renal, and hepatic or hematologic dysfunction. Mucous membrane inflammation, CNS, or musculoskeletal hyperemia are signs of the condition. Full thickness desquamation involves the hands and feet in 1-2 weeks. Hair and nail loss occur 1-2 months later.

C. **DDX:** Kawasaki's disease, Rocky Mountain Spotted Fever, scarlet fever, TEN, drug reactions, Staphylococcal Scalded Skin Syndrome, and meningococcal sepsis.
D. **Work-up:** Order CBC, cultures, SMA-7, LFTs, calcium, PT and PTT.

3.2 RX:
A. Start IV with nafcillin, vancomycin, or clindamycin.
B. Initiate drainage of staphylococcal infection and remove any foreign bodies.
C. Prescribe corticosteroids.
D. Complications include coagulopathy, respiratory depression, and myocardial depression.
E. **Disposition:** Admit all symptomatic patients.

4. Erythema Multiforme / Stevens-Johnson Syndrome:

Erythema Multiforme is an acute, self-limited hypersensitivity reaction involving the skin and mucous membranes. Stevens-Johnson Syndrome is similar to erythema multiforme but with systemic involvement. The mortality rate is 50%.

4.1 Clinical Evaluation:
A. **Symptoms:** Exposure to drugs, herpes, hepatitis, influenza, fungal infections, collagen vascular disease, and flu-like prodrome. Stevens-Johnson syndrome is bullous lesions with systemic and mucous membrane involvement.
B. **Signs:**
Erythema multiforme: Target lesions- papule or vesicle surrounded by normal skin, followed by a halo of erythema on hands and wrists. Macules bullae involving the soles, palms, extensors of extremities, and back of hands and feet may be evident.
Stevens-Johnson syndrome (potentially fatal): Mucous membrane and multisystem involvement. Also headache, tachycardia, tachypnea, hematuria, diarrhea, bronchitis, and pneumonia are displayed.
C. **DDX:** Toxic epidermal necrolysis, urticaria, necrotizing vasculitis, drug reaction, contact dermatitis, viral exanthems, Rocky Mountain Spotted Fever, Meningococcemia, and syphilis.
D. **Work-up:** Order CBC, cultures, SMA-7, LFTs, calcium, PT and PTT.

4.2 RX:
A. Support ABC's, IV O_2, and monitor as indicated.
B. Discontinue offending agent.
C. Mild form resolves in 2-3 weeks.
D. For severe cases, use 80-120 mg of prednisone q day, wet compresses of potassium permanganate solution, or 0.05% silver nitrate.
E. Consult an ophthalmologist for corneal lesions.
F. **Disposition:** Admit severe cases, usually to the ICU and consider transfer to a burn center.

BACTERIAL INFECTIONS

1. Scarlet Fever:

Scarlet Fever is a Streptococcal sore throat accompanied by a rash which is induced by Group A β-hemolytic *Streptococcus*. Scarlet fever is commonly contracted by children.

1.1 Clinical Evaluation:
A. **Symptoms:** Fever, sore throat, and malaise followed by a rash in 12-24 hours are typical symptoms.
B. **Signs:** Papular eruptions occur in the hyperemic base of the chest that have a paper like texture and pinhead sized lesions. Pharynx injected, petechiae on palate (red strawberry tongue), and desquamation result with circumoral pallor.

C. **DDX:** Measles, rubella, infectious mononucleosis, roseola, syphilis, Toxic Shock Syndrome, Staphylococcal Scalded Skin Syndrome, Kawasaki disease, and drug hypersensitivity.
D. **Work-up:** Order a throat culture and antistreptolysin-O titer.

1.2 RX:
A. Treat with penicillin VK po 25-50 mg/kg/day divided qid for children, 250 mg qid for adults for 10 days, **or** erythromycin, 40 g/kg/day for children divided qid, 250 mg po qid for 10 days for adults, **or** Bicillin, CR 600,000 units for children, 1,200,000 units for adults IM.
B. Complications include glomerulonephritis, rheumatic fever, pneumonia, otitis, and lymph node infection.
C. **Disposition:** Discharge.

2. Impetigo:

Impetigo infects primarily children with the number of cases increasing in the summer months. This type of infection is caused by *Staphylococcus aureus* or Group A β-hemolytic *Streptococcus*. However, the bullous form is induced by *Staphylococcus aureus*.

2.1 Clinical Evaluation:
A. **Symptoms:** Rare fever.
B. **Signs:** Painful lesions on face, buttocks, and extremities. The condition begins as papules and vesicles that erode into honey colored crusts. The bullous form has flaccid bulla.
C. **DDX:** Herpes, tinea, scabies, and contact dermatitis.

2.2 RX:
A. Administer dicloxacillin, 12-25mg/kg/day divided qid, **or** erythromycin, 40 mg/kg/day divided qid.
B. Complications include glomerulonephritis which affects almost 1% of patients with this condition. However, rheumatic fever is not a complication. Antibiotics do not prevent glomerulonephritis.
C. **Disposition:** Discharge.

3. Rocky Mountain Spotted Fever:

Rickettsia rickettsii is transmitted by female ticks. In the southeast, it is carried by the *Dermacentor variabilis* (dog tick) and in the west by the *Dermacentor andersoni* (wood tick). With treatment, the mortality rate is almost 5% overall.

3.1 Clinical Evaluation:
A. **Symptoms:** Abrupt high fever, headache, nausea, myalgias, and rash on second through fourth digits.
B. **Signs:** Red macules that blanch on wrists and ankles. Macules spread to the trunk and face and become petechial lesions on the palms and soles. The spleen may also enlarge.
C. DDX: Drug eruptions, infectious mononucleosis, rubeola, Mycoplasma, roseola, enteroviruses, erythema infectiosum, drug eruptions, and anaphylactoid purpura.
D. **Work-up:** Determine Weil-Felix reaction. Obtain CBC, SMA-7, and blood culture.

3.2 RX:
A. The treatment of choice is Tetracycline 25-50 mg/kg qid or doxycycline 100 mg Bid for >-10 days
B. If patient appears seriously ill or is less than 9 years of age, use chloramphenicol, 100 g/kg/day up to 3 g/day divided q 6 hours.
C. **Disposition:** Treat until afebrile for 4 days usually as an outpatient.

4. Meningococcemia:

Patients with Meningococcemia can progress to shock and death within hours. Meningitis cases occur primarily in the late winter and early spring. Meningitis has a 50% mortality rate.

4.1 Clinical Evaluation:

A. **Symptoms:** Fever, headache, malaise, myalgias, and arthralgias.

B. **Signs:** Maculopapular tender lesions. Ecchymosis and purpura indicate DIC and shock- mucous membranes involvement. Altered mental status, focal neurologic signs, tachycardia, tachypnea, hypotension, cyanosis, petechiae, arthritis, and tenosynovitis are other signs of the condition.

C. **DDX:** Sepsis, Rocky Mountain Spotted Fever, Henoch-Schönlein, Gonococcemia, endocarditis, hemolytic uremic syndrome, and influenza.

D. **Work-up:** Obtain CXR, CBC, PT, PTT, SMA-7, ABG, cultures and LP. Expect thrombocytopenia, lactic acidosis, prolonged PT and PTT, low fibrinogen, and elevated fibrin degradation products.

4.2 RX:

A. For adults, use penicillin G, 24,000,000 units/day divided q 2-4 hours IV. For pediatric patients, administer penicillin G, 250,000 units/kg/day divided q 2-4 hours IV up to 20 MU, **or** ampicillin, 200-400 mg/kg/day divided qid IV. Some initiate treatment with ceftriaxone.

B. Treat penicillin-allergic individuals with chloramphenicol, cefuroxime, or 3rd generation Cephalosporin.

C. Initiate inotropic support and IV fluids. Steroids and heparin are controversial.

D. **Disposition:** Admit to ICU. Prescribe prophylaxis with rifampin, 10 mg/kg q 9-12 hours for 8 doses in children, and 600 mg q 9-12 hours for 8 doses in adults working in the household, nursery, daycare, or for those in contact with oral secretions.

5. Erythema Nodosum:

Erythema Nodosum presents with multiple bilateral cutaneous inflammatory non-ulcerating, non-scarring eruptions that initially begin as erythematous nodules and become bruise-like areas. Outbreaks occur on the extensor surfaces of the shins, thighs, and forearms.

5.1 Clinical Evaluation:

A. **Symptoms**: Affects mainly women in their third to fifth decade. Etiologies include oral contraceptives, collagen vascular disease, and infections. Complaints of fever, malaise, chills, and arthralgias are typical.

B. **Signs**: Raised, warm, tender, brightly erythematous nodules are located on the anterior shins. The diameter of the lesions is 1-15 cm. Hilar adenopathy and episcleral lesions are present.

C. **DDX:** Superficial thrombophlebitis, cellulitis, septic emboli, erythema induratum, nodular vasculitis, cutaneous polyarteritis nodosa, lymphoma, and sarcoidosis granulomata.

D. **Work-up:** Determine elevated sedimentation rate. Obtain CBC, a throat culture, and a stool culture. Perform a skin test for Mycobacteria if indicated.

5.2 RX:

A. Advise bed rest, elevation of legs, and the use of elastic stockings. Prescribe aspirin, 600 mg po q 4 hours, or indomethacin, 75-150 mg per day, divided tid.

B. Resolves in 3 to 8 weeks.

C. For severe pain, treat with 400-900 mg of potassium iodide q day, divided bid-tid for 3-4 weeks.

D. Administer corticosteroids for severe, refractory cases.

E. **Disposition**: Manage as an outpatient.

6. Lyme Disease:

Borrelia burgdorferi is transmitted by the deer tick Ixodes scapularis. This is a multiseptemic disorder with three clinical stages.

6.1 Clinical Evaluation:

A. **Symptoms:** Fever, malaise, lethargy anorexia, headache, stiff neck, and arthralgias.

B. **Signs:** Initially a small red papule forms which expands to a large lesion (>15 cm) consisting of a bright red outer border with central clearing. Regional lymphadenopathy, Kernig and Brudzinski's signs, focal neurological deficits, altered mental status, conjunctivitis, papilledema and joint swelling.

C. **DDX:** Meningitis, hepatitis, erythema multiforme, erythema nodosum, myocarditis, acute rheumatic fever, and Guillan-Barré's syndrome.

D. **Work up**: Obtain CBC, SMA-7, PT, PTT, ECG, cultures and LP.

6.2 RX:

A. Doxycycline 100 mg bid or Amoxicillin 25-50 mg/kg/day tid for 10-21 days.

B. Use Ceftriaxone 75-100 mg/kg/day IV for Lyme meningitis, arthritis or carditis.

C. **Disposition**: Most patients can be treated as an outpatient but those with neurological or cardiac complications require admission.

ENDOCRINE

For an algorithm approach to treating a patient with altered mental status and in whom an endocrine etiology is possible, refer to the section on "Change in Mental Status" within the Neurology section.

1. Alcoholic Ketoacidosis:

Alcoholic Ketoacidosis is defined as anion gap acidosis with high levels of ketoacids that are secondary to increased mobilization of free fatty acids and enhanced liver conversion of substrates to ketones.

1.1 Clinical Evaluation:

A. **Symptoms:** Chronic alcoholic with recent debauchery and decreased food intake. Complains of abdominal distress with nausea and vomiting that leads to decreased alcohol consumption. Patients often present 1-2 days after last alcohol use.

B. **Signs:** Tachycardia, ketotic breath, dehydration, Kussmaul respirations, tachypnea, and abdominal findings are variable. Neurological signs are normal to lethargic or stupor.

C. **DDX:** Pancreatitis, peptic ulcer disease, gastritis, hypoglycemia, and other causes of an anion gap metabolic acidosis.

D. **Work-up:** Order CBC, SMA-7, phosphate, serum ketone and lactate level, ABG, and possibly LFTs.

1.2 RX:

A. Administer thiamine, 100 mg IV, before administering glucose.

B. Replace fluid loses by using D_5NS or NS, and specific electrolytes. Insulin is not required.

C. Treat with sodium bicarbonate when pH is < 7.10.

D. **Disposition:** Admit the patient to a floor or unit depending on his/her stability.

2. Adrenal Crisis:

Acute insufficiency (crisis) occurs in patients with or without chronic adrenal insufficiency. This condition is precipitated by acute infection, sepsis, adrenal hemorrhage, acute stress or illness, including trauma, myocardial infarction, hypothermia, surgery, and burns. An abrupt withdrawal of steroids from a patient on chronic steroids may also result in adrenal crisis.

2.1 Clinical Evaluation:

A. **Symptoms**: Weakness and confusion with appropriate medical history. GI symptoms are prominent, such as anorexia, nausea, vomiting and abdominal pain.

B. **Signs**: Acutely ill with hypotension and circulatory collapse. Elevation in the patient's temperature may occur with hyperpigmentation, disorientation, confusion, or unconsciousness.

C. **DDX**: Myocardial infarction, heart failure, hypovolemia, sepsis, pulmonary embolism, and shock.

D. **Work-up**: Order SMA-7, CBC, ECG, CXR, Foley, and a CT prn. Determine adrenal insufficiency simultaneously with treatment.

2.2 RX:

A. Support airway, IV, O_2, and monitor.

B. Simultaneous treatment and confirmation of adrenal insufficiency may be achieved.

C. Obtain plasma cortisol and ACTH level before and after infusion as described below. Redraw cortisol between 6-8 hours if therapy is indicated. Collect urine for 24 hours to determine 17-hydroxycorticosteroid level.

D. Administer cosyntropin (synthetic ACTH), 0.25 mg IV.

E. Infuse over 1 hour, D_5 NS 1 L IV containing dexamethasone (Decadron), 4 mg or Hydrocortisone 100 mg IV.

F. Continue D_5 NS IV to restore blood pressure, 2-3 L over next 8 hours.
G. Avoid treatment of hyperkalemia with insulin. It will resolve with IV fluids and glucocorticoid replacement.
H. **Disposition**: Admit patient to the ICU.

3. Diabetic Ketoacidosis:

Diabetic Ketoacidosis is a relative deficiency of insulin with concurrent excess of stress hormones.

3.1 Clinical Evaluation:

A. **Symptoms:** Omission of daily insulin and/or stress, such as infection, cerebrovascular accident, myocardial infarction, trauma, pregnancy, hyperthyroidism, nausea, vomiting, abdominal pain, pancreatitis, and emotional upset.
B. **Signs:** Dehydration, hypotension, and tachycardia, gastric dilation, paralytic ileus, and abdominal tenderness. Neurological signs are normal orientation to coma.
C. **DDX:** Hypoglycemic coma, non-ketotic hyperosmolar coma, alcoholic ketoacidosis, and lactic acidosis.
D. **Work-up:** Order CBC, SMA-7, ABG, phosphorus, serum ketones, and urinalysis. Obtain ECG, CXR, and culture as appropriate. Glucose and serum ketones are usually elevated, K^+ will drop with treatment, and anion gap acidosis is present. Recheck SMA-7 q 2-4 hours or more frequently prn.

3.2 RX:

A. Support airway, IV, O_2, and monitor.
B. Start a NS IV at 1 L/hour for first 2-3 hours. Provide initial bolus prn.
C. Run 50 mL of insulin through tubing to saturate binding sites before administering to patient, then begin 10 units/hour IV for adults or 0.1 units/kg/hour for peds. When glucose is almost 250 mg/dL, slow infusion to 2-4 units/hour and change IVF to $D_5$1/2NS.
D. Administer sodium bicarbonate if the pH is < 7.0.
E. Consider potassium and phosphate replacement.
F. **Disposition:** Admit patient to the ICU.

4. Hypoglycemia:

A patient is considered hypoglycemic when his/her serum glucose level is below 35-55 mg/dL. Hypoglycemia may be caused by postprandial or reflex endogenous insulin release, fasting, hepatic disease, and drugs, including ethanol, propranolol, salicylates, insulin, sulfonylureas, and alcohol.

4.1 Clinical Evaluation:

A. **Symptoms:** Most common history is a diabetic using insulin who fails to eat after an insulin dose. Patients with this condition present complaints of fatigue, anxiety, hunger, confusion, and headache.
B. **Signs:** Diaphoresis, pallor, tremulousness, tachycardia, and palpitations. Neurologic manifestations range from mental confusion to coma. Moderate hypothermia may be present.
C. **DDX:** Ketoacidosis, drug interaction, islet cell tumor, hormonal deficiency states, and all potential causes of change in mental status.
D. **Work-up:** Perform a Dexi stick test. Determine serum glucose and SMA-7.

4.2 RX:

A. Administer 50 mL of D_{50} solution IV.
B. Consider continuous 5, 10, or 20% glucose infusion.
C. Treat with glucagon, 2 mg IM, if IV is unavailable.
D. Provide complex carbohydrates, i.e., like a sandwich.
E. **Disposition:** Discharge home unless the patient has prolonged hypoglycemia. Admit if there are indications of sulfonylurea ingestion.

5. Hypothyroidism and Myxedema Coma:

Hypothyroidism is a clinical condition resulting from decreased circulating levels of free thyroid hormone. Myxedema coma is severe hypothyroidism. Myxedema commonly occurs in elderly females with hypothyroidism in conjunction with a precipitating event, such as hypothermia, shock from any cause, hypoglycemia, and sepsis. The mortality rate is as high as 50% with treatment.

5.1 Clinical Evaluation:

A. **Symptoms:** History of hypothyroidism, treated Graves disease, and stoppage of thyroid replacement. Patients may complain of weakness, cold intolerance, constipation, muscle cramps, arthralgias, paresthesias, weight gain, menorrhagia, depression, and hoarseness.

B. **Signs:** Dry skin, dull facial expressions, husky voice, bradycardia, hypothermia, decreased BP, increased DBP, periorbital puffiness, swelling of the hands and feet, reduced body and scalp hair, delayed relaxation of DTRs, macroglossia, anemia, hyponatremia, and enlarged heart.

C. **DDX:** Nephrotic syndrome, chronic nephritis, depression, neurasthenia, CHF, amyloidosis, dementia, and nephritis.

D. **Work-up:** Order CBC, SMA-7, thyroid function tests (TSH & free T_4), and ABG, examining especially for hypercarbia. ECG may show low voltage.

5.2 RX:

A. Support airway, IV, O_2, and monitor.
B. Start IVF and glucose.
C. Initiate passive rewarming for hypothermia.
D. For thyroid replacement, use levothyroxine (T_4), 300-500 μg slow IV.
E. Consider hydrocortisone, 100-300 mg. Adrenal insufficiency is often a concomitant finding.
F. Treat precipitating causes.
G. **Disposition:** Admit patient to the ICU.

6. Non-Ketotic Hyperosmolar Coma:

Non-Ketotic Hyperosmolar Coma is a syndrome of profound dehydration caused from osmotic diuresis. The condition typically occurs in young adults or elderly patients, two thirds of which do not have a diabetic history. However, individuals with this condition are predisposed to a diabetogenic stressor, such as drugs, infection, surgery, or myocardial infarction. Fluid deficits are high, 9-12 L. The mortality rate is 50%.

6.1 Clinical Evaluation:

A. **Symptoms:** Antecedent polyuria and polydipsia, altered mental status from lethargy to coma frequently progresses over hours to days.

B. **Signs:** Signs of dehydration, postural hypotension, and reflex tachycardia due to cardiovascular collapse. Neurologic findings include seizures, change in mental status, focal deficits, aphasia, nystagmus, tremors, and hyperreflexia.

C. **DDX:** Diabetic ketoacidosis and other causes of change in mental status, i.e., hepatic failure, sepsis, drug ingestion, dehydration, uremia, and cerebrovascular accident.

D. **Work-up:** Order chemistries (glucose average values about 1000 mg/dL), CBC, U/A, ABG, CXR, ECG, blood and urine culture, amylase, liver enzymes, and coagulation studies. Calculate serum osmolarity = 2(Na) + glucose/18 + BUN/2.8.

6.2 RX:

A. Support ABCs, IV, O_2, and monitor.
B. Initiate fluid resuscitation with 1-2 L NS for the first hour followed by 1 L/hour over the next few hours.
C. Replace potassium if the patient is not hyperkalemic or is not in renal failure.

D. Hyperglycemia will decrease with fluid resuscitation; however, consider a low dosage of insulin for patients who are hyperkalemic, acidotic, or in renal failure. Administer regular insulin, 0.1/kg/hour, until glucose levels drop to 250 mg/dL.

E. **Disposition:** Admit the patient to the ICU.

7. Thyroid Storm:

Thyroid Storm is caused by the undiagnosed or undetected thyrotoxic Graves' disease or a toxic multinodular goiter. The abrupt onset of this condition is usually precipitated by infection, trauma, vascular accident, or diabetic complications.

7.1 Clinical Evaluation:

A. **Symptoms:** Severe weakness proceeding weight loss a few weeks prior to presentation. Heat intolerance and eye complaints may be displayed from bulbar palsy. The patient probably has a history of thyroid disease. Nervousness, increased sweating, palpitations, dyspnea, increased appetite, tremor, and emotional lability may also be exhibited.

B. **Signs:** Temp > 38.7 °C (100 °F), wide pulse pressure, neurologic manifestations from restlessness to coma, increased DTRs, and cardiovascular effects, including atrial fibrillation and congestive heart failure. Ophthalmopathy, goiter, warm moist skin, and weight loss may be present.

C. **DDX:** Heat stroke and drug toxicity, including neuroleptic malignant syndrome and withdrawal syndromes, psychosis, pheochromocytoma, and congestive heart failure.

D. **Work-up:** Obtain CBC, SMA-7, and LFTs. The calcium levels are often elevated. Order TFTs to include T4-RIA and free T4 index.

7.2 RX:

A. Support airway, IV, O_2, monitor.

B. Block effects with propranolol, 1-2 mg IV q 15 minutes prn to a 10 mg total dose.

C. Block release with SSKI, 3-5 gtt po/ng q 8 hours.

D. Block synthesis with PTU, 900-1200 mg po/ng load.

E. Treat hyperthermia with acetaminophen and a cooling blanket.

F. Treat congestive heart failure.

G. Provide stress-dose corticosteroid, such as hydrocortisone, 100-500 mg/day IV.

H. **Disposition:** Admit patient to the ICU.

8. Wernicke-Korsakoff Complex:

Wernicke-Korsakoff Complex is a potentially fatal disorder caused by a thiamine deficiency. Wernicke's encephalopathy has one or more findings of a triad of global confusion, ataxia, and ophthalmoplegia. Korsakoff's psychosis consists of irreversible memory deficit marked by amnestic apathy and confabulation. The mortality rate is between 15-20%.

8.1 Clinical Evaluation:

A. **Symptoms:** Chronic alcoholics and patients with history of genetic defect in transketolase are most common. Administration of glucose in thiamine deficient person can precipitate symptoms.

B. **Signs:** Nystagmus and ophthalmoplegia followed by disorientation and ataxia. Abnormal mental status includes progression to coma, hypotension, hypothermia, and circulatory collapse.

C. **DDX:** Alcohol intoxication or withdrawal, acute or chronic subdural hematoma, intracranial trauma, metabolic or drug induced encephalopathy's, CNS infection, vascular accident, tumor, demyelinating disease, and hypothermia.

D. **Work-up:** Diagnosis clinical. Concomitant magnesium deficiency is common. Order lab tests to eliminate the possibility of other pathologic etiologies.

8.2 RX:

A. Administer 100 mg of thiamine IV.
B. Monitor cardiac responses and vital signs. Evaluate serial Neuro exams.
C. Advise alcohol abstinence and an adequate diet.
D. **Disposition:** Admit patient to an acute care service.

ENVIRONMENTAL

1. Bee, Wasp, and Ant Stings (Hymenoptera):

Hymenoptera stings originate from bees, wasps, hornets, yellow jackets, and ants. Stings may result in local inflammatory reactions, immediate and delayed hypersensitivity reactions, atypical reactions, and direct systemic toxicity.

1.1 Clinical Evaluation:

A. **Symptoms:** Pruritus, pain, slight erythema and edema at the sting site.

B. **Signs:**

Local reaction: Redness and edema is apparent at sting site. Stinger or venom sac may be present.

Toxic reaction: Ten or more stings are present that results in vomiting, diarrhea, light headedness, syncope, headache, fever, muscle spasms, and edema.

Anaphylactic reaction: Generalized urticaria, facial flushing, itching eyes, dry cough, chest or throat constriction, wheezing, dyspnea, cyanosis, abdominal cramps, diarrhea, nausea and vomiting, vertigo, fever, chills, pharyngeal stridor, shock, loss of consciousness, involuntary bowel and bladder action, and bloody frothy sputum. Reaction may be fatal.

1.2 RX:

A. Support airway, IV, O_2, and monitor.

B. For a local reaction, remove stinger, if present, but do not squeeze. Wash the affected area with soap and water to minimize the risk of infection. Analgesics may be indicated. Apply an ice pack to the site and elevate the limb to delay absorption and limit edema. Administer 20-40 mg of prednisone po q day for 3 days, to reduce swelling. Treat with Benadryl, 25-50 mg po q 6-8 hours, or Zantac, 150 mg po bid, for pruritus.

C. For a systemic reaction, administer epinephrine HCl, 1:1000 0.3-0.5 mL sq for an adult, **or** 0.01 mL/kg sq for a child but no more than 0.3 mL. A second injection may be given for more severe reactions. This injection should be given in 10-15 minutes in conjunction with diphenhydramine, 25-50 mg IM/IV. If bronchospasm develops, administer albuterol, nebulized 2.5 mg in 3 mL and repeat. Oxygen, via mask, or ETT should be administered as indicated. If hypotension develops, give crystalloid infusions. Persistent hypotension requires dopamine, 200 mg in 250 mL of NS at 5 μg/kg/minute, titrated to effect. Administer Solu-Medrol, 90-120 mg IV initially, followed by prednisone, 10-40 mg po every day for 5-7 days, to limit urticaria and edema.

D. For a delayed reaction, 10-14 days after the sting, treat with po steroids. Administer brompheniramine maleate, 2-4 mg qid for adults, 1-2 mg qid for a child, **or** diphenhydramine, if needed. Antibiotics may be necessary if a secondary infection occurs.

E. **Disposition:** If treatment requires epinephrine, the patient should be monitored in the ED for several hours to ensure that the symptoms do not intensify. Monitor all severe reaction cases for 24-48 hours and examine the patient for cardiac problems, bleeding, and neurologic complications.

2. Black Widow Spider Envenomation:

Latrodectus mactans females are characterized by a globular abdomen, leg spans of 2.5 cm, and a red hourglass design on the ventral surface of the abdomen. These spiders are poisonous.

2.1 Clinical Evaluation:

A. **Symptoms:** A brief, sharp pain is noted. Over the next 30 minutes, pain is described as deep, burning, aching, or numbing which may begin near the bite location, such as in an arm or leg. Pain may be located in the back, neck, chest, abdomen, or flanks. Vomiting, headache, chest tightness, hypertension, salivation, and lacrimation may occur.

B. **Signs:** Two minor puncture wounds are present. No necrosis or significant swelling is apparent. A halo lesion consisting of a circular area of pallor surrounded by a ring of erythema may be exhibited. Rigid and tender muscles, diaphoresis, hypertension, and periorbital ecchymosis may be displayed.

C. **DDX:** Almost any illness that causes pain must be considered. Therefore, eliminate the possibility of myocardial infarction and acute abdomen.

D. **Work-up:** Obtain ECG, CXR, CBC, SMA-7, U/A, and CPK.

2.2 RX:

A. Support airway, IV, O_2, and monitor.
B. Initiate tetanus prophylaxis.
C. Relieve pain.
D. Indications for antivenin (I vial IM/IV) are severe pain or dangerous hypertension. Antivenin is contraindicated in patients allergic to horse serum. In addition, it is not recommended for patients taking β-blocking agents. Perform a skin test before administration of antivenin.
E. Control hypertension with nitroprusside, nifedipine, and/or hydralazine.
F. Use of calcium and methocarbamol is of questionable value.
G. **Disposition:** Patients with mild to moderate symptoms who are controlled by oral analgesics may be discharged. If the patient treated with antivenin shows no complications and is asymptomatic, he/she may go home after 8-10 hours of observation. Admit victims of ages < 14 and > 65 years, individuals with history of hypertension, women who are pregnant, and patients requiring parenteral narcotics.

3. Brown Recluse Spider Envenomation:

The *Loxosceles reclusa* spider measures 1-5 cm leg to leg. It is fawn to dark brown and has a violin-shaped, dark brown to yellow marking on its cephalothorax with the larger end pointed toward the head. The spider has three pairs of eyes rather than the typical four pairs present in other spiders.

3.1 Clinical Evaluation:

A. **Symptoms:** The bite feels like a pin prick that itches, tingles, and swells. The affected area becomes red, tender, and blanches within a few hours after the bite. Weakness, nausea, arthralgias, and myalgias may occur. Systemic loxoscelism presents with severe illness, high fever, rash, and hemolytic anemia with hemoglobinuria

B. **Signs:** Fever, chills, malaise, rash, blebs or purpura form may result. Necrosis with induration and eschar may be displayed within hours.

C. **DDX:** Other bites and stings, erythema multiforme, diabetic ulcer, herpes simplex, and poison oak and ivy.

D. **Work-up:** Order CBC, U/A coagulation studies, LFTs, serum amylase, and SMA-7.

3.2 RX:

A. Provide standard initial wound care and apply ice compresses to the affected area.
B. The best treatment is not known. However, a controversial treatment includes the administration of dapsone, a leukocyte inhibitor, 100 mg po bid, and erythromycin, 250 mg po qid.
C. Treatment of systemic arachnidism consists of platelet or RBC administration.
D. Use of methylprednisolone, 1-2 mg/kg IV qid, is of questionable benefit.
E. Primary treatment is "benign neglect."
F. Antipruritic or antianxiety drugs are comforting.
G. Prescribe analgesics for pain.
H. NSAIDS are contraindicated.
I. Corrective surgery is delayed 6-8 weeks when necrosis is clearly demarcated.
J. **Disposition:** Consult the regional Poison Control center or a toxicologist. Recheck patient daily for 3-5 days after he/she is discharged. Refer to plastic surgery. Admit patients with significant systemic symptoms.

4. Cat Bites:

Cat bites tend to be puncture wounds with infection rates of 50%. Long, narrow teeth often produce wounds that are at high risk for producing tenosynovitis. Typical organisms that cause the infections are *Staphylococcus aureus, Streptococcus* species, *Klebsiella, Enterobacter* species, anaerobes, *Pasteurella multocida*, and small gram-negative rods.

4.1 Clinical Evaluation:

A. **Symptoms:** Headache, fever, malaise, and tender regional lymphadenopathy may be displayed one week after a cat scratch or bite. Transient macular or vesicular rash may be present. Determine immunization and health status of the animal.
B. **Signs:** Lymphadenopathy, possible rash, and suppurative lymph nodes. Local extremity wound may be red, swollen, and digit partially flexed with tenderness or passive extension.
C. **DDX:** Plague, syphilis, lymphogranuloma venereum, sporotrichosis, anthrax, fungal infection, mononucleosis, sarcoid, lymphoma, and bacterial adenitis.

4.2 RX:

A. Copiously irrigate the affected area.
B. Debride devitalized tissue.
C. Normal hosts with relatively clean lacerations, especially of the face, can be safely sutured especially if the bite is treated within a few hours of injury. Hand bites should not be closed.
D. Delayed primary closure and healing by secondary intention are less apt to result in an infection.
E. Use Augmentin, 500-875 mg bid or 250-500 mg tif for 7 days, or penicillin, 500 mg tid plus plus dicloxacillin 500 mg qid for 7 days, as the first drugs of choice in cat bites. Secondary choices consist of doxycycline, 100 mg bid for 7 days, or tetracycline, 500 mg qid for penicillin-allergic patients plus clindamycin 300 mg qid for 7 days..
F. Implement tetanus prophylaxis.
G. Cat scratch disease resolves spontaneously in 1-2 months. Antibiotics are not effective for this disorder.
H. **Disposition**: Admit patients who are septic, immunocompromised, or who show infectious signs of CNS, head, joint, or deep structure involvement for IV antibiotics. All patients who are discharged should be re-examined in 24-48 hours.

5. Cold-Induced Tissue Injuries:

Frostbite is the destruction of tissue by freezing. Immersion foot is tissue injury at temperatures between 32-50 °F with prolonged exposure to a wet environment.

5.1 Clinical Evaluation:

A. **History/Signs**: Initially the skin is pale, waxy white, or mottled blue, and may range from rock-solid to firm on palpation. Frozen tissue is cold and lacks sensation. Check for a superimposed burn injury due to rewarming. Vesicles or bullae with clear to bloody fluid may be present. Patients with immersion foot complain of numbness, pain, and paresthesias. Early findings include coolness, pallor, sensitivity, and edema. Later cyanosis, mottling, or erythema may be exhibited. Maceration with secondary bacterial or fungal infection may also be present.
B. **DDX**: Devascularizing injury, envenomation, and thermal or chemical burn.

5.2 RX:

A. Ensure that the patient does not rub, warm, or manipulate the affected part on transport to ED.
B. Remove all wet nonadherent apparel and place patient under a warm blanket.
C. Implement tetanus prophylaxis.
D. Rapidly thaw frostbitten part in a 40 °C water bath.
E. Administer an analgesic for pain control.
F. Remove clear blisters but leave hemorrhagic blisters intact.
G. Apply aloe vera every 6 hours.
H. Treat pain with ibuprofen, 400 mg po bid, and ascorbic acid, 1 g po bid.

I. Advise patient to stop smoking.
J. Treat Immersion Foot by rewarming and elevation. Avoid manipulation and pressure.
K. Provide local skin care, including cleansing, topical antibiotics, such as Neosporin and silver sulfadiazine cream, and dressing for denuded areas.
L. **Disposition:** Admit all patients except very mild cases. A surgical consultation should be obtained. If patient is discharged, re-examine him/her within 24 hours.

6. Dog Bites:

Dog bites usually present as crush-type lacerations with devitalized adjacent tissue. Approximately 10% of all dog-bite wounds become infected with a much higher rate involving full thickness bites. The organisms that are typically contracted are the same as those cited for "cat bites".

6.1 Clinical Evaluation:

A. **Symptoms:** Details of the biting event, including time, offending animal, immunization and health status, captured status, and nature of attack, provoked vs. unprovoked, should be obtained.
B. **Signs:** Check for wound infection, septic arthritis, and osteomyelitis. If a wound infection occurs within 24 hours after the bite, assume *Pasteurella multocida* as the causative agent.

6.3 RX:

A. Irrigate wound, debride devitalized tissue, and initiate tetanus prophylaxis.
B. Cleanse small puncture wounds and lacerations. Do not bandage the wounds.
C. Close most lacerations with the exception of those in the hand with a potential for joint or tendon involvement.
D. Carefully evaluate hand wounds.
E. Obtain a culture if the wound is infected.
F. Treat with Augmentin 500-875 mg bid or Cephalexin 50 mg qid for 7 days. Alternative antibiotics are clindamycin 300 mg qid plus doxycycline 100 mg bid for penicillin allergic patients.
G. **Disposition:** Patient can usually be discharged. However, if there are signs of serious infection the patient must be admitted, particularly if there is any hand involvement.

7. Electrical Injuries:

7.1 Clinical Evaluation:

A. **Symptoms:** Nausea, vomiting, paresthesias, and pain.
B. **Signs:** Pallor, ileus, burned and necrotic tissue, skeletal fractures, joint dislocations (especially post. shoulder), and spinal compression fractures. CNS manifestations include amnesia, altered mental status, irritability, depression, emotional lability, motor deficits, seizures, and coma. Arrhythmias and respiratory depression may occur. Small entrance wounds are commonly found on hands and upper extremities and may demonstrate charring, depression, edema, and inflammatory changes. Large exit wounds may be multiple and have an explosive appearance. Compartment syndrome can occur.
C. **Work-up:** Support airway, IV, O_2, and monitor. Order an ECG. Provide standard trauma evaluation as appropriate. Order CBC, SMA-7, CPK, including isoenzymes to evaluate for cardiac injury, and rhabdomyolysis. Check for rhabdomyolysis with urine dip (positive for RBC in presence of myoglobin). If positive, send for U/A to include urine myoglobin. Consider coagulation studies, LFTs, amylase, lipase, and calcium.

7.2 RX:

A. Support ABCs while immobilizing the c-spine.
B. Use standard ACLS and advanced trauma life support protocols as indicated.
C. Position an indwelling urinary catheter, place on O_2, and monitor ECG continuously.
D. Treat rhabdomyolysis with aggressive fluid resuscitation, mannitol and diuretics to enhance urinary output. Add sodium bicarbonate to IV in order to alkalinize the urine and prevent myoglobulin precipitation in the renal tubules, usually 3 amps in 1 L of D_5W run at 250 mL/hr.
E. Initiate NG suctioning, tetanus prophylaxis, and consider treating with an antibiotic, such as Ancef.

F. **Disposition:** All patients exposed to > 1000 V will probably require admission to a monitored bed or ICU. Intermediate voltage exposures also can cause serious injury. Patients with low- voltage nonsystemic injuries may be discharged after evaluation, observation, and management in the ED. For all serious injuries, consultation and/or transfer to a burn center is essential.

8. Heat Illnesses:

Heat illness is the inability of the normal regulatory mechanism to cope with heat stress. A spectrum of symptoms occur, including loss of the ability to sweat, cramps that result from sweat induced hyponatremia without volume depletion, and heat exhaustion resulting from volume depletion, and heatstroke involving CNS temperature elevation with CNS findings.

8.1 Clinical Evaluation:

A. **History/Signs:**

Signs for heat exhaustion are weakness, dizziness, anxiety, muscle incoordination, agitation, confusion, palpitations, oliguria, elevated temperature, headache, vomiting, muscle cramps, and diarrhea. Skin is cool and clammy. Tachycardia and hypotension may occur.

Signs of heatstroke are confusion, coma, seizures, tachypnea, tachycardia, ataxia and high core temperature (> 40 °C). Malaise or flu-like prodrome are also displayed.

B. **DDX:** Meningitis, thyroid disease, drug intoxication, and neuroleptic malignant syndrome.

C. **Work-up:** Acquire medication history and determine any underlying medical problems. Obtain orthostatic vital signs, rectal temperature, ABG, CBC, SMA-7, CPK levels, U/A, liver enzymes, coagulation studies, calcium, magnesium, phosphorous, and uric acid. Consider ECG and CXR. Order urine myoglobin.

8.2 RX:

A. Support airway, IV, O_2, and monitor.
B. Cool patient rapidly by spritzing with lukewarm water and blowing air over him/her with a fan. Continue cooling process until the patient's core temperature drops to 38.5 to 39 °C.
C. Insert a Foley catheter.
D. Correct acid-base, electrolyte, and coagulation abnormalities.
E. Treat with alkaline diuresis, 3 amps $NaHCO_3$ in 1 L of D_5W run at 250 mL/hr, if rhabdomyolysis is present.
F. Treat shivering with midazolam, 2.5-10.0 mg IV.
G. Treat seizures with diazepam or phenobarbital. However, phenytoin is ineffective.
H. **Disposition:** Admit heat exhausted patient to floor. Admit all patients with heatstroke to the ICU.

9. High Altitude Illness:

Symptoms associated with High Altitude Illness can begin at elevations > 8000 feet. Rapid altitude gain and pre-existing cardiopulmonary disease result in a higher incidence of symptoms. There are a spectrum of syndromes ranging from mild Acute Mountain Sickness (AMS), accompanied by headache and insomnia, to High Altitude Pulmonary Edema (HAPE), and High Altitude Cerebral Edema (HACE). Death may occur. Acetazolamide is useful in prevention.

9.1 Clinical Evaluation:

A. **Symptoms:** Headache, anorexia, nausea/vomiting, malaise, insomnia, and lassitude for AMS. In addition, cough, hemoptysis, shortness of breath, dyspnea on exertion for HAPE, and confusion, ataxia, and change in mental status for HACE may be exhibited.
B. **Signs:** Confusion, poor judgment, coma, tachycardia, tachypnea, cyanosis, peripheral and periorbital edema, rales, papilledema, and retinal flame hemorrhages.
C. **DDX:** Upper respiratory infection, gastroenteritis, hypothermia, hypovolemia, asthma, exacerbation of COPD, noncardiogenic pulmonary edema (due to medication or neurologic problem), pneumonia, and meningitis. The differential of CNS manifestations also includes metabolic, psychiatric, toxic, and traumatic disorders.
D. **Work-up:** Order CBC, SMA-7, ABG, CXR, and ECG. Consider pulmonary function tests.

9.2 RX:

A. If AMS is severe, a descent to below 2500 m (8100 feet) is required. Administer oxygen, diuretics, and fluid therapy.
B. Descent is the primary treatment. Consider endotracheal intubation, ventilatory support, continuous positive airway pressure, or PEEP for HAPE and HACE.
C. Consider use of a Ganow bag if available.
D. **Disposition:** A patient who does not have an underlying illness and have experienced mild to moderate AMS may be discharged if he/she has improved. Those with underlying cardiopulmonary or cerebrovascular disease, severe AMS, HAPE, HACE, or complications, such as ECG changes, should be admitted.

10. High Pressure Injection Injuries:

High pressure injection injuries appear innocuously but can have devastating consequences if treatment is delayed or inadequate. Consultation with a hand or plastic surgeon is always warranted.

10.1 Clinical Evaluation:

A. **Symptoms:** High pressure exposure.
B. **Signs:** Extremity or body part is initially pain-free, followed by an acute inflammatory process that causes swelling and intense pain. Usually a small pinhole entrance wound is present and a drop of injectate can be expressed from the wound. The index finger is the most commonly injured extremity. Pallor, pulselessness, and paresthesia may be also be displayed.
C. **DDX:** Envenomation by reptiles, insects, arachnids, tenosynovitis, and foreign body.
D. **Work-up:** Conduct a detailed peripheral neuro/motor/sensory exam to the affected part. Evaluate peripheral pulses and palmar arches by Doppler. Perform an Allen's test and order an X-ray to rule out a foreign body and gas. Obtain preoperative labs.

10.2 RX:

A. Place hand in a soft, bulky dressing without undue compression. Splint in neutral position and elevate injured area with pillows.
B. Administer a broad-spectrum antibiotics.
C. Administer tetanus toxoid.
D. DO NOT start an IV or obtain blood pressures in the affected arm.
E. Consult a hand or plastic surgeon.
F. **Disposition**: Admit the patient for possible surgical exploration.

11. Human Bites:

A human bite may result in a dangerous wound, especially when distal extremities are involved. Aerobic and anaerobic bacteria from mouth become embedded in the wound potentially leading to tenosynovitis, septic arthritis, or osteomyelitis if untreated. The infection rate is > 20%.

11.1 Clinical Evaluation:

A. **Symptoms:** Suspect a human bite when the wound is over the knuckles, ears, nose, tongue, nipples, fingertips, or penis.
B. **Signs:** Erythema, swelling, warmth, and purulence. There is more pain than normally expected. Lymphangitis and adenopathy indicate a risk for sepsis.
C. **Work-up:** Determine immunologic status of patient. If immunocompromised, obtain CBC and SMA-7. Consider a blood culture if there is evidence of an infection. X-ray all significant hand wounds and wounds that overlie bones and joints.

11.2 RX:

A. Copiously irrigate the wound.
B. Implement tetanus prophylaxis.

C. Close facial wounds if there is no infection. Wounds of the hands and wounds with tendon injury or joint space involvement should be referred to a surgeon.
D. Treat fractures as open fractures.
E. Use an antibiotic to cover *Staphylococcus, Streptococcus, Eikenella corrodens* and other gram-negative organism infections. If patient is sent home, treat him/her with Augmentin 500-875 mg bid or 250-500 mg po tid for 5-7 days, for prophylactic coverage. Prescribe erythromycin, 500 mg po qid, if patient is allergic to penicillin. Another alternative is penicillin, 500 mg po qid, with dicloxacillin, 500 mg po qid.
F. **Disposition:** If patient is sent home, ensure that the wound is rechecked in 24 hours. Patients with signs of soft tissue infection, including lymphangitis, adenopathy, or symptoms of systemic infection, such as fever, chills, and rigors, should receive IV antibiotics in the ED and be admitted. In addition, admit individuals who are immunocompromised.

12. Hypothermia:

The hypothermic patient typically has a core temperature of less than 35 °C (95 °F). Several mechanisms may contribute to the cause of hypothermia, including conduction (loss of heat by direct contact), convection (body to air loss), radiation (loss to air), and evaporation (sweating).

12.1 Clinical Evaluation:

A. **History/Signs:** Apathy, confusion, lethargy, fatigue, incoordination, shivering, slurred speech, tachycardia, and tachypnea occur in mild hypothermia. With progressive hypothermia (< 86 °F), shivering stops, pulse rate, blood pressure, and respiratory rate decrease. Disorientation, stupor, inappropriate behavior, polyuria, rhonchi, and wheezing may be noted. ECG shows A-fib, PAT, T wave changes, PVCs, or Osborne waves. In severe hypothermia, the patient experiences coma, dilated unreactive pupils, absent or weak pulses, barely detectable respirations, absent reflexes, muscle rigidity, hypotension, decreased EEG amplitude, or an ECG showing bradycardia, asystole, or V-fib.
B. **DDX:** Hypothermia may occur with endocrine, metabolic, toxic, traumatic, or vascular conditions which cause CNS depression.
C. **Work-up:** Order ECG, CXR, ABG, CBC, amylase, SMA- 7, coagulation profile, urinalysis, serum calcium, magnesium, phosphate, lactate, cardiac enzyme levels, liver and thyroid function tests, and toxicology screening as indicated. Determine oxygen saturation.

12.2 RX:

A. Support airway, IV, O_2, and monitor.
B. Monitor temperature continuously with a rectal probe.
C. Remove wet nonadherent clothing and cover the patient with warm blankets.
D. Warm IV fluids to 45 °C.
E. Actively rewarm neonates and adults with moderate and severe hypothermia by providing warm IV fluids and humidified O_2 heated to 42-45 °C.
F. Actively rewarm the core for patients with severe hypothermia by performing a peritoneal lavage with 45 °C fluid. Warm the blood by hemodialysis or by using a femorofemoral cardiopulmonary bypass pump. Perform a pleuromediastinal lavage by way of thoracostomy or thoracotomy.
G. Correct underlying metabolic derangements.
H. Consider stress-dose steroid or thyroid hormone if patient is unresponsive to aggressive warming or underlying endocrinopathy exists.
I. **Disposition:** Observe a patient with mild hypothermia until he/she is asymptomatic and normothermic. Individuals who are very young, very old, or those with underlying pathology should be admitted. Admit patients with moderate to severe hypothermia to the ICU.

13. Lightning Injuries:

13.1 Clinical Evaluation:

A. **Symptoms:** History of lightning strike or location are consistent with injuries sustained. Hair standing on end is evident.

B. **Signs:** Cardiopulmonary arrest, prolonged apnea, altered mental status, antegrade or retrograde amnesia, hemiparesis, hemiplegia, flaccid paralysis, altered autonomic function, c-spine fracture and associated spinal cord injury, and lateralizing neurologic signs. Extremities may appear cold, mottled, and pulseless. Ocular lesions may be present, including hyphemia, uveitis, iridocyclitis, and vitreous hemorrhage may occur. Less common signs are transient unilateral or bilateral blindness, choroid rupture, chorioretinitis, retinal detachment, and optic atrophy. Mydriasis is unresponsive to light. Sensorineural hearing deficit, hemotympanum, CSF otorrhea, tympanic membrane rupture, or basilar skull fracture are common signs.

C. **DDX:** Cerebrovascular accident, seizure disorders, neuro-trauma, Stokes-Adams attack, toxic ingestion, envenomations, myocardial infarction, cardiac arrhythmias, physical assault, hypertensive crisis with intracranial hemorrhage, acute narrow angle glaucoma, and traumatic iritis.

D. **Work-up:** Provide standard trauma evaluation as appropriate. Order ECG, CBC, SMA-7, CPK, and isoenzymes to evaluate for cardiac injury and rhabdomyolysis. Check for rhabdomyolysis with urine dip (positive for RBC in presence of myoglobin). If positive, send for U/A to include urine myoglobin. Consider PT, PTT, LFTs, amylase, lipase, and calcium. Complete an ocular exam.

13.2 RX:

A. Support airway, IV, O_2, monitor. Provide standard burn care.

B. Administer tetanus toxoid.

C. Treat myoglobinuria, (refer to the "Electrical Injuries" section) with IV of 0.9% sodium chloride.

D. Treat cardiac arrhythmias in the standard fashion.

E. Administer 100 mg of thiamine, 50 mg of dextrose, and 2 mg of naloxone IV to patients with altered mental conditions.

F. Monitor: continuously and place on supplemental O_2. ACLS and advanced trauma life support protocols should be followed.

G. **Disposition:** Admit the patient for continuous monitoring.

14. Snake Envenomation:

Appropriate snake bite treatment is often determined by the type of snake that was encountered. When this information is not available, the patient's symptoms may be the only way to evaluate the severity of the bite or the type of snake involved. References that describe the snakes that are indigenous to the area may be helpful.

14.1 Clinical Evaluation:

A. **Symptoms:** Encounter with a venomous snake, which is usually alcohol related (on the patient's side).

B. **Signs:** One or 2 fang marks are present that result in pain, edema, and erythema at site. Systemic effects may include increased or decreased temperature, nausea, vomiting, diarrhea, pain, restlessness, and increased or decreased heart rate. Neurotoxic symptoms consist of dysphagia, convulsions, psychosis, muscle weakness, paresthesia, fasciculation, and in extreme cases, paralysis. Hemopathic manifestations, such as local bleeding, ecchymosis, bleeding from kidneys, peritoneum, rectum, or vagina, are seen with pit viper bites.

C. **Work-up:** Order T&C, CBC, PT, PTT, SMA-7, U/A, and wound culture.

14.2 RX:

A. Support airway, IV, O_2, and monitor.

B. Place supine to rest and decrease metabolism. Position injured body part in a dependent position.

C. Administer a tetanus booster.

D. If there is severe bleeding, transfuse as needed.

E. Treat arrhythmias per ACLS.
F. Treat itching or urticaria with antihistamines.
G. Administer antivenin as determined by the type of snake encountered. Antivenin should generally be given within 4 hours of the bite. After 12 hours, the value is uncertain. Check for hypersensitivity.
H. Copperhead snake bites are self-limited and do not require antivenin unless the snake is unusually large, multiple bites are present, or the victim is small or debilitated.
I. Compartment syndrome may develop in injured extremity. Perform a fasciotomy at a pressure of 30 mm Hg or higher.
J. **Disposition:** Asymptomatic patients may be discharged after 8-12 hours of observation. Admit the patient to ICU if the he/she is receiving antivenin and/or if the bite is severe. Mild to moderate envenomation patients may be admitted to a floor bed.

15. Submersion Injuries:

Drowning is death from suffocation due to submersion in a fluid. Near-drowning implies that the victim survived, at leas temporarily, such an experience.

15.1 Clinical Evaluation:

A. **Symptoms:** History of coughing, choking, or vomiting after submersion.
B. **Signs:** Various stages of resuscitation. The patient may be awake, lethargic but is arousable, combative, comatose or in cardiac arrest. Signs include increased pulse, blood pressure, and respiratory rate. If severe hypoxia is present, vital signs are decreased or absent. Hypothermia may be present. Vomitus, water, or a foreign material is present in the mouth. Rhonchi, rales, or wheezing is displayed. Gastric distention is common. Decorticate or decerebrate posturing or flaccid paralysis, unreactive pupils and other cranial nerve findings with severe hypoxia are exhibited. Loss of brain stem and deep tendon reflexes may also be observed.
C. **DDX:** Head and/or spinal trauma, drug or chemical intoxication, cardiac arrest, stroke, cerebral air embolus, attempted suicide or murder, and hypothermia.
D. **Work-up:** Obtain ECG, ABG, CBC, electrolytes, U/A, glucose, platelet count, liver function tests, BUN, creatine, coagulation studies, and cardiac enzymes. Consider CXR, c-spine, X-ray, a CT of the head, and an alcohol and drug screen.

15.2 RX:

A. Early resuscitation is the most important factor influencing morbidity and mortality.
B. Provide ACLS, advanced trauma life support, and change in mental status treatment.
C. Administer bronchodilators prn, such as albuterol, 2.5 mg per nebulizer.
D. Treat hypotension with isotonic crystalloid solution IV.
E. Insert a Foley, a CVP, and a NG tube.
F. Treat agitation and seizures pharmacologically.
G. Treat increasing ICP with hyperventilation, elevation of head to 30°, osmotic diuretics and barbiturates.
H. Intubate on 100% O_2 for full arrest, coma, inability to protect airway, combativeness, or when the pO_2 is < 50 mm Hg, or a pCO_2 is > 50 mm Hg is displayed.
I. Place on PEEP.
J. Consider extracorporeal membrane oxygenation in patients unresponsive to 100% oxygen and PEEP.
K. **Disposition:** Asymptomatic patients, or those who become so after 4-6 hours of observation, with a normal physical exam, room air ABG analysis, and CXR may be sent home. However, ensure that the patient is discharged in the care of a friend or relative. Admit all others. The level of care for admits, floor vs. ICU, depends on severity and progression of clinical and laboratory findings. Indication for transfer include lack of ICU facilities and the unavailability of a pulmonary specialist capable of performing bronchoscopy.

GASTROINTESTINAL

1. Acute Abdominal Pain:

The most common cause of abdominal pain in a large series is not known (42%), followed by gastroenteritis (31%), gastritis, peptic ulcer disease, gallbladder disease, diarrhea, and pancreatitis. Visceral abdominal pain from the autonomic fibers is crampy, intermittent, and colicky. Somatic abdominal pain resulting from pain fibers in parietal peritoneum is constant, sharp, and localized. Generally, abdominal pain lasting longer than 6 hours or abdominal pain in the elderly requires a surgical consultation.

1.1 Clinical Evaluation:

A. **Symptoms:** Location, onset, duration, quality, and severity of pain should be recorded. Associated symptoms, including nausea, vomiting, diarrhea, urinary difficulties, vaginal discharge or bleeding should also be noted. Previous episodes with drugs, alcohol, should be determined and a menstrual history must be obtained.

B. **Signs:** Check VS and temperature. Evaluate for pallor, shock, rales, diminished breath sounds (lower lobe pneumonia may mimic abdominal pain), splinting, guarding, and pulsatile masses. Auscultate for bowel sounds and percuss for peritoneal irritation. Palpate all four quadrants, initially away from most tender region. Check for masses, rebound, point tenderness, Murphy's sign, iliopsoas sign, and obturator sign. Examine back for costovertebral angle tenderness. Check for hernias. Rectal for masses, tenderness and blood. In males, scrotal masses and tenderness are evident. Females experience vaginal discharge, bleeding, cervical motion tenderness, adnexal fullness, and focal tenderness.

C. **DDX:** Common emergencies requiring immediate surgical intervention are perforated viscus, ruptured abdominal aortic aneurysm, acute appendicitis, bowel ischemia, or infected, ectopic pregnancy, and strangulated hernia. Small-bowel obstruction and acute pancreatitis must also be identified to prevent morbidity.

Common causes of visceral, colicky pain are early appendicitis, bowel obstruction, and renal colic.

Common causes of somatic pain are late appendicitis, liver disease, and peritonitis. Other common causes of abdominal pain are UTI, diverticulitis, PID, gastroenteritis and diabetic ketoacidosis. Irritable bowel syndrome is a diagnosis of exclusion. Gastroenteritis is associated with vomiting (gastritis) and diarrhea (enteritis).

Common etiologies for tenderness according to abdominal regions are:

⇒ **RUQ** - Hepatitis, Cholecystitis, and Cholangitis.
⇒ **LUQ** - Gastritis and PUD.
⇒ **EPIGASTRIC** - PUD and Pancreatitis
⇒ **RLQ** - Appendicitis, PID, and Ectopic.
⇒ **LLQ** - Diverticulitis, PID, and Ectopic.
⇒ **SUPRAPUBIC** - Cystitis, Hernia, and Torsion.
⇒ **DIFFUSE/OR ANY QUADRANT** - Aneurysm, pancreatitis (mostly periumbilical), bowel obstruction, ureteral calculus, perforation/peritonitis, irritable bowel syndrome, gastroenteritis, and inflammatory bowel disease.
⇒ **CVA/FLANK** - ureteral calculus and pyelonephritis.

D. **Work-up:** Order CBC, U/A, and SMA-7. Order LFT'S, amylase and lipase if indicated. Obtain an ECG, chest and abdominal series, X-rays, cardiac enzymes, and CT of abdomen as needed. Special CT evaluation of appendix may be appropriate. Bedside or formal ultrasound may be performed.

1.2 RX (refer also to specific cause):

A. Support airway, IV, O_2, and monitor prn. Insert a NG tube for obstruction or bleeding cases.
B. Order NPO.
C. Provide analgesia per local custom or per previous consultation with surgical colleagues.

D. Obtain appropriate consultation with surgery or obstetrics.
E. **Disposition:** Admit all patients except those with the mildest problems.

2. Appendicitis:

Appendicitis usually arises as an outcome of hyperplasia of the lymphatic tissue or fecaliths which induce luminal obstruction. Mucus accumulates, intraluminal pressure increases, and an obstruction of lymphatic drainage occurs resulting in severe pain. Peak incidence of appendicitis occurs in the second and third decades.

2.1 Clinical Evaluation:

A. **Symptoms:** A typical case exhibits diffuse abdominal pain lasting several hours, low-grade fever, followed by pain localizing to the right lower quadrant and is accompanied by anorexia, nausea, and occasional vomiting.

B. **Signs:**

Temperature is rarely above 100 °F without perforation.
Abdomen: Guarding, maximum tenderness at McBurney's point, sometimes hyperesthesia, percussion, rebound, psoas sign (tenderness on hyperextension of right hip), obturator sign (tenderness on internal rotation of flexed hip).
Rectal: Tenderness in the right lower quadrant.
Pelvic: Rule out PID, torsed ovarian cyst, or ectopic pregnancy.

C. **DDX:** Most common misdiagnoses, listed in a descending order of frequency, are mesenteric lymphadenitis, PID, torsed ovarian cyst, mittelschmerz, and gastroenteritis. Less common erroneous causes include diverticulitis, perforated ulcer, cholecystitis, ectopic pregnancy, kidney stone, bowel obstruction, pyelonephritis, endometriosis, and mesenteric infarction.

D. **Work-up:** Order CBC (WBC shows slight elevation with left shift), U/A, X-ray (plain film of abdomen may show appendicolith), and βHCG. Consider obtaining a focused "appendicitis CT" or an ultrasound if the technician is experienced. Obtain SMA-7. Order LFTs amylase and lipase if fishing.

2.2 RX:

A. Support airway, IV, O_2, and monitor prn.
B. Order NPO.
C. **Disposition:** If the diagnosis is definite, obtain a surgical consultation and transfer the patient to surgery. If the diagnosis is unclear, admit the patient for observation or inform him/her to return in 8 hours for a re-examination if the pain increases.

3. Cholecystitis:

Ninety five percent of cholecystitis is caused by gallstone(s) (cholelithiasis) attempting to pass through the cystic duct. Biliary colic is pain lasting less than 6 hours. Longer pain, fever, and obstruction with secondary infection are typically displayed as a result of cholecystitis. This condition is common in females over 40 as well as in the obese and multiparous patients.

3.1 Clinical Evaluation:

A. **Symptoms:** Common presentation is a sudden onset of pain in the right upper quadrant after a fatty meal. Pain is initially colicky, then constant and radiating to the back and/or the right scapular region. The pain is accompanied by nausea and vomiting.
B. **Signs:**
C. Vitals: Low grade fevers are common. Patients with biliary colic are restless whereas individuals with cholecystitis avoid motion.
D. Abdomen: Decreased bowel sounds and right upper quadrant tenderness with guarding and rebound are typical signs. Occasionally the gallbladder is palpable.
E. Murphy's sign: Arrest of inspiration on palpation of RUQ.

F. **DDX:** Appendicitis, perforated ulcer, acute pancreatitis, hepatitis, and RLL pneumonia. Also, gastric, PUD, and myocardial infarction.

G. **Work-up:** Order CBC (WBC 10,000 to 15,000), chemistries (increased bilirubin, mild elevation of SGOT, SGPT, and alk phosphatase). Amylase elevation suggests pancreatitis secondary to biliary tract disease. Obtain U/A, ultrasound, or a radionuclide scan (hepato-iminodiacetic acid - HIDA) if the ultrasound is normal.

3.2 RX:

A. Support airway, IV, O_2, and monitor prn. Insert a NG tube for decompression.

B. **Disposition:** A patient with a resolved uncomplicated biliary colic may be sent home. However, those individuals with acute cholecystitis should be admitted and surgical consult should be obtained.

4. Cirrhosis:

The most common cause of cirrhosis is the destruction of the liver by the consumption of large quantities of alcohol. The metabolism alters, coagulopathy occurs, and the detoxifying ability of liver is lost. Because of fibrosis, blood is shunted from the hepatic artery to the portal vein, resulting in portal hypertension and varices. Complications include bleeding esophageal varices, hepatic encephalopathy, hepatorenal syndrome and spontaneous bacterial peritonitis. Typical presentations are altered mental status, jaundice, and/or bleeding.

4.1 Clinical Evaluation:

A. **Symptoms:** Malaise, lethargy, weight loss, fluid retention, pruritus, weakness, muscle wasting, anorexia, nausea, vomiting, diarrhea, and fever. Large quantities of alcohol are consumed over a given period of time. Viral, gall bladder, inflammatory bowel diseases, and other chronic or childhood diseases may be involved. Coagulopathy may occur. Exposure to hepatotoxic agents, such as carbon tetrachloride, and the ingestion of drugs, including acetaminophen, allopurinol and phenytoin, may be coincident to pathology.

B. **Signs:**

Vitals are important and variable.
Skin: Spider angiomas, palmar erythema, hyperpigmentation, and jaundice.
Chest: Gynecomastia.
Abdomen: Ascites and hepatosplenomegaly.
Rectal: Bleeding.
Extremities: Asterixis ("liver flap"), pedal edema, and polyneuropathy.
Neuro: Cerebellar dysfunction, tremors, and altered mental status.

C. **DDX:**

D. Jaundice: Hemolysis, obstructive jaundice, viral hepatitis, hepatotoxic ingestions, and septicemia.

E. Altered mental status: Hepatic encephalopathy, viral hepatitis, Reye's syndrome, hepatotoxic/other drug ingestions, and intracranial bleed.

F. **Work-up:** Order CBC (anemia and thrombocytopenia), chemistries (elevated bilirubin, alk phosphatase, hyponatremia, hypokalemia, and decreased albumin), coagulation studies (elevated PT), serum ammonia, CXR, and ECG. Obtain a toxicology screen and a CT of the brain as needed.

4.2 RX:

A. Correct fluid and electrolyte abnormalities. Rehydration and protein restriction may be necessary.

B. Support ABCs. Administer thiamine, 100 mg IV, and glucose, if the patient has decreased mental status.

C. For bleeding esophageal varices, use 2 large bore IV lines, replace volume with NS and packed cells, suction with NG, start an IV vasopressin drip, 20 units in 200 cc NS at 0.5 units/minute, and tamponade with a Sengstaken-Blakemore tube or an emergency portal decompression if needed.

D. For hepatic encephalopathy, administer neomycin, 1g po or by NG q 6 hours, to suppress bacteria responsible for ammonia production. Prevent ammonia from diffusing from the bowel by administering lactulose, 30 cc po/PR tid. Lactulose in contact with colonic bacteria produces a low pH which traps ammonia in the colon as non diffusible ammonium ions.

E. For spontaneous bacterial peritonitis, administer ampicillin 102 g IV q 4-6 hours plus gentamicin 5-7 mg/kg IV q 24 hours..

F. **Disposition:** Admit all patients except those exhibiting the mildest symptoms. Admit patients with complications to the ICU. Obtain a surgical consultation for bleeding varices.

5. Diarrhea:

Diarrhea is characterized by an increase in stool liquidity, frequency, and urgency. Most acute cases originate from viral agents or from toxins of *Staphylococcus* or *Clostridium* organisms.

5.1 Clinical Evaluation:

A. **Symptoms**: The patient may have been exposed to family members or friends with diarrhea. Also, obtain a history of the types of food, drugs (particularly antibiotics), and/or alcohol that were consumed. Determine whether the patient has had any previous episodes, a history of surgery, systemic illnesses, traveled recently and/or lost weight..

B. **Signs:** Check temperature and orthostatics. Dehydration or cachexia are signs of severe or chronic diarrhea.

- Abdomen: Bowel sounds are increased except in the surgical abdomen. Tenderness is localized or diffuse. Mass may be present.
- Rectal: Tenderness and blood.

C. **DDX:** Viral, bacterial (commonly *Shigella, Salmonella, or Campylobacter*), parasites (amebiasis and *Giardia*), inflammatory bowel disease (Crohn's disease or ulcerative colitis), food poisoning, acute surgical abdomen (small bowel obstruction, perforated appendicitis, ulcer, diverticulitis, and mesenteric infarction), and drugs.

D. **Work-up:** Order CBC, SMA-7, U/A, KUB, and stool specimen for wet mount, Gram/Wright stain for WBCs, which suggests a bacterial etiology, ova/parasites, and culture as needed.

5.2 RX:

A. Start IV fluids and electrolytes for dehydration.

B. **Disposition:** A patient may be discharged home with instructions to consume clear liquids for 48 hours. They should then be reevaluated. If a bacterial cause is indicated consider treatment with trimethoprim-sulfamethoxazole (Septra or Bactrim), one DS tab BID or Cipro, 500 mg po bid for 7 days. Admit the severely dehydrated or the surgical abdomen patient (refer also to the "Acute Abdominal Pain" section).

6. Diverticular Diseases:

Diverticula is the herniation of mucosa/submucosa through the muscular layer of the colon (usually sigmoid) near the vasculature. This condition is prevalent in the elderly. Diverticulosis is defined as the presence of diverticula with or without symptoms. Diverticulitis is the inflammation of diverticula with significant signs and symptoms. Complications of diverticular disease include perforation, bleeding, obstruction, and abscess and fistula formation.

6.1 Clinical Evaluation:

A. **Symptoms:** Left lower quadrant pain is intermittent, crampy, and worsens after eating. The pain is relieved by bowel movement or flatus but may be accompanied by constipation or diarrhea (diverticulosis). Constant severe left lower quadrant pain with altered bowel habits, anorexia, nausea, vomiting and fever (diverticulitis). Previous attacks, bloody bowel movements, and dark colored stools are also prevalent.

B. **Signs:**

Vital signs: Hypotension, tachycardia and orthostatic changes.
Abdomen: Tenderness LLQ and mass. Signs of peritonitis.
Rectal: Blood and presence of a mass.
Pelvic: Mass.

C. **DDX:** Irritable bowel syndrome, inflammatory bowel disease, colon/rectal cancer, appendicitis (rare), sigmoid volvulus, tubo-ovarian abscess, ischemic colitis, and angiodysplasia (bleeding).
D. **Work-up:** Order CBC, SMA-7, flat upright, and decubitus abdominal x-ray. Obtain blood and urine cultures, PT, PTT, and T&C PRN.

6.2 RX:
A. For diverticulosis, order a high fiber diet and an anticholinergic, such as dicyclomine (Bentyl), 20 mg po qid.
B. For mild diverticulitis, treat as described for diverticulosis, and order a clear liquid diet, begin aerobe/anaerobe antibiotic coverage with amoxicillin or cephalexin (Keflex), plus metronidazole (Flagyl), 500 mg po qid, or Cipro, 500 mg po bid for 7 days.
C. For severe diverticulitis, start an IV of LR, NG suction, and administer cefoxitin, 1 g IV q 6 hours.
D. For massive GI bleeding, start two large bore (16 g) IV lines of Ringer's Lactate, insert a Foley catheter, and treat with packed cells as needed (refer to the "GI Bleeding" section).
E. **Disposition:** For the diverticulosis and mild diverticulitis patient, discharge with a surgical follow-up. Admit the diverticulitis and GI bleeding patient and obtain a surgical consultation.

7. Gastrointestinal Bleeding:

Gastrointestinal bleeding may occur in the upper or in the lower GI tract depending on whether it is proximal or distal to the suspensory ligament of Treitz. The most common cause of upper GI bleeding is peptic ulcer disease. Typically, lower GI bleeding results from diverticulosis. GI bleeding may be occult, overt, or massive.

7.1 Clinical Evaluation:
A. **Symptoms:** Patient may cite a history of vomiting blood (hematemesis) with or without abdominal pain. Coughing up blood (hemoptysis), pharyngeal bleeding, and nosebleed (epistaxis) should be excluded. Black tarry stools (melena) suggest upper GI bleeding. Bright red bloody stools (hematochezia) indicate lower GI bleeding. Severe bleeding may be present with weakness, pallor, syncope, or if in shock as hypotension, tachycardia, and diaphoresis. Inquire about previous episodes, history of ulcers, alcohol abuse, liver disease, aspirin and antiinflammatory meds, bleeding problems and anticoagulants.
B. **Signs:**
Vitals: Check for hypotension, tachycardia, and orthostasis.
HEENT: Check nose and pharynx.
Skin: Stigmata of alcoholism.
Abdomen: Distention, bowel sounds, masses, tenderness, and rebound.
Rectal: Frank bleeding or occult blood.
C. **DDX:**
D. Upper: Peptic ulcer disease, erosive gastritis, erosive esophagitis, esophageal varices, Mallory-Weiss tears, and neoplasm.
E. Lower: Diverticulosis, neoplasm, polyps, infection, inflammation, vascular tectasia, hemorrhoids, and trauma.
F. **Work-up:** Order CBC, PT, PTT, T&C 4-6 units as needed, SMA-7, and NG. Examine NG aspirate for bright red blood or coffee-ground material.

7.2 RX:
A. Support airway, IV, O_2, and monitor prn.
B. Insert an NG tube and perform a saline lavage to control upper GI bleeding.
C. For hemodynamic instability, upper or lower bleeding, place on O_2 and a cardiac monitor. Start 2 large-bore IV lines, NS or LR wide open, and insert a Foley for measurement of I/O. If a Class III hemorrhage (30 to 40% blood loss), transfuse with packed cells. Use O^- blood if the patient is hypotensive after 2 L of NS and if type-specific blood is not available.
D. Consider use of vasopressin or octreotide IV.
E. **Disposition:** Admit all unstable cases and obtain an immediate surgical or GI consultation. Admit a patient with persistent bleeding and unstable vital signs to the ICU.

8. Inflammatory Bowel Disease:

Category	**Regional Enteritis**	**Ulcerative Colitis**
Name	Crohn's disease Regional enteritis Terminal ilcitis Granulomatous ileocolitis	Ulcerative colitis
Area	**Stem-to-stern** **Segmental** (skip areas) Most common area is ileum	95% rectosigmoid **Contiguous** (no skip areas)
Demographics	12-30 years 55-60 years Common in Europeans Jews White > Black 10-15% have family history	10-20 years 20-30 years 15 x greater risk with 1st° relative
Bowel	**ALL LAYERS** Thick Bowel Wall Narrow lumen Creeping fat - mesenteric fat over bowel wall "Cobblestone" mucosal appearance **Fissures** **Fistulas** **Abscesses**	**Mucosa and Submucosa** Mucosal ulceration Epithelial necrosis Mild - Mucosa is fine, granular and friable Severe - Spongy, red, oozing ulcerations Crypt abscesses **Toxic Megacolon**
Clinical	F, chronic D without gross blood, RLQ pain, fistula-fissure-abscess	Bloody D, Abdomen pain, ±V, F. If Toxic Megacolon- toxic appearance ± mass.
Treatment	Antidiarrheal meds.	NO Antidiarrheal meds.

Most emergency visits are for complications of an already diagnosed disease, including hemorrhage, intestinal obstruction, bowel perforation and toxic megacolon.

8.1 Clinical Evaluation:

A. **Symptoms:**

Both: Abdominal pain, fever, and weight loss.
Crohn's Disease: Chronic diarrhea and anorexia.
Ulcerative colitis: Occasional constipation, rectal bleeding, bloody diarrhea, and tachycardia. Inquire about frequency of bowel movements, severity of abdominal pain, rectal bleeding, past history of hospitalizations and a family history of a similar disease.

B. **Signs:**

Vitals: Fever, tachycardia, decreased BP and dehydration.
Abdomen: Distended, tender, tympanitic, rigid, rebound, and presence of mass (toxic megacolon). Rectal positive for blood.

C. **DDX:**

Bleeding: Bacterial diarrhea, i.e., *Shigella* or *Campylobacter*, amebiasis, gay bowel syndrome, HIV infection, ischemic colitis.

Abdominal pain: Gastroenteritis, appendicitis, cholecystitis, intestinal obstruction, aneurysm, mesenteric occlusive disease, and diverticulitis.

D. **Work-up:** Order CBC, chemistries, and abdominal series.

8.2 RX:

A. For both types of conditions, support airway, IV, O_2, and monitor prn. Correct volume and electrolytes. Consult with private M.D. about the patient's condition and admission requirements in cases of a known disease.

B. For patients with ulcerative colitis and fulminating symptoms and who are not being treated with steroids, give corticotrophin (ACTH) 120 units/day continuous IV. If the patient is taking steroids, prescribe hydrocortisone, 100 mg IV q 6-8 hours, or methylprednisolone, 20 mg IV q 6-8 hours.

C. For toxic megacolon, treat aggressively with fluids and NG decompression. If the patient is not fulminant, consider prednisone, 30 mg po bid. Admit patients with toxic megacolon, hemorrhage, obstruction, perforation to the ICU and obtain a surgical consultation.

D. For regional enteritis, such as Crohn's, administer sulfasalazine, 5 g per day, diphenoxylate (Lomotil), 5 mg po qid, and consider metronidazole, 10-20 mg/kg/day.

E. **Disposition:** Admit patients to control pain and individuals who are toxic.

9. Intestinal Obstruction:

The most common cause of mechanical obstruction of the small bowel is adhesions associated with previous surgery, followed by hernia, and carcinoma. Large bowel obstruction usually results from fecal impaction or carcinoma. Paralytic ileus, or decreased motility of intestine, is induced by dysfunction of structures touching the bowel, including ureteral distention or retroperitoneal hemorrhage.

9.1 Clinical Evaluation:

A. **Symptoms:** Most common symptoms are crampy abdominal pains and spasms lasting several minutes. Vomiting and abdominal distention are also common. Inquire about previous surgeries and any abdominal infections, such as PID.

B. **Signs:**

Abdomen: Inspect for scars and hernias. Bowel sounds are decreased, come in rushes, and are frequently high pitched or tinkling. Distention and tympany may be present.

Palpation: Tenderness is diffuse.

Rectal: May reveal impacted feces or tumor. Guaiac test for occult blood.

C. **DDX:** Perforated ulcer, pancreatitis, appendicitis with peritonitis, cholecystitis, renal and biliary colic. If distention present, uremia, mesenteric thrombosis, and peritonitis. Large bowel obstruction: Peritonitis, colitis with distention, ileus, i.e., postoperative, and uremia.

D. **Work-up:** Order CBC, SMA-7, upright CXR, and flat and upright abdominal films. For small bowel obstruction, examine for stepladder appearance of bowel gas with air-fluid levels. For large bowel obstruction, examine for a round or square shape of the bowel gas with haustra markings.

9.2 RX:

A. Support airway, IV, O_2, and monitor prn. Insert a NG tube to decompress stomach.

B. **Disposition:** Obtain a surgical consultation and admit the patient.

10. Pancreatitis:

Aberrant activation of enzymes in the pancreatic ducts resulting in the autodigestion of portions of the gland. The most common cause of pancreatitis is related to alcoholism with cholelithiasis coming in second. Ranson's criteria for predicting severity of the condition on admission are age > 55, WBC > 16,000, glucose > 200, LDH > 350, AST > 250.

10.1 Clinical Evaluation:

A. **Symptoms:** Constant severe abdominal pain, often radiating to the back because of retroperitoneal irritation. Leaning forward relieves the pain because it moves peritoneal organs away from retroperitoneum. Nausea and vomiting are common. Inquire about alcohol, drugs, gallbladder disease, endocrine disorders, and previous attacks.

B. **Signs:**

Vitals: Fever and tachycardia in severe cases. Observe for sequelae of alcoholism.

Abdomen: Guarding, decreased bowel sounds, diffuse tenderness, and often with signs of peritoneal irritation. Hemorrhagic pancreatitis shows periumbilical ecchymosis (Cullen's sign) and/or flank ecchymosis (Grey Turner's sign).

C. **DDX:** Acute cholecystitis, peptic ulcer disease, alcoholic gastritis, perforated viscus and bowel infarction. Serum amylase elevation occurs in cholecystitis, bowel obstruction, perforated peptic ulcer, mesenteric thrombosis, ruptured aortic aneurysm, ruptured tubal pregnancy and advanced renal insufficiency.

D. **Work-up:** Order CBC, because a low Hb and hematocrit may suggest hemorrhagic pancreatitis, as well as SMA-7, calcium (glucose elevation, calcium decrease secondary to precipitation of calcium soaps), and amylase and lipase elevation (lipase more sensitive). Obtain CXR, effusion and/or free air, and KUB, gallstones, calcifications in chronic pancreatitis, and localized ileus - "sentinel loop". If febrile, consider a CT or an ultrasound to evaluate for complications such as abscess.

10.2 RX:

A. Support airway, IV, O_2, and monitor prn. Maintain NPO.

B. Administer meperidine (Demerol), less spasms of ampulla of Vater compared to morphine, 50-100 mg IM q 4-6 hours prn.

C. Administer prochlorperazine (Compazine), 10 mg IM (5-10 mg IV) q 3 hours prn, or hydroxyzine (Vistaril), 50 mg IM q 2-3 hours prn vomiting.

D. Insert an NG tube if an ileus is present.

E. **Disposition:** Admit patient to general floor. Obtain an ICU or surgical consultation if the patient is hemorrhagic or other complications are present.

11. Peptic Ulcer Disease (PUD):

Peptic Ulcer Disease is the disruption of balance between the acid-pepsin and mucosal defense factors which causes ulceration of the gastroduodenal mucosa extending through the muscularis mucosa. Surgical complications include bleeding and perforation.

11.1 Clinical Evaluation:

A. **Symptoms:** Exacerbations of abdominal pain occur after eating when the acid increases in response to food (gastric ulcer), or at night/early morning when food or antacids bring rapid relief and "pain later" (duodenal ulcer). Risk factors include a positive family history, associated diseases, male gender, advanced age, smoking, and use of ASA or NSAIDS. Bleeding may have no symptoms. Inquire about hematemesis and dark stools. Sudden onset of severe constant abdominal pain radiating to back, chest, or shoulders indicates a perforation.

B. **Signs:** Few signs present unless complications occur.

Vitals: Bleeding or perforation may show tachycardia and hypotension. Orthostatic vital signs occur if bleeding suspected. Patient with perforation has shallow respirations and lies perfectly still.

Abdomen: Uncomplicated cases have bowel sounds with mild epigastric tenderness. Guarding, rebound, and abdominal rigidity signals a perforation.

Rectal: Guaiac.

C. **DDX:** Gastritis, gastroenteritis, biliary tract disease, esophagitis, pancreatitis, myocardial infarction, angina, and pneumonia.

D. **Work-up:** Order CBC, SMA-7, ECG (if in age group with high risk), and upright CXR and/or flat and upright abdominal films to detect free air. If bleeding or a perforation is suspected, obtain PT, PTT, T&C/type and screen, and place on a cardiac monitor.

11.2 <u>RX</u>:

A. Place on O_2 and monitor prn.

B. For uncomplicated cases, relieve pain with antacids, such as Maalox or Mylanta or combinations thereof, 30 cc po. For some cases, administer IV cimetidine (Tagamet), 300 mg bolus IVPB and continuous infusion 900 mg over 24 hours, or IV ranitidine (Zantac), 50 mg q 6 hours as necessary.

C. For "bleeding" cases, start O_2 and an IV of isotonic solution (LR or NS). Insert a NG tube and perform a nasogastric lavage with saline. (Refer also to the "Gastrointestinal Bleeding - Treatment" section.)

D. For "perforation" cases, place the patient on O_2, insert a NG tube, start large bore IVs, and insert a Foley catheter.

E. **Disposition:**

Uncomplicated: Discharge to home with a H_2 receptor antagonist, such as cimetidine, 800 mg, ranitidine, 300 mg, or famotidine (Pepcid), 40 mg qhs prn. May also prescribe OTC antacid, such as Mylanta, po qid (1° ac & qhs). May consider a proton pump blocker like lansoprazole (Prevacid) 30 mg qd or omeprazole (Prilosec) 40 mg qd x 4-8 wks.

Pain, bleeding, elderly or comorbid disease: Admit to a general floor.

Continued bleeding or perforation: Obtain an immediate surgical consultation and prepare the patient for the OR.

GYNECOLOGY

1. Ovarian Cysts:

Ovarian cysts often cause pressure, which results in pelvic or abdominal discomfort. Typically ovarian cysts are asymptomatic unless a rupture, hemorrhage, infection, or torsion occurs.

1.1 Clinical Evaluation:

A. **Symptoms:** Rupture causes acute pain, often unilateral after exercise or intercourse.
B. **Signs:** Ovaries of premenarchal and postmenopausal women should not normally be palpable. If so, rule out malignancy. Irritation of peritoneum can be absent, well localized, or diffuse. Sudden enlargement of adnexal mass signifies an intra-ovarian hemorrhage that requires surgery.
C. **DDX:** Dermoid cyst, serous cyst, endometrioma, malignancy, ectopic pregnancy and torsion.
D. **Work-up:** Order a pregnancy test. Perform an ultrasound and a culdocentesis.

1.2 RX:

A. A cyst rupture resolves spontaneously.
B. Perform a laparotomy for a ruptured endometrioma and corpus luteum cyst.
C. **Disposition:** Admit a patient with extreme pain or when there is evidence of severe infection or unusually severe hemorrhage. Otherwise outpatient management is recommended.

2. Ovarian Torsion:

Ovarian torsion is the twisting of the ovary which produces intense pain.

2.1 Clinical Evaluation:

A. **Symptoms:** Sudden onset, sharp, intermittent, and unilateral pain. Similar episodes in past probably represent spontaneous detorsion. Nausea, vomiting, low grade fever, and dysuria are also symptoms of ovarian torsion.
B. **Signs:** Cervical motion and adnexal tenderness, may indicate peritonitis is present.
C. **DDX:** Ectopic pregnancy, appendicitis, PID, and ovarian cyst.
D. **Work-up**: Order a pregnancy test, US, CBC, and a culdocentesis.

2.2 RX:

A. Perform a laparotomy.
B. Complications include infertility and an increased risk of ectopic pregnancy from a scarred tube. Infection and necrosis may lead to peritonitis and shock.
C. **Disposition:** Admit for surgery.

3. Pelvic Inflammatory Disease:

Minimum CDC criteria must be identified for diagnosis. A clear distinction between this condition and vaginitis/cervicitis must be made.

3.1 Clinical Evaluation:

A. **Symptoms:** Pelvic pain, fever, dysuria, nausea, vomiting, and abnormal vaginal bleeding post menses. The risk factors are IUD, recent instrumentation, and history of PID.
B. **Signs:** Must exhibit abdominal tenderness, cervical motion tenderness and adnexal tenderness. Friable cervix and purulent discharge are evident. Fitz-Hugh-Curtis Syndrome includes perihepatitis, inflammation around liver as a result of pus leaking from right Fallopian tube.
C. **DDX:** Ectopic pregnancy, appendicitis, ovarian cyst, cystitis, and pyelonephritis.

D. **Work-up:** Order CBC, U/A, pregnancy test, and cervical cultures for gonorrhea and Chlamydia. Consider ultrasound for severe tenderness or lack of response to antibiotics in 48-72 hours. One of the following conditions must be present for a diagnosis.

Temp > 38.3 °C (100.9 °F).
WBC > 10,000 mm^3.
Inflammatory mass by exam or US.
Culdocentesis yields WBCs or bacteria.
Gram's stain is positive for gonorrhea or antibody test (C-reactive protein) and culture is positive for *Chlamydia.*

3.2 RX:

A. Admit patients with the following conditions and treat with antibiotics: Tubo-ovarian abscess or pyosalpinx, fever > 100.4°, pregnant, unable to tolerate po, IUD present, peritonitis, uncertain diagnosis, failure on outpatient antibiotics for 48 hours, and nulli gravida.
B. For an outpatient regimen, prescribe ceftriaxone, 250 mg IM, or cefoxitin, 2 g IM or Cipro 500 mg P.O., for PCN allergic. Add to this, doxycycline, 100 mg po bid for 10-14 days.
C. For an alternate outpatient regimen, administer ofloxacin, 400 mg po bid for 14 days, **plus** either clindamycin, 450 mg po qid, **or** metronidazole, 500 mg po bid or doxycycline 100 mg po bid, for 14 days.
D. An inpatient regimen includes cefoxitin, 2 g IV q 6 hours, **or** cefotetan, 2 g IV q 12 hours. Add to the above treatment, doxycycline, 100 mg po/IV q 12 hours.
E. For an Alternate inpatient regimen, administer clindamycin, 900 mg IV q 8 hours, **and** gentamycin, 2 mg/kg IV loading dose, followed by 1.5 mg/kg q 8 hours IV.
F. After a patient is discharged from the hospital, continue treatment with doxycycline, 100 mg po bid to a 14 day total.
G. Complications include infertility, abscess, dyspareunia, chronic pelvic pain, and increased risk of ectopic pregnancy.
H. **Disposition:** Admit all but the mildest cases of PID.

4. Sexual Assault:

Rape is non-consensual. The victim is threatened and in fear of bodily harm. Sexual assault can range from fondling of genitals to oral, anal, or vaginal penetration with objects or any part of the assailants body. Fifty percent of victims know their attacker but only 1 in 4 rapes are reported. Facial and extremity trauma are more common than genital trauma. Child molestation is an illegal act performed on or with a child with lewd intent. Children are usually < 11 and the assailant is typically known by the child.

4.1 Clinical Evaluation:

A. **Symptoms:** Pertinent details about the event should be obtained, including time, date, place of the attack, description of the assailant, penetration area, ejaculation, threats, weapons, and alcohol/drug use. Also ask, "Did the victim shower, douche, brush teeth, go to the bathroom, or change clothes"? Determine the last consensual intercourse, last menstrual period, birth control method, medical history, and allergies.
B. **Signs:** Carefully document all trauma-related lacerations, bruising, bite marks, and scratches. Special attention should be paid to the neck, mouth, breasts, wrists, and thighs. Vagina and anus must be carefully inspected for trauma. Male victims of sodomy may have abrasions on the thorax or the abdomen.
C. **Work-up:** Obtain cervical cultures to test for *Chlamydia* and gonorrhea. Order a pregnancy test, RPR, hepatitis B, HIV serologies, and X-rays for fractures. Perform a wet mount to observe for sperm. Sperm motility is lost in 12 hours; however, non-motile sperm can be recovered in 72 hours. Conversely, acid phosphate decreases in 2-9 hours. Obtain the victim's underclothes, pubic hair combing, and fingernail clippings as evidence. Acquire rectal or buccal smears to determine whether penetration occurred at that site.

4.2 RX:

A. Advise rape counseling.

B. Provide STD prophylaxis with ceftriaxone, 125 mg IM, and doxycycline, 100 mg po bid for 10 days. Provide pregnancy prophylaxis with 2 tablets of Ovral and 2 additional tablets in 12 hours. Give tetanus if needed. Recommend re-evaluation by the GYN for STD and pregnancy. Consider an empiric antiviral prophylaxis for HIV.

C. **Disposition**: Arrange an outpatient follow up with the primary M.D. and an appropriate psychiatric follow-up. Consider a "safe-house", shelter, or other disposition as needed to ensure a safe environment.

HEAD AND NECK

1. Dental, Oral, and Salivary Gland Infections:

The key to the diagnosis and management of dental and space infections of the head and neck is an understanding of the fascial planes. Cellulitis of the odontogenic origin usually involves the middle and lower half of the face and neck. Ludwig's angina is an infection involving the submaxillary, sublingual, and submental space with elevation of the tongue. This is a serious infection that may potentially obstruct the airway.

1.1 Clinical Evaluation:

A. **Symptoms:** Pain, gingival swelling, massive facial swelling, a toxic appearance, and a compromised airway. Pain increases with eating.

B. **Signs:** Pain to percussion with a tongue blade indicates involvement at the apex of the tooth. Tender swelling over the gingiva adjacent to a tooth suggests either a periodontal abscess or an extension of a periapical abscess to the cortex of the bone into the subperiosteal space. This condition presents with board-like swelling, brawny induration, difficulty swallowing, stiffness of tongue movements, and trismus. Respiratory compromise may occur as the tongue is elevated and the oropharynx becomes occluded.

C. **DDX:** Tumor, tuberculosis, cervical lymphadenitis, submaxillary and parotid gland disease, and autoimmune disease.

D. **Work-up:** Obtain a lateral soft tissue radiograph of the neck. Consider a CT scan, CBC, and blood cultures. Determine electrolyte levels if the patient is severely dehydrated.

1.2 RX:

A. Administer penicillin, 15-20 million units daily, **or** clindamycin, 600-900 mg tid IV, **or** cefazolin, 1-2 g IV tid for serious infection. Simple caries and minor periodontal infections may be managed with Pen VK 500 mg PO qid and oral analgesics.

B. Admit all patients with evidence of extension of infection to the fascial planes of the head and neck.

C. Facial cellulitis with closure of the eye indicates the potential spread of an infection to the periorbital spaces and an increased risk for cavernous sinus thrombosis.

D. **Disposition:** Patients with extensive trismus, Ludwig's angina, or impending Ludwig's angina should be admitted.

2. Epistaxis:

Epistaxis is a hemorrhage from the nostril, nasal cavity or nasopharynx.

2.1 Clinical Evaluation:

A. **Symptoms:** Elucidate the nature, onset, duration, and amount of bleeding. Determine whether there is personal or family history of epistaxis or another type of bleeding disorder. Obtain a medication history, especially for Coumadin, and ascertain if the patient is chronically or acutely ill, or has experienced trauma. Eliminate the possibility of a foreign body insertion.

B. **Signs:** Ecchymosis, purpura, spider angiomas, hemarthrosis, hepatomegaly, and hypertension.

C. **Work-up:** Determine hemoglobin, hematocrit, and platlet count. Check PT and PTT if indicated. Consider plain radiographs or CT of facial bones if trauma is suspected.

2.2 RX:

A. For severe episodes, support airway, IV, O_2, and monitor.

B. Gown both you and the patient. Wear gloves and protective eyewear.

C. Maintain a direct external pressure for 5 minutes to stop the bleeding and then request the patient to gently blow his/her nose to clear out all clots. If bleeding is brisk, cocaine-soaked pledgets may be used in the affected nostril for 10-15 minutes before attempting another type of therapy.

D. Control focal areas of anterior epistaxis with application of silver nitrate or use a small amount of topical hemostatic agent.

E. For persistent bleeding, apply an anterior pack, which consists of a petroleum jelly-impregnated gauze strip smeared with an antibiotic ointment, by using the nasal speculum and bayonet forceps, in a stair-step manner, with the leading and terminal ends protruding from the nasal orifice. Once this is accomplished, tape a 2 X 2" piece of gauze over the involved nostril. A Merocel anterior nasal packing may also be used. This pack should be left in place for a minimum of 24-48 hours. Prescribe either penicillin or a first-generation cephalosporin to the patient.

F. Failure to control bleeding or the inability to visualize an anterior source denotes a posterior hemorrhage which mandates the application of a posterior pack. This can be accomplished with a posterior Merocel posterior pack or an epistax balloon. Patients require pain medication for this procedure.

G. **Disposition:**

Admit patients when a posterior pack is required.

Patients who are over-anticoagulated and those with a chronic, debilitating illness or a recurrent epistaxis are also candidates for admission.

For epistaxis that is unresponsive to the measures described above, obtain an otolaryngologic consultation.

Prescribe amoxicillin or penicillin to patients who are discharged with an anterior nasal packing. Advise the individual to consult an otolaryngologist within 1-2 days.

3. Foreign Bodies in the External Auditory Canal:

3.1 Clinical Evaluation:

A. **Symptoms:** In children, there is often a history of chronic otitis externa. Alternatively, the child simply pulls at his/her ears. In younger children, there is usually no definite history of the child inserting anything in his/her ears but the parents are concerned because the child is complaining of pain and there is drainage from the ear. The history should include the type of foreign body involved, the mechanism used, and any history suggestive of tympanic membrane perforation.

B. **Signs:** Once the patient has been provided with an anesthesia or an analgesia, place a speculum in the ear and with a good light source inspect the canal.

C. **DDX:** Chronic or acute otitis externa and cholesteatoma.

3.2 RX:

A. After adequate anesthesia/analgesia place a large ear speculum in the ear and visualize the canal by using a good light source. In the case of small foreign bodies, gently irrigate with a jet of lukewarm water and direct the stream behind the foreign object.

If the foreign body is vegetable material, irrigation may cause it to swell with subsequent occlusion of the canal. In this case, the foreign body can usually be removed with alligator forceps.

Smooth objects, such as beads, may be removed with a suction catheter interfaced with a soft funnel tip. For some cases, a right-angle hook can be passed behind the foreign body and then it can be carefully withdrawn.

B. **Disposition:** For young children with foreign bodies in the ear, consider an ENT consultation to discuss examination and treatment. Immediately refer any patient with small alkaline batteries in the external canal to an otolaryngologist for removal.

4. Foreign Bodies in the Upper Airway:

4.1 Clinical Evaluation:

A. **Symptoms:** An adult may swallow a piece of chicken or fish and then have the sensation of a bone being caught in his/her throat. In young children, cough, stridor, hoarseness, wheezing, choking, or respiratory distress may be displayed.

B. **Signs:** Patient is unable to speak with audible stridor and wheezes upon auscultation. A complete oropharyngeal examination should be performed to inspect for the presence of a foreign body.

C. **Work-up:** Order CXR, both inspiratory and expiratory. Obtain a lateral neck radiograph and consider fluoroscopy. Consider nasopharyngoscopy.

4.2 RX:

A. Immediate airway management must be the first priority.

Once the diagnosis of a hypopharyngeal or a subglottic foreign body has been established in a young child, obtain a consult for a laryngoscopy or bronchoscopy to remove the foreign body. Conduct this procedure with the patient under general anesthesia and in the OR.

In the adult, remove fish or chicken bones with indirect laryngoscopy by using a blade, curved clamp, or McGill forceps. If this technique is unsuccessful, remove the foreign body by employing a flexible bronchoscope with a channel for biopsy forceps. A consultation is usually required.

B. **Disposition:**

Obtain an otolaryngology consultation for children with subglottic foreign bodies and for adults with hypopharyngeal foreign bodies that cannot be removed by means of indirect laryngoscopy. After the foreign body is removed, discharge the patient if he/she is in no acute distress. Recommend follow-up as necessary.

5. Nasal Foreign Bodies:

5.1 Clinical Evaluation:

A. **Symptoms:** History of chronic rhinorrhea may be present. Also, one of the parents or the caretaker may have witnessed the insertion or the patient may confess to having inserted a foreign body in his/her nose. In many cases, there is no history of foreign body insertion and the patient presents with unilateral or bilateral purulent, foul-smelling rhinorrhea, unilateral nasal obstruction, epistaxis, or complications, including sinusitis, septal abscess, cellulitis, erosion of the soft palate, bronchial aspiration, or rarely, cerebral tetanus.

B. **Signs:** Nasal mucosa is red, swollen, and excoriated with possible signs of infection. Discharge may be foul-smelling and there may be facial swelling and pain to palpation. A fever may be present.

C. **DDX:** Unilateral or bilateral sinusitis, facial cellulitis, and septal abscess.

D. **Work-up:** Radiologic evaluation may be helpful in cases of radiopaque foreign bodies. Radiographs are also beneficial when complications arise due to foreign bodies, such as sinusitis. A CT scan may be necessary if the foreign body is not radiopaque or if the foreign body cannot be localized.

5.2 RX:

A. First attempt to occlude the uninvolved nares and place your mouth over the child's mouth. Blow until a resistance of the closed glottis is felt. Exhale forcibly into the patient's mouth until the foreign body is expelled from the nose.

B. If the forced air technique does not clear the nares, anesthetize and vasoconstrict the patient with 4% cocaine and attempt to remove the foreign body. Many smaller objects may be amenable to removal with either a bayonet or alligator forceps. Round, hard objects, such as beads, can often be removed with a phalange-tipped suction catheter.

C. A #4 Fogarty catheter may be inserted above and posterior to the foreign body. Inflate the balloon with 1 mL of water and apply traction to the catheter until the balloon is lodged against the foreign body. Care must be taken not to dislodge the foreign body into the nasal pharynx when inserting the catheter.

D. Attempting to push the foreign body posterior into the nasal pharynx should not be initiated under any circumstances because aspiration may occur.
E. **Disposition:**
If above techniques are unsuccessful, obtain an otolaryngologic consultation.
Request a consultation when there are complications because of the foreign body, including cellulitis or sinusitis.
If the foreign body is a small alkaline battery and it has been in the nares for longer than 1-2 hours, immediately refer to an otolaryngologist.
Treat sinusitis with antibiotics and arrange close outpatient follow-up.
If the patient has facial cellulitis, admit him/her and treat with parenteral antibiotics.

6. Peritonsillar Abscess:

6.1 Clinical Evaluation:

A. **Symptoms:** Pain, dysphagia, muffled voice, progressive inability to swallow, drooling, dyspnea, and earache are evident.
B. **Signs:** Dehydration, unilateral enlargement of a tonsil, and trismus. Erythematous soft palate and uvula pushed toward the opposite side of the abscess are common signs.
C. **DDX:** Squamous cell carcinoma, lymphoma, leukemia, or vascular lesion.
D. **Work-up:** Obtain a Monospot, CBC, serum electrolyte determination, and a throat culture. Consider a soft tissue X-ray of the neck.

6.2 RX:

A. Administer penicillin, 1-2 million units IV q 4 hours, or clindamycin, 600 mg IV tid.
B. Consult an otolaryngologist to assist in determining the definitive management for all cases.
C. Treat peritonsillar cellulitis with the same antibiotics. IV rehydration should be started in the ED.
D. **Disposition:** Admit patients unless early peritonsillar cellulitis exists. Treat these patients with oral antibiotics and hydration. Advise a follow-up with an otolaryngologist within 24 hours.

7. Red Eye:

The most common causes of red painful eye are trauma, via a foreign body, and conjunctivitis. Conversely, iritis is a less common condition. Atypical causes include corneal inflammation, iritis, and acute glaucoma. Conjunctivitis is the inflammation/infection of the conjunctiva arising from viral agents, such as adenoviruses, allergins, or bacteria, including *Staphylococcus*, *Streptococcus*, *H. influenzae, N. gonorrhea.* Iritis is the inflammation of the anterior uveal tract, which consists of the iris, ciliary body, and choroid. The iris is the anterior extension of ciliary body. Acute angle-closure glaucoma is the obstruction of the outflow of aqueous humor from the anterior chamber with an increase in intraocular pressure.

7.1 Clinical Evaluation:

A. **Symptoms:**
Conjunctivitis: Symptoms are gradual with vague discomfort, burning, itching, tearing, and photophobia. A discharge is usually present. Other family members may also be affected. The patient may have recently been swimming. Allergic conjunctivitis is exhibited in asthmatics and in individuals with hay fever. Occupational hazards include exposure to toxins.
Iritis: The onset is gradual and is accompanied by moderate pain, photophobia, and blurred vision. Trauma is common and the condition may be associated with collagen vascular disease.
Glaucoma: The onset is abrupt, often at night, with extreme monocular pain and blurred vision. Nausea, vomiting, headache, and halos around lights are frequently associated with this condition. Previous episodes may have occurred. May be precipitated by anticholinergic drugs.
B. **Signs:** Mandatory visual acuity with Snellen chart. Examine periorbital area and lids for cellulitis and chemosis in allergic conjunctivitis. Purulent discharge is evident with a bacterial infection and the discharge is watery with viral and allergic reactions. In glaucoma cases, the cornea is "steamy" and the pupil is mid-dilated and unresponsive. Alternatively, the pupil is constricted with redness surrounding the pupil, ciliary flush, and light reflex causes pain in cases of iritis.

C. **DDX:** Conjunctivitis, iritis, angle- closure glaucoma, trauma, allergic/toxic reactions, and corneal infection (keratitis). Other causes include meds, vascular conditions, neoplasia, mucocutaneous syndromes, immunologic diseases, and dry eye syndromes.

Finding	Conjunctivitis	Iritis	Glaucoma
Onset	Gradual	Gradual	Sudden
Pain	Mild	Moderate	Severe
Vision	Normal	Blurred	Blurred
Injection	Diffuse	Ciliary	Diffuse flush
Pupil	Normal	Small	Mid-dilated
Cornea	Clear	Clear	Hazy
Discharge	Watery or purulent	Minimal	Minimal
Pressure	Normal	Normal	Increased

D. **Work-up:** Order a Gram stain and tonometry because the intraocular pressure is elevated, usually > 50 mm Hg, in glaucoma. Fluorescein staining may indicate a dendritic pattern in HSV and scleral scratches with a foreign body. Finally, a slit-lamp will reveal the anterior chamber with inflammatory cells and flares in cases of iritis and as hazy with glaucoma.

7.2 RX:

A. For allergic conjunctivitis, apply cold compresses and provide instructions to avoid the causative allergen. Treat bacterial, viral, and unclear cases with sulfacetamide, (Bleph-10, Sulamyd) or gentamicin, Genoptic, Garamycin, Gentacidin to prevent a secondary infection. Prescribe eye drops, 2 drops q 4 hours for 2 days, followed by qid for 5 days.

B. For iritis, dilate the affected pupil with 2 drops of 1% cyclopentolate (Cyclogyl) once. Before discharge, administer 1 drop of 2% homatropine.

C. For glaucoma:

Apply a cholinergic agent, such as 2% pilocarpine, to the pupil, 1 drop every 15 minutes until the pupil constricts, followed by 1 drop q 6 hours.

Prescribe a β-blocker timolol (Timoptic sol), 0.5% sol 1 drop at 10 minute intervals for three doses, followed by 1 drop q 12 hours.

Administer prednisolone acetate 1%, 1 drop every 30 minutes to 1 hour.

Administer a 20% solution of mannitol, a hyperosmotic agent, at 50 g IV over 60 minutes.

Administer acetazolamide (Diamox), (inhibits aqueous humor formation), 500 mg IV q 12 hours.

D. Corneal ulceration: Often a secondary *Pseudomonas* infection will arise in contact lens users. In these cases, obtain an immediate ophthalmologic consultation for corneal scraping. If he/she is not available, culture the infection and start an aggressive topical antibiotic, up to q 30 minutes. Consider a broader coverage antibiotic, such as ciprofloxacin. If secondary iritis presents, consider dilation, pain medication, and very close ophthalmology follow up.

E. **Disposition:**

For conjunctivitis cases, discharge the individual with outpatient follow-up and ophthalmologic consultation as needed.

For iritis, obtain an ophthalmologic consultation.

For glaucoma patients, admit and request immediate ophthalmologic consultation.

8. Sudden Visual Loss:

8.1 Clinical Evaluation:

A. **Symptoms:** Pain, location, trauma, onset symptoms, and previous episodes.
   Glaucoma: Halos around lights.
   Iritis: Photophobia and tender eye.
   Vitreous hemorrhage: "Cobwebs", "floaters", and peripheral light flashes.
   Retinal detachment: "Shade being drawn" and decrease in peripheral visual field.
   Macular dysfunction: Distortion, and spot in center of field.
   TIA: Transient visual loss.
   Vascular obstruction: Sudden, painless, and unilateral loss of vision.
   Temporal arteritis: Headache and pain in temporal region.
   Hypertension, diabetes, leukemia, and thrombocytopenia.

B. **Signs:**
   Temporal arteritis: Tenderness over temporal artery.
   Optic tract radiation impairment: Visual fields confrontation technique, homonymous hemianopsia in contralateral field.
   Hyphema: Blood in anterior chamber.
   Pupils: Accommodation, light, and consensual response.
   Retinal artery occlusion: Pale retina with "cherry red spot" at macula.

C. Retinal artery occlusion, retinal vein occlusion, uveitis, retinal detachment, glaucoma, macular dysfunction, TIA, cerebrovascular accident, neoplasm, temporal arteritis, and ischemic optic neuropathy.

D. **Work-up:** Order CBC, chemistries, and sedimentation rate. Determine visual acuity via Snellen eye chart and intraocular pressure by a tonometer. Perform a slit lamp exam and a CT of the brain as indicated.

8.2 RX:

A. To lower the intraocular pressure for a retinal artery occlusion,, gently digital massage on the closed eye, administer acetazolamide (Diamox), 500 mg IV, and make the patient breath into paper bag to increase CO_2 and to dilate arterioles.
B. To treat glaucoma, refer to "Red Eye" section.
C. For temporal arteritis, give prednisone, 40 mg bid.
D. **Disposition:** Obtain an immediate ophthalmologic consultation and, in most cases, admit the patient.

9. Tonsillitis:

9.1 Clinical Evaluation:

A. **Symptoms:** Sore throat, fever, headache, dehydration, dysphagia, and myalgias.
B. **Signs:** Erythema of the soft palate and tonsils, possible exudates, ulcerative lesions, petechiae, swollen cervical lymph nodes, and palpable liver and spleen.
C. **Work-up:** Order a throat culture and a rapid screen for Group A β-hemolytic *Streptococcus*. Obtain CBC and Monospot. Ascertain electrolyte levels when dehydration is present. Acquire lateral neck films if an abscess is suspected.

9.2 RX:

A. If the cause of tonsillitis is likely Group A *Streptococcus*, use penicillin V, 250-500 mg po qid for 10 days, **or** erythromycin, 250-500 mg po qid for 10 days, **or** Bicillin LA, 1.2 million units IM.
B. If the rapid screen for Group A β-hemolytic *Streptococci* is negative, await the throat culture results. Treat symptomatically.
C. **Disposition:**
   If the patient is not toxic and no suppurative complication is suspected, arrange an outpatient follow up with the patient's primary physician.
   Consider admission anytime a complication of tonsillitis is identified, such as a peritonsillar abscess or cellulitis. If these signs occur, an ENT consultation is required.

10. Vertigo:

A subjective sensation of motion either of the self or of the external environment. The two types that exist are central and peripheral vertigo.

10.1 Clinical Evaluation:

A. **Symptoms:** Sensation of motion, faintness, near syncope, and unsteady gait.

For central vertigo, the onset is insidious and the symptoms are mild, continuous, and may last days to years. Headache, visual disturbances, facial numbness, dysarthria, dysphasia, extremity weakness, and unilateral ataxia suggest a central cause.

Peripheral vertigo begins suddenly, lasts for minutes to hours, is intense and paroxysmal. The relation of symptoms to head motion, drug ingestion, medication use, alcohol, nicotine, caffeine, stress, dental work, and head or neck trauma is important. Tinnitus, hearing loss, ear pain, or fullness, and discharge from the external canal suggest a peripheral cause.

B. **Signs:** Visually inspect the auricle and mastoid area, specifically examining for discoloration, erythema, and disfigurement. Palpate and pull the auricle testing for pain. Check for perforation of the tympanic membrane. Check hearing loss to determine if it is conductive or sensory neural.

Perform the Fistula test by placing the head 60° backwards and applying pneumatic otoscopy to the external canal. Exert a positive pressure and examine the eyes for movement. The test is positive if vertigo or nystagmus are produced.

Perform the Hall-Pike maneuver examining for nystagmus and a sensation of vertigo. The nystagmus for central vertigo has no latency period or fatigability, is not suppressible, and there is no positional component. With peripheral vertigo, nystagmus is not continuous, there is a latency period of 2-25 seconds, shows fatigability, is usually suppressed by fixation, and has a definite positional component. Perform a neurologic examination examining for any focal deficits. Certain cranial nerve abnormalities may suggest a specific disease or an area of involvement. Assess cerebellar function.

Periheral	**Central**	**Systemic**
Otitis media	Acoustic neuroma	Diabetes mellitus
Acute labyrinthitis	Encephalitis	Thyroid disorder
Ménière's disease	Meningitis	Anemia
Trauma	Vertebral basilar insufficiency	Polycythemia
Benign positional vertigo	Multiple sclerosis	Hypertension
Medications	Trauma	Psychogenic
Motion sickness	Drugs	
	Tumor	
	Toxins	

C. **DDX:**

D. **Work-up:** Due to the broad differential, the recommended selective screening tests are CBC and SMA-7. Also consider an ECG. Labs may be useful for evaluation outside of the ED, including RPR and thyroid function tests. Perform appropriate radiographs where indicated, such as for trauma cases. Also, consider CT and MRI if a central cause for the vertigo is suspected.

10.2 RX:

A. Start meclizine, 25 mg po qid prn, **or** dramamine, 50 mg po q 4 hours, **or** a scopolamine transdermal patch, 0.5 mg behind the ear q 3 days, **or** diphenhydramine, 25-50 mg qid.
B. Parenteral antiemetics are helpful, especially if persistent nausea and vomiting occur.
C. Implement an antibiotic treatment program for infectious causes of vertigo in the ED.
D. Obtain a surgical consultation for a cholesteatoma, perilymphatic fistula, otosclerosis, acoustic neuroma, or other accessible CNS masses.

E. Physical therapy has been shown to improve symptoms associated with benign positional vertigo by desensitization with repetitive head motion.
F. Vascular insufficiency syndromes and nonhemorrhagic cerebrovascular accidents may require antiplatelet or anticoagulation therapy.
G. **Disposition:** consult an otolaryngologist for many cases of peripheral vertigo. Patients with a positive fistula test, trauma, mastoiditis, and purulent labyrinthitis require an immediate otolaryngologic consultation. Admit all patients with central vertigo for a full evaluation.

HEMATOLOGY/ONCOLOGY

TRANSFUSION PRODUCTS:

Cryoprecipitate: Used for the replacement of fibrinogen and factor VIII. Each unit contains approximately 200 mg of fibrinogen and 100 units of factor VIII in a final volume of 10-15 mL. Transfuse to achieve a fibrinogen level of 100 mg/dL, i.e., approximately 10 units. Each unit of cryoprecipitate should increase the fibrinogen level by an increment of 5-10 mg/dL.
Fresh Frozen Plasma: Used as a source of factors V and VIII as well as other clotting factors. Transfuse 2 units at a time and repeat if bleeding persists.
Platelets: Used to correct the prolonged bleeding time associated with factor V deficiency as well as thrombocytopenia. Platelets should also be considered when bleeding time is prolonged (> 9 minutes). Each unit of platelets should increase platelet count to 5000-10,000/μL.

1. Anemia:

Anemia can be induced by a large variety of diseases. In general, it is described as a decrease in hemoglobin or hematocrit. Symptoms vary based on the cause.

1.1 Chemical Evaluation:

A. **Symptoms:**

Production: Abnormalities of Hgb, Fe, and globin.
Destruction: Secondary to synthesis anomaly (e.g., sickle cell, etc.), extrinsic destruction, or sequestration.
Hemorrhagic: Past medical history of bleeding risks include cirrhosis, PUD, variceal hemorrhage, malignancy, infection, bleeding, and diatheses.
Chronic anemia: Occurs from blood loss or production abnormality. Commonly presents with gradual onset malaise, DOE, and fatigue. Previously existing underlying disease may become symptomatic- angina, claudication, GI symptoms, syncope/near syncope, and focal neuropathy secondary to ischemia.
Acute hemorrhage: Symptoms include history of sudden onset, ± previous history of bleeding disorders. Examine for hypovolemia, shock, and determine the source.

B. **Signs:** Pallor, tachycardia, orthostasis, wide pulse pressure, murmur, icterus, petechiae, ecchymosis, and hepatosplenomegaly.

C. **DDX:**

Production: Insidious onset of symptoms and low reticulocyte count.
Hypochromic/microcytic (low MCV): Iron deficiency, thalassemia, and sideroblastic (lead poisoning).
Macrocytic (elevated MCV): B_{12}, folate deficiencies, cirrhosis, and thyroid disorders.
Normocytic (normal MCV): Production disorder in marrow, including fibrosis which leads to aplasia and metaplasia. Endocrine disorders, uremia, cirrhosis and chronic inflammation may contribute.
Destruction (high reticulocyte count, hemolysis): Intrinsic: Glucose-6-phosphate dehydrogenase deficiency, pyruvate kinase deficiencies, membrane anomalies, including spherocytosis and spur cells, hemoglobinopathies, such as Thalassemia and sickle cell. Extrinsic: Antigen/ab, autoantibody immune hemolysis, mechanical cell shearing on valve, environmental sources, such as drugs, toxins, hyperthermia, drowning, and sequestration.
Hemorrhagic: Acute or chronic. Search for source. A past medical history of heparin/Warfarin is helpful.

D. **Work-up:** CBC with differential. If anemia is not secondary to a known recent hemorrhage, a reticulocyte count and a peripheral smear may be useful. Additional diagnostic tests are usually not useful in the ED. If hypochromic/microcytic anemia is determined, further laboratory evaluation may include iron, TIBC, and/or ferritin. If the smear indicates hemolysis, additional testing may include Coombs' test, serum bilirubins, and urine for free hemoglobin. Bone marrow biopsy may be required if cause remains unknown. An endoscopic evaluation should be considered.

1.2 RX:

A. Resuscitate patients presenting with hypovolemic shock. Ongoing GI hemorrhage or DIC may require ED transfusion of appropriate blood products.
B. Chronic anemia and anemia secondary to chronic disease or iron deficiency is usually tolerated well and outpatient management may be appropriate.
C. **Disposition:** Admit for active bleeding, severe hypovolemia, shock, ischemia from low blood volume, or when a transfusion is required. Follow on out-patient status to determine chronic picture.

2. Deep Vein Thrombosis (DVT):

A deep vein thrombosis is the development of single or multiple clots within the deep veins of the pelvis or extremities. The most important concern is embolization, most commonly to the lung, which results in a life-threatening pulmonary embolism. Isolated calf DVT is a low risk for embolization, although up to 20% may propagate proximally.

2.1 Clinical Evaluation:

A. **Symptoms:** Risk factors consist of stasis such as travel, sedentary/debilitated etc.; hypercoagulability, such as cancer, surgery, gravid, BCPs, and tobacco); vessel pathology, such as vascular disease, surgery, and trauma; and previous DVT.
B. **Signs:** Edema is the most reliable sign. Palpable cords, calf firmness, warmth, tenderness, and Homan's sign may suggest DVT but are not reliable.
C. **DDX:** Cellulitis, lymphangitis, ruptured Baker's cyst, muscle strain, and edema (congestive heart failure and pregnancy).
D. **Work-up:** Obtain PTT, PT, ECG and CBC. The type of tests ordered is based on suspected location.

   Doppler ultrasound (~ 85% sensitivity and specificity (s&s)) is noninvasive and particularly useful at detecting popliteal and femoral thrombi. It is not effective however at detecting calf vein thrombi.

   Impedance plethysmography (s&s ~ 95% above knee) is unreliable for detecting calf vein thrombi.

   Contrast venography is the gold standard test. It is the most specific and sensitive test for DVT. There is some discomfort and a risk of morbidity.

2.2 RX:

A. Administer heparin, 80 units/kg IV bolus, followed by a 18 units/kg/hour IV drip. Aim for a PTT of 1.5-2.5 normal. Alternative medication is enoxaparin (Lovenox) 1.0 mg/kg sc bid or 1.5 mg/kg qd.
B. **Disposition:** Admit and treat a proximal DVT patient.

3. Disseminated Intravascular Coagulation (DIC):

Disseminated Intravascular Coagulation is the generation of fibrin in the blood and the consumption of procoagulants and platelets. DIC is always associated with a severe underlying disease or an injury. No single parameter is diagnostic of DIC. Repeated measures of coagulopathy are often required. The mortality rate is as high as 70%.

3.1 Clinical Evaluation:

A. **Symptoms:** Infection, (30%), surgery/trauma, (25%), CA, (20%), hepatic disease, obstetric, and other symptoms, such as myocardial infarction, environmental injuries, snakebite, and pancreatitis.

B. **Signs:** Hemorrhage ± thrombotic manifestations. Bleeding from IV sites, hematuria and blood in NG aspirate, bloody sputum, ecchymosis, and petechia are displayed. Thrombotic manifestations include renal failure, bowel infarction, pulmonary insufficiency, cyanosis, hypoxemia, and change in mental status.

C. **DDX:** Massive hepatic necrosis, vitamin K deficiency, hemolytic-uremic syndrome, and thrombocytopenic purpura.

D. **Work-up:** A peripheral smear shows evidence of microangiopathic hemolysis with schistocytes. Thrombocytopenia is a result of consumption in microvascular clots and platelet activation by circulating thrombin. A persistently normal platelet count nearly excludes the diagnosis of acute DIC. Platelet counts of 50,000-100,000 are consistent with DIC. PT, PTT, and Thrombin time are generally prolonged and fibrinogen levels are depleted, i.e., < 150 mg/dL; fibrin degradation products are elevated, i.e., > 10 mg/day, and D-dimer is elevated, i.e., > 0.5 mg/dL.

3.2 RX:

A. Treat underlying disorder. Manage severe hemorrhage with fluids, blood, and platelets. Evacuate uterus in a septic abortion. Treat hypovolemia, sepsis, acidosis, and hypoxia.

B. For a patient at high risk of bleeding or actively bleeding with biochemical evidence of DIC, replace fibrinogen, platelets, and clotting factors with cryoprecipitate (fibrinogen & factor VIII), FFP (clotting factors), and platelets (maintain platelets > 50,000/μL) as appropriate. Provide whole blood if necessary. Consider aminocaproic acid for refractory DIC, 5-10 g slow IV push, followed by 2-4 g/hour for 24 hours or until bleeding stops. Use concurrent heparin treatment.

C. Consider management of thrombotic complications with heparin **except** for common ED presentations of DIC after surgery or trauma, with abruption, or when other bleeding risks are present. Administer heparin at low-doses, 500 units/hour, ± 500-1000 units bolus. After 2-3 hours of infusion, consider 2-3 units of FFP, and 6-8 units of platelets.

D. Monitor fibrinogen. If < 100 mg/dL, consider cryoprecipitate. Each unit of cryoprecipitate should increase fibrinogen by an increment of 5-10 mg/dL.

E. Consider obtaining a hematology consultation.

F. **Disposition:** Admit to ICU.

4. Heparin Overdose:

4.1 Clinical Evaluation:

A. **Symptoms:** Patient develops hemorrhage or requires reversal of anticoagulation.

B. **Work-up:** Order CBC, including platelets, PT, and PTT.

4.2 RX:

A. Protamine sulfate forms a heparin-protamine complex and reverses the anticoagulant effect of heparin. Protamine neutralizes heparin within 5 minutes. Protamine should be considered if heparin (bolus or infusion) was given within 4 hours of the onset of bleeding. The plasma half-life of heparin is 1-2 hours and protamine is unlikely to be beneficial more than 4 hours after last heparin dose.

B. Dosing:

For a recent heparin bolus, administer 1 mg protamine sulfate IV for each 100 units of heparin.
For a continuous heparin infusion administer 1 mg protamine sulfate IV for each 100 units of heparin given over the preceding 4 hours.
If heparin has been discontinued for more than 30 minutes, reduce protamine dosage by 50%.
Doses should be infused slowly over 1-3 minutes and should not exceed 50 mg in any 10 minute period.

C. Adverse effects include mild hypotension, although anaphylactic reaction is uncommon. There is also a risk of allergic reactions in diabetic patients exposed to protamine through some insulin preparations.
D. **Disposition:** Admit, usually to ICU.

5. Sickle Cell Crisis:

Sickle Cell Disease occurs when Hgb S replaces Hgb A. Hgb S patients are at a higher risk for deoxygenation, polymerization of Hgb, and sickling of RBC. SS disease occurs when the hepatitis B surface antigen of 90% RBCs are sickled. Conversely SA Trait arises when the HBs < 60% of RBCs are sickled. SA disease may present with painless gross hematuria, priapism, anemia. This condition is rarely crisis. SS disease has a higher incidence for sickle crises resulting in bony, visceral infarcts, hemolytic/aplastic anemia, and infection.

5.1 Clinical Evaluation:

A. **Symptoms:** Patients who are suspected or known to have this disease may present with severe pain in the back, abdomen, chest, or extremities, ± associated fever, and jaundice. A recent illness, such as URI, gastroenteritis, may precede the symptoms. With recurrent splenic infarction there is an increased risk for underlying infection.
B. **Signs:** Assess for evidence of underlying infection, organomegaly, joint effusion, and for cardiothoracic or abdominal catastrophe.
C. **DDX:**

Chest: Myocardial infarction, pulmonary embolism, pneumonia, and bony infarct.
Abdomen: Visceral infarct, obstruction, and infection.
Head: Infection, cerebrovascular accident, and bony infarct.
Extremity: Infection, trauma, and bony infarct.

D. **Work-up:**

For a patient with a fever > 38°C, determine the source by obtaining a CBC with differential and reticulocyte count, T&C, blood culture, U/A with C&S, CXR, abdominal X-rays, or CT prn.
Vaso-Occlusive Crisis: For a patient with a stable hematocrit and reticulocyte, obtain U/A and C&S, CXR prn to exclude infection.
Hemolytic Crisis: For a patient who is ill and jaundiced, with a low hematocrit and reticulocyte count, order a type and screen/cross, as well as a U/A with C&S, and CXR prn to exclude the

Sequestration Crisis: For children < 8 years with abdominal pain, shock, and hepatosplenomegaly, order the labs cited above as well as a CBC to reveal low Hgb and pancytopenia.
Aplastic Crisis may follow acute infection: For a patient who is ill and/or in shock, order the labs listed above to reveal a low hematocrit and reticulocyte count, and any evidence of infection.

5.2 RX:

A. For patients with vaso-occlusive crisis, place on O_2 if hypoxic, hydrate with 0.9 NS IV fluid, and administer analgesics (NSAIDS, narcotics), folic acid, and antibiotics prn.
B. For hemolytic patients, treat as described above and transfuse with packed red blood cells.
C. For sequestration, treat as described above and consider surgery, i.e., possibly a splenectomy.
D. For aplastic patients, treat as described above and transfuse as needed.
E. **Disposition:** Admit the patient for transfusion, antibiotics, hydration, and pain control.

6. Warfarin Overdose:

6.1 Clinical Evaluation:

A. **Symptoms:** Patient develops hemorrhage or requires reversal of anticoagulation. Coumarins are present in many rodenticides.
B. **Work-up:** CBC, platelets, PT, and PTT.

6.2 RX:

A. Recent oral ingestion: Perform elimination measures by gastric lavage and administering activated charcoal.

B. Coumadin Anticoagulation: Rapidly or slowly correct coagulopathy, depending on the severity, risk of bleeding, or the necessity for reinstitution of anticoagulation.

C. Emergent Reversal:

Replace Vitamin K dependent factors with FFP, 15-20 mL/kg, followed by 5-7 mL/kg every 8-12 hours.

Administer Vitamin K, 10-50 mg for adults and 0.2-0.6 mg/kg peds IV or IM. Dilute if given by IV in 50 cc NS. Do not infuse faster than 1 mg/minute because slow infusion minimizes risk of anaphylactoid reactions and shock. Some prefer **test dose IM** to avoid anaphylaxis.

D. Reversal over 24-48 hours: Administer Vitamin K, 10-50 mg for adults, and 0.2-0.6 mg/kg for peds IM. Full reversal of anticoagulation will result in resistance to further Coumadin therapy for several days.

E. Temporary correction: Prescribe lower doses of Vitamin K, 0.5-1.0 mg, to reduce the prothrombin time without interfering with reinitiation of Coumadin.

F. **Disposition:** Admit patients with hemorrhage to the ICU.

INFECTIOUS DISEASES

1. Acquired Immune Deficiency Syndrome:

HIV is a retrovirus that infects the CD4 (T Helper Cells). This type of infection causes cell death and a decline in immune function which in turn allows malignancies and opportunistic infections to occur. HIV is transmitted through blood and blood products, including semen, vaginal secretions, etc. HIV is also transported through the placenta.

1.1 Clinical Evaluation:

A. **Symptoms:** Presentations include fever, chronic infections, persistent lymphadenopathy, opportunistic infection, weight loss, malignancies, and mental status changes, including encephalopathy.

B. **Work-up:** Customize for symptoms. Consider CXR, ABG, CBC, SMA-7, and LFTs. Blood C&S x 2. Sputum for Gram stain, C&S, & AFB. Obtain a CT, with and without contrast, followed by a LP. Include C&S, India ink for *Cryptococci* and the *Cryptococcal* antigen. Order Giemsa and immunofluorescence, or silver stain for *Pneumocysti*s and fungal C&S. Obtain fecal cells, O&P, and culture. Determine VDRL, serum *Cryptococcal* antigen and sulfadiazine levels. Perform a UCG and a U/A.

1.2 RX:

A. The treatment for HIV infections and exposures are changing rapidly. Currently, multiple antiviral agents are prescribed but the specific treatment is dependent upon with the type of exposure. Consult current guidelines and/or an infectious disease specialist prior to initiating a therapy.

B. For oral or esophageal candidiasis, prescribe fluconazole (Diflucan) 200-400 mg IV/po, **or** itraconazole (Sporanox) 200 mg 200 mg IV/po **or** ketoconazole, 5-10 mg/kg/day.

C. For CNS Toxoplasmosis, administer pyrimethamine, 200 mg load then 75-100 mg/day, plus sulfadiazine, 100 mg/kg/day and folic acid 5 mg/day.

D. For *Cryptococcal* meningitis, give amphotericin B, 0.5 mg/kg/day IV over 2-6 hours. May add flucytosine (5-Fluorocytosine) 50-150 mg/kg/d po q 6 hours.

E. For herpes simplex, administer acyclovir, 5 mg/kg IV over 1 hour q 8 hours **or** 200 mg po 5 x q day.

F. For herpes zoster, prescribe acyclovir, 10-12 mg/kg IV q 8 hours. Infuse over 1 hour.

G. Pneumocystis carinii pneumonia affects almost 80% of patients with AIDS. For patients with this condition, treat with trimethoprim/sulfamethoxazole (TMP/SMX, Septra, Bactrim), 15-20 mg/kg/day (based on TMP) IV in 3-4 divided doses for 21 days. Consider prednisone, if room air $pO_2 \leq 70$ mm Hg, or A-a gradient $\geq$ 35 mm Hg, **or** pentamidine (Pentam), 4 mg/kg IV q day for 21 days, (4 mg/kg/d inhaled), **or** dapsone, 100 mg po q day for 21 days. Consider prednisone, if room air $pO_2 \leq$ 70 mm Hg, or A-a gradient $\geq$ 35 mm Hg.

H. Arrange PCP prophylaxis for patients with a history of PCP and a CD4 < 200 by administering TMP/SMX D, 160/800 mg po q day, **or**pentamidine, 300 mg in 6 mL sterile water via nebulizer over 20-30 minutes q 4 weeks. May pretreat with albuterol, 2.5 mg in 5 mL NS.

I. For post-exposure prophylaxis consult current recommendations, usually with 3 agent therapy.

J. For HIV patients infected with TB, first isolate the causative agent and then treat with isoniazid, 5 mg/kg/day up to 300 mg/kg/day, **plus** rifampin, 10 mg/kg/day up to 600 mg/day po, **plus** pyrazinamide, 25 mg/kg/day to a maximum of 2.0 g/day po. Consult an infectious disease specialist because additional drugs may be required.

K. **Disposition:** Admit patients with clinical signs of sepsis or respiratory distress to the ICU. Most HIV patients with infections require at least admission to a medical bed for IV therapy.

2. Cellulitis:

Cellulitis is a subcutaneous infection that is most commonly caused by *Staphylococcus* or *Streptococcus* organisms. It usually involves deeper, dermal layers to fascia than the epidermal involvement of erysipelas. In healthy patients, pathogen isolation incidence is more probable, (80-90%), with known open lesion, pustule or broken skin (80-90%). For 10-40% of cellulitis patients, no known source can be identified by the skin/blood cultures. Thus, most patients are initially treated with antistaph/streptococcus antibiotic because the culture may be of little value.

Healthy individuals: *Staphylococcus* and *Streptococcus*.
Children: *Staphylococcus, Streptococcus*, and *H. influenzae*.
Diabetes Mellitus, Alcohol, Immunosuppression: *Staphylococcus, Streptococcus, Enterococcus, Enterobacter*, anaerobes, *Pseudomonas a.*, bacteroides, *Clostridium perf.,* and MRSA.

2.1 Clinical Evaluation:

A. **Symptoms:** ± fever, ± pain, warm, red region on skin, possibly surrounding a primary lesion, ± lymphangitic streaking, tender adenopathy, and ± induration followed by suppuration.
B. **Signs:** Erythema, edema, and warmth and tenderness of skin.
C. **DDX:** Erysipelas, local abscess, fasciitis, myositis, thrombophlebitis, gout, foreign body, and herpetic/viral exanthem.
D. **Work-up:** Obtain CBC, open wound culture, and ± aspiration skin.

2.2 RX:

A. Treatment in the ED will usually be empiric; causative organisms will be suspected only.
B. For *Streptococcal* origins, treat with aqueous penicillin G (600,000 units), followed by IM procaine penicillin, 600,000 units q 8-12 hours.
C. For *Staphylococcus* origins or unknown etiology, prescribe a penicillinase-resistant penicillin, such as oxacillin, 0.5-1.0 g po q 6 hours.
D. For patients with severe infections, treat with a penicillinase-resistant penicillin, such as nafcillin, 1.0-1.5 g IV q 4 hours, **or** vancomycin, 1.0-1.5 g/day IV.
E. For gas forming cellulitis, administer aqueous penicillin G, 10-20 million units/day IV, **or** metronidazole, 500 mg IV q 6 hours, **or** clindamycin, 600 mg IV q 8 hours.
F. For animal bites, treat with penicillin or nafcillin, IV for 7 days, before switching to oral antibiotics.
G. For human bites, treat with amoxicillin-clavulanic acid, or IV antibiotic.
H. For facial cellulitis caused by *H. influenza B*, treat with cefotaxime IV.
I. For diabetes mellitus, treat with cefoxitin or, if the patient is toxic, prescribe clindamycin and gentamicin.
J. For a compromised host, administer clindamycin and gentamicin.
K. For IV drug abusers, treat with vancomycin and gentamicin.
L. **Disposition:** Discharge healthy individuals with a simple infection and treat via an outpatient protocol. Admit individuals who display signs of systemic toxicity, extension of infection, or poor host resistance for IV antibiotic and observation.

3. Cystitis and Pyelonephritis:

E. coli is responsible for almost 80% of uncomplicated UTI in women and *S. saprophyticus* is the cause of about 10% of the cases. In complicated UTIs, such as abnormality of urinary tract, *E. coli* accounts for ~ 35%, *Enterococcus faecalis* for ~ 16%, *Proteus mirabilis* and *S. epidermidis* for ~ 13% each, and *Klebsiella* and *Pseudomonas* for ~ 5% each. Eighty percent of the uncomplicated pyelonephritis is caused by uropathogenic *E. coli*.

3.1 Clinical Evaluation:

A. **Symptoms:** Fever, dysuria, frequency, urgency, retention, and hematuria. High fevers, nausea, vomiting, and back pain suggest pyelonephritis. Examine for recent or ongoing catheterization.

B. **Signs:** Fever, tachycardia, dehydration, and costovertebral angle tenderness. Debilitation and mental status changes can occur particularly in elderly patients with urosepsis.

C. **DDX:** Cystitis vs pyelonephritis, PID, vaginosis, urethritis, renal calculus, renal infarction, renal thrombosis, glomerulonephritis, pancreatitis, cholecystitis, splenic infarct, appendicitis and other causes of abdominal pain. Always consider AAA for the elderly with symptoms of pyelonephritis.

D. **Work-up:** For cystitis without complicating factors, obtain additional studies, including urine dip or microscopic analysis of sediment. Positive findings consist of elevated WBCs, nitrites or bacteria. Order a culture for patients with diabetes, with symptoms > 1 week, and with recurrent urinary tract infections. Also, order cultures from pregnant, elderly, and pyelonephritis patients. Determine CBC and SMA-7 as indicated for toxic and pyelonephritis patients.

3.2 RX:

A. For uncomplicated cystitis, treat with a 3 day po course of TMP-SMX, 160/800 mg bid, **or** trimethoprim, 100 mg bid, **or** a quinolone bid. Quinolones are suggested for recurrent infections and recent treatment failures.

B. For uncomplicated cystitis in a pregnant patient, treat 3-7 days with nitrofurantoin, 100 mg qid, **or** amoxicillin, 250 mg tid.

C. For complicated cystitis, treat with a 10-14 day course of quinolones.

D. For uncomplicated pyelonephritis, such as cases not involving the debilitated, indigent, immune-suppressed, septic, or the dehydrated, and patients able to tolerate po, treat for 14 days with TMP-SMX DS bid **or** quinolone. Rule out AAA as indicated.

E. For pyelonephritis or UTI patients requiring admission, many IV regimens are available, including ampicillin, 1 g q 6 hours, plus gentamicin, 1 mg/kg q 8 hours, **or** ofloxacin **or** ciprofloxacin, 200-400 mg q 12 hours, **or** ceftriaxone, 1-2 g q day.

F. For candida cystitis, irrigate bladder continuously with Amphotericin B, 50 mg/1000 mL sterile water via 3-way Foley catheter at 1 L/day for 5 days, **or** fluconazole (Diflucan), 100 mg po or IV for 1 dose, followed by 50 mg po or IV q day for 5 days.

G. For patients with severe symptoms prescribe phenazopyridine (Pyridium), 100-200 mg po tid to relieve spasm.

H. **Disposition:** Admit patients with complicated pyelonephritis. Consider admission for individuals with complicated UTI and those who are debilitated, dehydrated, unable to tolerate po, and appear toxic.

4. Encephalitis:

Encephalitis is inflammation of the brain caused by a viral or bacterial source. This condition occurs in about 2000 individuals per year within the US. Many of these cases are treatable. However, an early ID consultation is recommended.

4.1 Clinical Evaluation:

A. **Symptoms:** Symptomatic individuals may have antecedent viral syndrome or vaccination, or may have traveled to an area with a high incidence of encephalitis. Usual presentation is HA, fever and change in mental status. More developed symptoms include severely decreased MS, seizures, and focal neurologic deficits. Immune compromise predisposes to encephalitis, particularly due to Mycobacteria, *Cryptococcus, Listeria,* and herpes.

B. **Signs:** Assess mental status while carefully documenting deficits. Seek focal neurologic findings, papilledema. Check for meningitic involvement, such as photophobia, neck stiffness, Kernig's & Brudzinski's signs.

C. **DDX:** Includes change in mental status differential diagnosis, particularly DKA, hyperosmolar hyperglycemic nonketotic coma, hypoglycemia, drug intoxication or toxidrome, metabolic encephalopathy, Reye's, Addisonian crisis, brain abscess, and cerebrovascular accident.

D. **Work-up:** Order CBC and SMA-7+. Consider calcium, magnesium, phosphate, osmolality, ammonia level, LFTs, ABG, CXR, pan-culture, and a toxicology screen. Obtain CT and perform LP. It is advisable to perform the CT prior to LP. Nonetheless, a CT must ALWAYS be performed before LP with suspected increased ICP. A CSF with encephalitis will show elevated protein levels with low levels of glucose in cases of bacterial and tubercular infections and pleocytosis. Generally, increased levels of lymphocytes suggest a viral etiology. An elevation in neutrophils indicate a bacterial or a non-viral etiology while increased monocytes suggest an infection arising from a bacteria and Mycobacteria source.

4.2 RX:

A. Support airway, IV, O_2, and monitor. Arrange ICP management that includes hyperventilation, steroids, and mannitol prn.
B. For most cases, do not delay antibiotics for LP. Refer to separate sections which cite recommendations for treating "Meningitis", "Lyme's Disease", "Rocky Mountain Spotted Fever", "Toxoplasmosis", and "TB".
C. For treatments of arthropod-borne viruses, refer to "Rocky Mountain Spotted Fever" and "Lyme's Disease" sections.
D. For herpes simplex encephalitis, treat with acyclovir, 10 mg/kg IV q 8 hours for 10-21 days.
E. Treat varicella-zoster associated symptoms similar to the program cited for HSV encephalitis.
F. **Disposition:** Usually admit the patient to the ICU.

5. Endocarditis, Infectious:

Endocarditis is an infection of the endocardial lining of the heart and valves. High risk groups include IV drug abusers, particularly cocaine, and individuals with prosthetic heart valves. Other high-risk groups consist of patients with mitral valve prolapse who undergo dental or surgical procedures and/or individuals with pre-existing rheumatic valvular disease. *Streptococcus* and *Staphylococcus aureus* account for 46% and 20% of the reported cases, respectively. However, *Pseudomonas, Serratia marcescens*, and *Candida albicans* are increasing at a greater incidence as the primary cause of this infection in drug abusers.

5.1 Clinical Evaluation:

A. **Symptoms:** Low grade fever persisting for weeks to months, non-specific complaints, myalgias, arthralgias, IV drug abuse, heart disease and recent GI, GU, or dental procedures.
B. **Signs:**
    Chronically ill: Skin track marks, Osler's nodes (painful red nodules on fingers), Janeway lesions (nontender plaques on the palms and soles), and subungual splinter hemorrhages.
    Fundus: Cotton-wool exudates, retinal hemorrhages, and Roth's spots (retinal white spots surrounded by hemorrhage).
    Lungs: Rales and other signs of congestive heart failure.
    Cardiac: Murmurs.
    Abdomen: Tenderness and splenomegaly.
    Neuro: Altered mental status and meningismus.
C. **DDX:** Septicemia, rheumatic fever, pericarditis, pneumonia, TB, meningitis, intra-abdominal infection, glomerulonephritis, cerebrovascular accident, SLE, cancer, congestive heart failure, multiple pulmonary embolisms, and DIC.
D. **Work-up:** Order CBC, SMA-7, PT, PTT, UA, oximetry or ABG, blood culture x 3, ECG, and CXR.

5.2 RX:

A. Support ABCs, IV, O_2, and monitor.
B. For valve disease and IV drug abuse cases, treat with nafcillin, 2 g IV q 4 hours, plus gentamicin, 1.5 mg/kg IV, followed by 1 mg/kg q 8 hours.
C. For prosthetic valve patients, administer vancomycin, 1 g IV q 12 hours, plus gentamicin plus rifampin, 300 mg po q 12 hours.

D. **Disposition:** Admit, usually to the ICU.

6. Epiglottitis:

Epiglottitis is an acute inflammation of the supraglottic, epiglottic, vallecula, aryepiglottic folds, and arytenoids. In children, the primary cause of epiglottitis is *H. influenzae* type b. Fewer cases occur as a result of *S. aureus, B. catarrhalis, Streptococci* and *Pneumococci.* The typical ages of children who contract epiglottitis are about 2-6 years. *H. influenzae* type b is also a common cause for epiglottitis in adults. Group A *Streptococcus* and some other types of viral agents have also been implicated.

6.1 Clinical Evaluation:

A. **Symptoms:**

Peds: Acute onset of illness, rapidly progressive with fever, sore throat, dysphagia, and drooling late in the course of illness.

Adults: Usually less fulminant progression as compared to children. Adults or children can deteriorate suddenly. Presents with sore throat, dysphagia, "hot potato" voice, and respiratory compromise.

B. **Signs:** Support ABCs for any patient in extremis.

In pediatric patients use caution by allowing patient to stay in a parent's arms. Examine without causing any undue agitation. Patients often appear ill, toxic, and/or anxious. They are usually sitting up with their head in a "sniffing" position. Inspiratory stridor may also occur.

Adults may appear very ill with signs of airway compromise similar to that exhibited by children.

C. **DDX:** Pharyngitis, peritonsillar abscess, retropharyngeal abscess, diphtheria, laryngotracheobronchitis, tracheitis, uvulitis, and FB.

D. **Work-up:** H&P may be adequate to make diagnosis. True diagnosis takes place with direct visualization. Portable cross-table lateral soft-tissue neck to check for thumb sign and vallecular blunting may be appropriate. In adults who appear mildly ill with symptoms that have progressed over several days and who have no evidence of potential airway compromise, consider direct nasopharyngolaryngoscopy with appropriate preparation in the ED. All other patients should have diagnosis and treatment performed in the OR.

6.2 RX:

A. Support ABCs, including bag-valve-mask, emergent intubation or placement of needle cricothyroidotomy, if immediately necessary. Otherwise intubation may take place in more controlled manner within the OR. Instruct all team members, including the surgeon skilled in tracheostomy and the parents of the pediatric patient to assemble and proceed to the OR.

B. Start antibiotics after definitive airway management. Treat with cefuroxime, 75-100 mg/kg/day IV/IM q 8 hours with a maximum of 9 g/day, **or**ceftriaxone, 50-75 mg/kg/day IV/IM q 12-24 hours, maximum 4 g/day, **or** cefotaxime, 100-150 mg/kg/day IV/IM q 6-8 hours, maximum 12 g/day, **or** ampicillin, 100-200 mg/kg/day IV q 6 hours, maximum 12 g/day, **and** chloramphenicol, 50-75 mg/kg/day IV q 6 hours.

C. **Disposition:** Transfer the patient to the OR or to the ICU.

7. Erysipelas:

Streptococcus a, c, d, and *Staphylococcus a* commonly infect children and the elderly. The source is often an unnoticed skin wound. With bacteremia, the range of illness is from localized to extensive.

7.1 Clinical Evaluation:

A. **Symptoms:** Small wound, local infection to widespread involvement, and ± fever.

B. **Signs:** Red, warm, tender skin, and no fluctuance. Lesion edge is raised and well demarcated.

C. **DDX:** Cellulitis, sinusitis, erysipeloid (hands), contact dermatitis, angioneurotic edema, lupus, and necrotizing fasciitis.

D. **Work-up:** Exam, ± punch biopsy. Skin aspiration is not usually helpful.

7.2 RX:

A. Treat outpatients with penicillin VK as follows.
   Provide children with 25-50 mg/kg/day divided q 6 hours.
   Administer adults 250-500 mg/dose q 6 hours.

B. For severe inpatient cases, administer parenteral antibiotics, such as cephalosporin, penicillinase-resistant penicillin, clindamycin, or vancomycin.

C. **Disposition:** Admit patients with widespread infection, clinical toxicity, and nonresponsive to po antibiotic. If nontoxic, discharge as an outpatient with po regimen and a close follow-up.

8. Hepatitis:

Hepatitis generally manifests as a large group of systemic infections that involve the liver. Similar clinical symptoms are exhibited; however, these systemic infections may be caused by several different viruses. Non-viral infectious and toxic cases can also be displayed by patients with hepatitis.

8.1 Clinical Evaluation:

A. **Symptoms:** Malaise, low-grade fever, and other constitutional symptoms, followed by abdominal pain, pigmented urine, icterus, and jaundice. Ascites, urticaria, arthralgias, bleeding problems, and a change in mental status may also be exhibited.

B. **Signs:** Change in mental status, scleral icterus, jaundice, hepato and splenomegaly, ascites, spider angiomas, gynecomastia, and testicular atrophy may be present in advanced hepatitis.

C. **DDX:** Cirrhosis, cholecystitis/cholangitis, alcoholic ketoacidosis, infectious mononucleosis, hepatic malignancy, Wilson's disease, and pancreatitis.

D. **Work-up:** Order CBC, SMA-7, LFTs, including AST (SGOT, measures hepatocellular injury/necrosis), ALT (SGPT, necrosis), alkaline phosphatase and bilirubins for signs of cholestasis and LDH. PT and PTT can help in evaluating hepatic function as do protein and albumin, which probably will not change ED diagnosis or management. Amylase, lipase, acetaminophen, and ammonia levels may assist in determining the cause and complications. Ascertain alcohol level and send toxicologic screen. Obtain CXR, ECG, C&S, ultrasound and paracentesis prn.
   Ascitic Fluid- Tube 1: Protein, albumin, specific gravity, glucose, bilirubin, amylase, lipase, triglyceride, LDH, fibrinogen, and fibronectin, 3-5 mL, red top tube.
   Tube 2: Cell count & differential, 3-5 mL, purple top tube.
   Tube 3: C&S, Gram stain, AFB, and fungal, 5-20 mL. Inject 20 mL into blood culture bottles.
   Tube 4: Cytology, > 20 mL.
   Syringe: pH, 2 mL.

8.2 RX:

A. Start IV fluids and antiemetics to relieve nausea, vomiting, and dehydration. Administer thiamine, 100 mg IM/IV, folate, 2 mg IM/IV, and multivitamins, 1 amp IV or 1 po to the alcoholic patient.

B. For signs of GI bleed or gastritis, treat with ranitidine, famotidine, or cimetidine IV.

C. For patients with prolonged PT, provide Vitamin K, 10 mg sq.

D. Treat per tox section for *amanita*, acetaminophen, arsenic, or isoniazid toxicity. Stop hepatotoxic meds, including isoniazid, acetaminophen, NSAIDS especially diclofenac, phenytoin, α-methyldopa, lovastatin, and nitrofurantoin.

E. Consider initiating lactulose and neomycin treatment for hepatic encephalopathy.

F. Refer to reference text for a detailed decision algorithm for exposure to known hepatitis patients.

G. Treat sexual and household HAV contacts with hepatitis immune serum globulin (ISG), 0.02 mL/kg IM.

H. Treat a person exposed to HBV by sexual contact, needle stick, or mucosal exposure with hepatitis B immune globulin, 0.06 mg/kg IM, and initiate active immunization. An exposed person who has been previously vaccinated should have anti-HBs drawn unless he/she is a known non-responder. In that case, the individual should receive hepatitis B immunoglobulin.

I. Consider ISG 0.06 mL/kg IM for parenteral HCV exposure.
J. Treat HDC as described for HBV.
K. A vaccine antibody against Hepatitis A virus may be available soon.
L. **Disposition:** Admission is not routinely required. However, admit patients with severe dehydration, intractable nausea and vomiting, a change in mental status, dangerous toxic etiologies, and other signs of acute or dangerous illnesses.

9. Meningitis:

Meningitis is caused by a variety of pathogens that have the potential of infecting different age groups. However, the incidence of *H. influenzae* is decreasing because of the Hib vaccine. Cephalosporins are not effective against *Listeria*; therefore, use ampicillin in ages ranging between 0-3 months and > 7 years. There is a 90% mortality rate when bacterial meningitis is not promptly treated. Atypical presentations are common.

9.1 Clinical Evaluation:

A. **Symptoms:** HA, fever, nuchal rigidity, photophobia, may have prior exposure. Late findings can include nausea, vomiting, and changes in mental status.
B. **Signs:** Patients often appear ill. Kernig's and Brudzinski's signs, photophobia, nuchal rigidity, papilledema, petechia are associated with meningococcus. A change in mental status may occur, including confusion, lethargy, coma, seizure, cranial nerve, or other focal neurologic findings.
C. **DDX:** Change in mental status differential diagnosis, viral syndromes, encephalitis or brain abscess, bacteremia, sepsis, seizures and acute narrow-angle glaucoma.
D. **Work-up:** Perform LP; CT may be obtained prior to LP if papilledema or other signs of increased ICP are present. Do not delay antibiotic treatment for this study. Also obtain CBC and any other studies appropriate to the presentation, i.e., sinus films, blood culture, U/A, and SMA-7.

CSF Tube 1: Cell count & differential, 1-2 mL.
CSF Tube 2: Glucose, protein, 1-2 mL.
CSF Tube 3: Gram stain of fluid or sediment, if fluid is clear, and C&S for bacteria, 1-4 mL.
CSF Tube 4: Cell count & differential and special studies. Latex agglutination or counterimmunoelectrophoresis antigen tests for *S. pneumoniae, H. influenzae* (type B), *N. meningitides, E. coli*, Group B *Streptococcus, Cryptococcus*, viral cultures, VDRL, 8-10 mL. Add India ink and AFB for immune compromised or exposed patients.

CSF results reveal hypoglycorrhachia, glucose < 50 mg/dL or CSF/Serum glucose < 0.5; elevated protein, often > 100 mg/dL; and elevated WBC or any granulocytes unless WBC < $5/mm^3$. Counterimmunoelectrophoresis detects bacterial antigens whereas Gram's stain detects bacterial organisms. Viral meningitis is associated with elevated levels of neutrophils in the CSF, normal glucose levels, and normal or only slightly elevated protein.

9.2 RX: Sample treatment regimens are provided below.

A. Treat patients who are < 1 month old and infected with Groups B&D *Streptococcus, E. coli, Listeria* as follows:

0-7 days: Ampicillin, 150/kg/day IV q 8 hours.
> 7 days: Cefotaxime, 200 mg/kg/day IV q 6 hours.
0-7 days old: An alternative is ampicillin + gentamicin, 5-7 mg/kg/day IM/IV over 30 minutes q 12 hours.
> 7 days: Ampicillin plus gentamicin, 5-7 mg IM/IV q day **or** use amikacin in place of gentamicin, if gentamicin resistance is likely.

B. Treat patients who are 1-3 months old (often infected with *H. influenzae, Pneumococci, Meningococci*, Group B *Streptococcus, E. coli*) as follows:

Ampicillin, 200 mg/kg/day IV q 6 hours, **and either** cefotaxime or ceftriaxone.
An alternative is chloramphenicol plus gentamicin.
Dexamethasone, 0.4 mg/kg IV given 15 minutes BEFORE an antibiotic to decrease incidence of hearing loss.

C. Treat patients who are 3 months-7 years old (often infected with *H. influenzae*, *Pneumococci*, *Meningococci*) as follows:
   Cefotaxime, 200 mg/kg/day IV q 6 hours, maximum 12 g/day, **or** ceftriaxone, 100 mg/kg/day IV q 12-24 hours, maximum 4 g/day.
   And alternative is ampicillin, 200 mg/kg/day IV q 6 hours, maximum 12 days.
   Dexamethasone (see above).

D. Treat patients who are 7 years-50 years old (often infected with *Pneumococci, Meningococci, Listeria* as follows:
   Ampicillin, 200 mg/kg/day IV q 6 hours, maximum 12 g/day.
   Penicillin G, 20 M units/day, **and either** cefotaxime, 200 mg/kg/day IV q 6 hours, maximum 12 g/day or ceftriaxone, 100 mg/kg/day IV q 12-24 hours, maximum 4 g/day.
   An alternative is third generation cephalosporin alone **or** chloramphenicol plus TMP/SMX.
   Consider dexamethasone.

E. Treat patients who are > 50 years old, debilitated, alcoholic, and are likely infected with *Pneumococci* as follows:
   Vancomycin plus third generation cephalosporin plus rifampin.
   An alternative is chloramphenicol plus TMP/SMX.

F. Treat HIV+ patients likely infected with *Cryptococcus neoformans, M. tuberculosis, Syphilis, Listeria, and Pneumococci* as follows:
   Treat as cited above for the > 50 year old age group.
   For *Cryptococcus neoformans*, prescribe amphotericin B test dose of 0.1 mg/kg with a maximum of 1 mg, followed by the remainder of first day dose, if tolerated.
   The initial dose should be 0.25 mg/kg/day **or,** if less severe, fluconazole (Diflucan), 3-6 mg/kg/day po q day, usually 400 mg po q day in adult.

G. Administer prophylactic medication to health professionals in very close contact with a symptomatic meningitis patient. Treat family members with rifampin, 600 mg po q hours for a total of 4 doses.

H. **Disposition:** Admit to ICU if necessary.

10. Myonecrosis (Gas Gangrene):

Myonecrosis manifests as an extensive tissue necrosis and edema that is complicated by infection of the muscle. This infection is caused by a *Clostridium* organism, i.e., primarily *Clostridium perfringens*. As the infection develops, exotoxins can produce the onset of sepsis, diffuse edema, and RBC hemolysis. The mortality rate of patients with myonecrosis is > 20%.

10.1 Clinical Evaluation:

A. **Symptoms:** Extensive and contaminated initial wounds. Compounding problems, such as compartment syndrome or immune compromise, may be displayed. There is a swift onset of pain, traditionally greater than expected for the injury, rapidly progressive edema, followed by sepsis.

B. **Signs:** Initially edema, later palpable emphysema, erythema, and bullae.

C. **DDX:** Compartment syndrome, thrombophlebitis, cellulitis, and necrotizing fasciitis.

D. **Work-up:** Check for Gram + bacilli. Obtain an X-ray and exam for gas along tissue planes.

10.2 RX:

A. Treat the patient with penicillin G as follows:
   For adults, administer 5-10 million units IV q 6 hours.
   For peds, give 0.2-0.5 million units IV q 4 hours.
   Alternatives include clindamycin, cephalothin, ceftriaxone, and erythromycin.

B. Immediate surgical intervention is necessary for fasciotomy and debridement.

C. Treat with hyperbaric oxygen.

D. **Disposition:** Transfer the patient directly to the OR. Alternatively, treat patient with hyperbaric oxygen and then transfer him/her to the OR.

11. Necrotizing Fascitis:

Necrotizing Fascitis is a rapidly progressive infection characterized by local skin, subcutaneous, and fascial involvement that are complicated by systemic toxicity. The disease has a polymicrobial origin, primarily caused by *Bacteroides*, *Clostridia,* and aerobes.

11.1 Clinical Evaluation:

A. **Symptoms:** A warm, edematous, painful infected wound that rapidly worsens. Fever, septicemia, acidosis, shock, and DIC are also exhibited.

B. **Signs:** Patients are ill to toxic in appearance with potentially unstable VS, shock, DIC, and hemolysis. Wounds develop necrosis of skin and underlying fascia with progression along fascial planes and local bulla. The wounds may have crepitance. No resistance to probing along the fascial plane is indicative of the diagnosis.

C. **DDX:** Myonecrosis, cellulitis, erysipelas, and phlegmasia cerulea dolens.

D. **Work-up:** Obtain an X-ray of affected area. Order wound Gram's stain and C&S, including anaerobic C&S, BC, CBC, and SMA-7. Add, as appropriate, tests for DIC, ABG, ECG, and CXR.

11.2 RX:

A. Start an antibiotic IV and transfer the patient to surgery for debridement. Administer ampicillin/sulbactam (Unasyn), 1.5-3 g q 6 hours, **or** ticarcillin clavulanate (Timentin), 3.1 g q 3-6 hours. Alternate with PRSP plus antipseudomonal aminoglycoside plus clindamycin, i.e., nafcillin, 2 g q 4 hours, plus gentamicin 2.0 mg/kg load, plus clindamycin, 600-900 mg q 8 hours.

B. **Disposition:** Transfer the patient to OR for debridement and then admit him/her to ICU.

12. Pneumonia:

Pneumococcus is responsible for 90% of all pneumonia cases. Predisposing factors consist of congestive heart failure, COPD, smoking, bronchiectasis, sickle cell disease, hypogammaglobulinemia, mental status change, seizures, aspiration, and the immunocompromised. Common etiologies of pneumonias are provided by age group and by medical association.

Neonates-12 wks:	**4 wks-4 years:**
Group B *Streptococcus*	RSV(to 6 months)
Coliforms	*Streptococcus pneumonia,* *H. influenzae*
Listeria m.	Viral, (para/influenza, adeno., EBV)
Herpes simplex	*B. pertussis*
Rubella	*Streptococcus pyogenes*
Chlamydia	*Staphylococci a.*
CMV	Gram negative bacteria, PCP
5-12 years	**12-Adult**
Pneumococcus	*Pneumococcus*
H. influenzae	*H. influenzae*
Mycoplasma	Mycoplasma
Viral	Viral
TB	Group A *Streptococcus*
	P. auruginosa
	Staphylococcus aureus
	E. coli
	Klebsiella
	Legionella
	Anaerobes
	TB
	Q fever
	Tularemia

Associated Illnesses: Bacterium.
COPD/Smokers: *H. influenzae* and *Klebsiella.*
Diabetics: *Klebsiella*, *E. coli*, and Gram negatives.
Alcohol abusers: *Klebsiella*, anaerobes, Gram negatives, and TB.
Sicklers: *Salmonella.*
IV drug abusers: *Staphylococcus aureus.*
Cystic Fibrosis: Resistant *Pseudomonas a.*

11.1 Clinical Evaluation:

A. **Symptoms:** URI symptoms, cough, sputum, wheezing, progressive dyspnea, fever, malaise, pleuritic chest pain/abdominal pain, anorexia n/v, and obtundation may all occur.

B. **Signs:** A fever that is > 40 °C suggests a bacterial source. Congestion, tachypnea, retractions, splinting, cough, hoarseness, stridor, wheezing, rhonchi, consolidation, friction rub on auscultation, dullness to percussion, ± egophony, ± exanthem, and obtundation (depressed gag) may be found.

C. **DDX:** Congestive heart failure, tumor, pulmonary contusion, effusion (from cirrhosis, congestive heart failure, uremia, and trauma), pleural/parenchymal thickening/scarring, and atelectasis. Causes include:

Pneumococcus is the primary culprit in 90% cases, especially when community acquired. All ages exhibit rusty/currant jelly sputum, and leukocytosis. The CXR reveals single lobular infiltrate to patchy infiltrates.

H. influenzae is the secondary bacterial cause of pneumonia. It is common in the young and the old. CXR shows patchy infiltrate, no effusion, Gram- pleomorphic rod that are ± encapsulated.

Mycoplasma is most common nonbacterial pneumonitis in adults. Associated symptoms include URI (50%), earache, such as bullous myringitis (10%), conjunctivitis, cervical nodes, pharyngitis, low WBC, and high ESR, CXR- unilateral lower lobe infiltrate, reticulonodular infiltrate (20%), and effusion (20%).

Viral causative agents are most common for all patients. In infants less than < 6 months, URI symptoms and exanthem are typically evident. Also seen in the 3-5 year old age group are fever, cough, coryza, poor feeding, wheezing, and retractions. CXR indicates hyperinflation, patchy infiltrate. Eighty percent have superimposed bacterial pneumonia and 40% have a normal CXR.

Klebsiella gives rise to a toxic manifestation, leukocytosis, and currant jelly sputum. The CXR reveals RUL infiltrate, AFL classic, bulging fissure (30%), perihilar and patchy infiltrate, and Gram-encapsulated rods may be found on Gram's stain of sputum.

Anaerobic causative agents are usually community acquired anaerobes. Nosocomial, Gram- aerobes and leukocytosis are evident. CXR shows classic RLL infiltrate but may also indicate a diffuse pattern which may lead to AFL.

Legionella is contracted from domestic water systems mainly during the summer and fall months. Adults, smokers, and the immunocompromised are at the greatest risk for acquiring this type. There is a rapid progression of the disease process. Symptoms may include tachypnea with relative bradycardia, abdominal pain, vomiting, diarrhea; leukocytosis, elevated ESR, ± LFT elevation, Gram stain reveals few polys, and no preponderant bacterium. CXR shows unilateral infiltrate (70%) to bilateral patchy infiltrate, ± consolidation, and effusion (10%). RAI and ELISA screens outside ED are specific but their sensitivity is low. Elevated ab titers, 1:128, suggest infection, 1:256, suggest acute infection.

Aspiration is caused by an unprotected airway leading to inflammation. The severity of the infection is based on 3 factors: 1) pH and volume of aspirate; pH < 2.5 associated with chemical and bacterial pneumonitis, 2) particulates, such as food or foreign bodies, can lead to an obstruction, persistent hyperexpansion of the lung on CXR, and chronic granulomatous changes, and 3) bacterial contamination by anaerobic pneumonia.

A **Work-up:** Order CBC with differential (left shift suggests bacterial process), O_2 saturation/ABG for suspected hypoxemia, sputum gram stain and culture, blood/urine culture for fever. Consider thoracentesis fluid analysis to rule out empyema as well as selected serologies and agglutinin studies based on index of suspicion outside of ED.

11.2 RX:

A. Treat infant patients who are 0-2 weeks with ampicillin and gentamicin.
B. Treat 2 week-2 month infants with erythromycin **or** cefotaxime.
C. Treat 2 months-8 year olds with erythromycin or a 2nd or 3rd generation cephalosporin.
D. Treat young children and adults with erythromycin or a 2nd generation cephalosporin.
E. Treat AIDs patients with Bactrim and erythromycin or a 2nd or 3rd generation cephalosporins.
F. Treat diabetics or alcoholics with cefazolin and aminoglycoside.
G. Treat the elderly with erythromycin or a 2nd or 3rd generation cephalosporin.
H. Treat patients exposed to the condition via the hospital with a 3rd generation cephalosporin. If pseudomonas is possible use ceftazidine, cefoperazone, or Zosyn. Use a macrolide if legionella is suspected
I. **Disposition:** Admit patients with hypoxia, volume depletion, toxicity, and serious PMH (diabetes, coronary artery disease, PVD, immunocompromised). Discharge a patient only if adequate follow up has been arranged and he/she can be cared for properly at home.

12. Sepsis:

Bacteremia is the presence of microorganisms in the blood. Sepsis is bacteremia with a systemic response to the presence of microorganisms in blood. Highest risk groups include neonates, the debilitated, the immunocompromised, drug abusers and the elderly. The most common organisms that elicit a sepsis response are as follows.

Neonates: Group B *Streptococcus* and *E. coli.*
Infants/Adults: *H. influenzae, N. meningitidis*, and *S. pneumoniae.*
Sicklers: *S. pneumoniae* and *Salmonella.*
IV drug abusers: *Staphylococcus aureus.*

Consider also Group A *Streptococcus*, *N. gonorrhea*, *Pseudomonas aeruginosa, E. coli*, and fungal septicemia in differential.
Rule of 2s: Children < 2, rectal temp > 102 °F, WBC > 20k are at 20% risk of bacteremia.

12.1 Clinical Evaluation:

A. **Symptoms:** Patient's complaints may indicate the primary focus of the infection, although vague symptoms of fever, malaise, headache, and arthralgias/myalgias are quite common. Recent history of illness/infection, and antibiotic use is also very helpful.
B. **Signs:** Variable, insidious to fulminant illness. Based on studies, fever, (70%), shock, (40%), hypothermia, (4%), rash- maculopapular, petechial, nodular, vesicular with central necrosis, (70% with meningococcemia), and arthritis, (8%). Fever occurs in < 60% of the affected infants < 3 months and in adults > 65 years.
C. **DDX:** Viral exanthems, Rocky Mountain Spotted Fever, typhus, typhoid fever, endocarditis, vasculitis (polyarteritis nodosa, Henoch-Schönlein purpura), toxic shock, and rheumatic fever.
D. **Work-up:** Order CBC with differential, blood and urine culture, consider CSF analysis for suspicious symptoms, CXR, CT prn, and bacterial/viral/fungal serologies as based upon clinical suspicion.

12.2 RX:

A. Bacteremia/sepsis probable by clinical suspicion, ± supportive lab data but no organism is identified.
   For neonates (4 weeks), treat with ampicillin, 200 mg/kg/day, and cefotaxime, 50 mg/kg/day IV, **or** ampicillin, 200 mg/kg/day, and gentamicin, 2.5 mg/kg/day IV.
   For children who are 2 months-15 years old, treat with ceftriaxone, 50-75 mg/kg/day, or ceftazidime, 100 mg/kg/day IV, **or** ampicillin, 200 mg/kg/24 and chloramphenicol, 50-100 mg/kg/day.
   For adults who are 15-60 years old, treat with penicillin G, 6-12 million units IV q d, or ampicillin, 200 mg/kg/day, **or** gentamicin, 2.5 mg/kg IV q 8 hours, and metronidazole, 7.5 mg/kg IV q 6 hours.
   For adults > 60 years or for alcoholics, treat with ampicillin, 200 mg/kg/day, and ceftriaxone, 50 mg/kg/day, **or** ampicillin, 20 mg/kg/day, and gentamicin, 2.5 mg/kg IV q 8 hours.
B. **Disposition:** Admit patients with clinical toxicity, unclear progression of symptoms, unclear follow-up, suspected meningitis and/or meningococcemia, and significant underlying medical problems. Discharge patients with minimal signs and symptoms, and in whom clinical suspicion is low and cultures are pending. Ensure that the patient is provided with clear, detailed discharge instructions, and follow-up arrangements, and that he/she can be reached by the phone.

13. Septic Arthritis:

Consider septic arthritis when any painful monarthritis is exhibited. Most common origin is hematologic. Other sources include inoculation through a laceration or bite, extension from adjacent infection. This condition is associated with FB or surgical hardware and indwelling central venous access. *Staphylococcus*, *Streptococcus*, and *H. influenzae* are most common organisms that elicit septic arthritis.

13.1 Clinical Evaluation:

A. **Symptoms:** Fever, chills, previous infection with potential for hematogenous seeding, especially gonorrhea and meningitis. Occurs primarily in the immune compromised host, the IV drug abuser, trauma patients, and in individuals with prior chronic arthritis.
B. **Signs:** Large joints are most commonly affected. Warm, erythematous, tender joint with decreased ROM 2° to pain, and often with an effusion.
C. **DDX:** Noninfectious arthritis, including crystalline disorders, inflammatory disorders with SLE and polymyalgia rheumatica, and trauma.
D. **Work-up:** Perform arthrocentesis avoiding overlying cellulitis if possible. Expect opaque fluid with WBC counts > 50,000/mm^3 in developed pyogenic arthritis. If necessary, perform arthrocentesis under fluoro. Send synovial fluid for Gram's stain and C&S. Plain X-rays are usually normal in

early infection and erosion occurs later. Order CBC, blood C&S, and examine for other, possibly causative, sources of infection.

13.2 RX:

A. Administer β-lactamase-resistant penicillins, such as nafcillin, methicillin or oxacillin IV. Add vancomycin if patient has a history of MRSA. Treat possible GC with ceftriaxone, cefotaxime or ceftizoxime.
B. For the neonate- 3 month old patient, treat with β-lactamase-resistant penicillins and either gentamicin or cephalosporin 3.
C. For the toddler-5 year old patient, prescribe β-lactamase resistant penicillins and Cephalosporin 3.
D. For patients who are > 5 years to an adult, treat with β-lactamase resistant penicillins and consider gentamicin.
E. Customize treatment for the compromised adults, such as an IV drug abuser, HIV patient, and the debilitated.
F. Consider surgical drainage for any FB involvement and foot involvement.
G. **Disposition:** Admit patient with orthopedic consultation. If unsure, admit and treat pending C&S.

14. Streptococcal Scarlet Fever:

Streptococcal Scarlet Fever commonly occurs in school age children especially in the winter and in the spring. For a Group A *Streptococcus* infection, there is a high risk of contracting rheumatic fever if it is not appropriately treated.

14.1 Clinical Evaluation:

A. **Symptoms:** Pharyngitis, URI symptoms, rash after onset of pharyngitis, and a 1-3 day duration.
B. **Signs:** Pharyngitis, exudate, red, blanching, papular, "sandpaper" texture, flushed face, more rash in hyperpigmented areas, joint creases, circumoral pallor, strawberry tongue, desquamation with resolution. Complications are the same as those cited for Streptococcus pharyngitis.
C. **DDX:** "Viral Exanthem"- measles, rubella, roseola, "fifth" disease, Rocky Mountain Spotted Fever, Kawasaki, Mycoplasma pneumoniae, adeno/enterovirus, and meningococcemia.
D. **Work-up:** Order leukocytosis, ASO serology +, throat culture.

14.2 RX:

A. Administer penicillin G, clindamycin, erythromycin, or ceftriaxone, po fluids.
B. **Disposition:** Admit dehydrated and/or toxic patients. Individuals who have pneumonia accompanied with respiratory distress must also be admitted. Outpatient follow-up is otherwise indicated.

METABOLIC DISORDERS

ACID-BASE DISTURBANCES

1. Metabolic Acidosis:

In metabolic acidosis cases, the pH is less than 7.35. (Refer also to "Anion Gap Metabolic Acidosis" within the Toxicology section.)

1.1 Clinical Evaluation:

A. Elevated AG: A MUDPILE CAT. (Refer also to "Anion Gap Metabolic Acidosis" within the Toxicology section.)

B. Normal AG: Hypochloremic- RTA, diarrhea, pancreatic fistula, ileostomy, ureteroenterostomy, TPN, NH_4Cl, and drugs, such as acetazolamide, Sulfamylon, cholestyramine, and spironolactone, etc.

1.2 RX:

A. Support ABCs, IV, O_2, and monitor.

B. Start NaCl or LR, 20 cc/kg boluses as needed, to restore blood pressure, followed by a maintenance rate to obtain a 0.5-1.0 cc/kg/hr urine output.

C. Implement a specific therapy for a given metabolic derangement or toxic ingestion.

D. Consider bicarbonate therapy when the pH is lower than 7.2.

2. Metabolic Alkalosis:

In metabolic alkalosis cases, the pH is greater than 7.40.

2.1 Clinical Evaluation:

A. NaCl Responsive: Contraction alkalosis, vomiting, NG suction, villous adenoma, penicillin and carbenicillin (large doses), diuretics, and rapid correction of chronic hypercapnia.

B. NaCl Unresponsive: Mineralocorticoid excess in primary hyperaldosteronism, hyperreninism, licorice ingestion, Cushing's syndrome, Barter's syndrome, and adrenal hyperplasia.

2.2 RX:

A. For NaCl Nonresistant cases:

Support ABCs, IV, O_2, and monitor.

Start 0.9% NaCl, 20 cc/Kg boluses, to establish blood pressure and then adjust rate to maintain a 0.5-1.0 cc/kg/hour urine output.

Add 20-40 mEq/L of KCl to maintenance fluid with urine output.

Consider arginine monohydrochloride and ammonium chloride for severe cases.

B. For NaCl Resistant cases:

Support ABCs, IV, O_2, and monitor.

Start 20-40 mEq/L KCl infusion with urine output to reduce cellular H^+ and enhance HCO_3 excretion.

Infuse spironolactone, an aldosterone antagonist, and/or acetazolamide to enhance HCO_3 excretion.

Consult for dialysis as indicated for renal failure.

3. Respiratory Acidosis:

For cases of respiratory acidosis, the pH is less than 7.35 with elevated pCO_2 (acute) and HCO_3 (compensation) concentrations.

Acute: Expect increase HCO_3^- = $(CO_2)/10$.

Chronic: Expect increase HCO_3^- = (CO_2)x 4.0.

3.1 Clinical Evaluation:

Acute airway obstruction, lung disease, pleural effusions, PTX, thoracic cage abnormalities, hypoventilation, hypokalemia, hypophosphatemia, hypomagnesemia, and muscular dystrophy.

3.2 RX:

A. Support ABCs, IV, O_2, and monitor.
B. Improve alveolar ventilation and oxygenation by using bronchodilators, postural drainage, noninvasive, and invasive respiratory support and antibiotics when necessary.
C. Metabolic acidosis may be coincident resulting from anaerobic metabolism.
D. Cautiously adjust oxygen supplements and assisted ventilatory rates in chronic acidosis to avoid CO_2 retention narcosis and posthypercapneic metabolic alkalosis, respectively.

4. Respiratory Alkalosis:

In respiratory alkalosis cases, the pH is greater than 7.35 with decreased concentrations of pCO_2 (acute) and HCO_3 (compensation).

1Acute: Expect HCO_3^- decrease = (pCO_2 x 0.2 (a drop of HCO_3^- of 2 for every decrease CO_2 of 10).

2Chronic: Expect HCO_{3-} decrease = (pCO_2 x 0.5 (a drop of HCO_3^- of 5 for every decrease CO_2 of 10).

4.1 Clinical Evaluation:

Hyperventilation, anxiety, pain, cerebrovascular accident, head trauma, early sepsis, fevers, pulmonary embolism, congestive heart failure, pneumonia, interstitial lung disease, hepatic insufficiency, pregnancy, ASA toxicity, thyrotoxicosis, hypoxemia, and ventilation-induced.

4.2 RX:

Treat underlying problem.

ELECTROLYTE DISTURBANCES

1. Hyperkalemia:

Causes of Hyperkalemia include acidosis, tissue necrosis, hemolysis, blood transfusion, GI bleed, renal failure, pseudohyperkalemia (leukocytosis), thrombocytosis, spironolactone, triamterene, amiloride, excess po potassium, RTA, high dose penicillin, β-blockers, Captopril, lab error, and decreased mineralocorticoid activity, such as Addison's hypoaldosteronism.

1.1 Clinical Evaluation:

A. **Symptoms:** Weakness, paresthesias, confusion, and paralysis.
B. **Signs:** Arrhythmias. The ECG shows peaked T-waves, ST depression, diminished R-wave, prolonged PR interval, small P-wave, sine waves, cardiac ventricular fibrillation, asystole, and cardiac arrest.
C. **Work-Up:** Treat with electrolytes, glucose, and magnesium. Monitor with ECG.

1.2 RX:

A. Consider discontinuing medication that may cause hyperkalemia. Treat as follows:

Calcium chloride, 5 mL of 10% solution, 13.6 mEq/10 mL, or 10 mL of 10% calcium gluconate, 4.6 mEq/10 mL, given over 2 minutes via peripheral vein and repeated in 5-10 minutes if necessary. If digitalis toxicity is suspected, administer over 30 minutes or omit entirely.

$NaHCO_3$, 44-132 mEq, 1-3 amps of 7.5%, IV over 5 minutes, repeat in 10-15 minutes, followed by infusion of 2-3 amps in D_5W titrated over 2-4 hours. Administer after calcium by using a separate IV.

Insulin, 10-20 units regular in 500 mL of $D_{10}W$ IV over 1 hour or 10 units IV push with 1 amp 50% glucose, 25 g, over 5 minutes, and repeat as needed.

Kayexalate, 15-50 g in 100 mL of 20% sorbitol solution po immediately and in 3-4 hours, up to 4-5 doses per day, or Kayexalate retention enema, 20-50 g in 200 mL of 20% sorbitol, retained for 30-60 minutes.

Furosemide, 40-80 mg IV every day.

Albuterol, for acute hyperkalemia, 10-20 mg in 3 cc normal saline by nebulizer.

Consider emergent dialysis if cardiac complications arise or if the patient is in renal failure.

Correct acidosis or hypovolemia.

A patient being treated for severe hyperkalemia requires continuous cardiac monitoring, frequent serial exams, and serum electrolyte determinations q 2 hours until the patient is out of danger.

B. **Disposition:** Admission to the ICU is mandatory.

2. Hypernatremia:

Excess free H_2O loss from renal (DI, osmotic diuresis-hyperglycemia, and mannitol); GI, skin and respiratory origins.

Inadequate free H_2O intake arising form coma, reset osmotic regulator, and poor po intake.

Excess Na^+ gain from iatrogenic agents ($NaHCO_3$, hypertonic saline, and exogenous steroids), hyperaldosteronism, Cushing's, and congenital adrenal hyperplasia.

2.1 Clinical Evaluation:

A. **Symptoms:** Confusion, muscle irritability, and weakness.

B. **Signs:** Flat neck veins, orthostatic hypotension, tachycardia, poor skin turgor, dry mucous membranes, seizures, coma, and respiratory paralysis.

C. **Work-up:** Obtain hematocrit, SMA-7, serum protein, and urine osmolality. Urine sodium concentration is useful primarily outside of the ED.

2.2 RX:

A. If volume is depleted, administer 0.5-3 L NS IV at 500 mL/hour until patient is no longer dehydrated, followed by D_5W, if hyperosmolar, or D_5NS, if not hyperosmolar. Provide by IV or po to replace half of body water deficit over the first 24 hours, 1 mEq/L/hour, then treat remaining deficit over next 1-2 days. Maintain a urine output at 0.5 mL/kg/hour or greater.

B. If correction is too rapid, CNS edema and seizures may result.

C. Body water deficit (L) = (0.6 x (weight kg) x ([serum Na]- 140))/140

D. **Disposition:** Most patients require admission.

3. Hypokalemia:

Hypokalemia occurs when the concentration of K^+ is less than 3.5 mEq/L. It is the most common electrolyte abnormality. The causes of hypokalemia are redistribution arising from alkalosis, insulin, B_{12} therapy, β-2-agonist, periodic paralysis; renal losses caused by diuretics, low magnesium, Batter's, RTA, vomiting, and glucocorticoid/mineralocorticoid excess; and GI losses due to gastric, diarrhea, bile, and fistula; and finally lab error. **K^+ is very dangerous, avoid overzealous administration.**

3.1 Clinical Evaluation:

A. **Symptoms:** Weakness, paresthesia, polyuria, and paralysis.

B. **Signs:** Areflexia, rhabdomyolysis, orthostatic hypotension, ileus, metabolic alkalosis, glucose intolerance, and paralysis. ECG: T-wave flattening or inversion, U-wave prominence, ST segment depression, and PVC's.

C. **Work-up:** Order electrolytes, BUN, Cr, Ca, magnesium, U/A, and an ECG.

3.2 RX:

A If serum potassium is > 2.5 mEq/L and ECG changes are absent, treat with KCl, 20-30 mEq/hour IV with saline. May combine with 30-40 mEq po q 4 hours in addition to IV. Total maximum dose is generally 100-200 mEq/day or 3 mEq/kg/day.

B If potassium is < 2.5 mEq/L and ECG abnormalities are present, treat with KCl, IV 30-40 mEq/hour and up to 80 mEq/L. May combine with po 30-40 mEq q 4 hours. Maximum daily dose IV is 3 mEq/kg/day. Administer half over 24 hours. Use K-Phos if phosphate is low.

C **Disposition:** Admit hypokalemic patients with any of the following conditions to the ICU for continuous monitoring: Malignant cardiac dysrhythmias, digitalis toxicity, profound weakness with impending respiratory insufficiency, serum potassium concentration of < 2.0 mEq/L, and rhabdomyolysis or hepatic encephalopathy.

4. Hyponatremia:

Hypovolemic Hyponatremia arises from renal losses due to diuretic excess, mineralocorticoid deficiency, salt losing nephritis, and renal tubular acidosis with bicarbonate urea; and extra renal losses as a result of vomiting, diarrhea, burns, pancreatitis, and traumatized muscle.

Euvolemic Hyponatremia is caused by glucocorticoid deficiency, hypothyroidism, pain, emotion, drugs, and syndrome with inappropriate ADH secretion.

Hypervolemic Hyponatremia develops from euphoretic syndrome, cirrhosis, cardiac failure, and acute/chronic renal failure.

4.1 Clinical Evaluation:

A. **Symptoms:** Lethargy, apathy, disorientation, muscle cramps, anorexia, nausea, and agitation.

B. **Signs:** Abnormal sensorium, depressed DTRs, hypothermia, pseudobulbar palsy, seizures, and Cheyne-Stokes respiration.

C. **Work-up:** Order serum electrolytes, serum glucose, urine sodium, urine osmolality, BUN, and creatinine.

4.2 RX:

A. For hypervolemic hyponatremia:

Restrict water to 0.5-1.5 L/day.

Administer furosemide, 40-80 mg IV or po q day.

Consider concurrent diuresis and sodium replacement for severe symptomatic hyponatremia.

B. For isovolemic hyponatremia:

Start furosemide, 80 mg, 1 mg/kg, IV q day-bid, and 0.9% saline with 20-40 mEq KCl/L at 65-150 mL/hour. The correction rate is < 0.5 mEq/L/hour.

Restrict water to 500-1500 mL/day.

C. For hypovolemic hyponatremia:

If volume is depleted, administer 0.5-3 L of 0.9% saline at 500 cc/hour until the patient is no longer orthostatic, followed by 0.9% saline, 125 mEq/L, with 10-40 mEq of KCl/L at 65-150 cc/hour or 100 cc 3% of hypertonic saline over 5 hours.

NEUROLOGY

1. Change in Mental Status and Coma:

1.1 Clinical Evaluation:

A. **Symptoms:** Progressive confusion, disorientation, stupor, obtundation to coma, ± fevers, medical compliance, and depressed mood/suicidal ideation. Search for significant PMH, including immunosuppression, endocrinopathy, CNS pathology, drug abuse, and trauma.

B. **Signs:**

Alcohol on breath: Alcohol intoxication, consider subdural hematoma.
Young, healthy patient: Consider an overdose.
Jaundice: Hepatic failure.
Petechial hemorrhage: ITP, DIC, leukemia, meningitis, and hepatic/renal failure.
Fecal/urine incontinence: Cerebrovascular accident and seizures that are not related to alcohol withdrawals.
Barrel chest/emphysematous, pursed lip breathing: Respiratory failure.
Healthy patients with pulmonary edema on CXR: Heroin, cocaine, or salicylate overdose.
Diaphoretic, cold, or hypothermic: Consider hypoglycemia, hypothermia, adrenal crisis, and sepsis.
Tachypnea: Respiratory failure and acidosis (respiratory, endocrine, or A MUDPILE CAT).
Meningismus, Kernig's/Brudzinski's: Meningitis, sepsis, and subarachnoid hemorrhage.
Rhinorrhea, otorrhea, Battle's sign, raccoon's eyes: Basilar skull fracture.
Needle tracks: IV drug abuser/overdose.
Tongue laceration: Seizure.
Broken bones with petechiae, respiratory distress: Consider fat emboli.

C. **DDX:**

Trauma (hypovolemia and head injury) and temperature.
Infection and intussusception.
Psychiatric: Space occupying lesions (cerebrovascular accident, SAH, and shock).
Alcohol: Endocrinopathy, exocrine, liver failure, and electrolytes.
Insulin: Oxygen.
Overdose: Uremia and hypertensive crisis. (A mnemonic is TIPS/AEIOU.)

D. **Work-up:** Perform an in-line c-spine immobilization for suspected trauma. Order CBC, SMA-7, calcium, magnesium, and serum toxicology screen. Consider urine toxicology, i.e., phencyclidine and lysergic acid, and an ECG. Obtain a rectal temperature, blood, urine and CSF culture prn, CXR, c-spines, and a head CT prn. Consider a laboratory evaluation for preeclampsia/eclampsia in the patient > 20 weeks pregnant with a change in mental status.

1.2 RX:

A. Support ABCs, IV, O_2, and monitor.
B. D-stick, D_{50}, 1-2 amps for adults. For Children < 8 years give D_{25} , 0.5-1.0 g/kg. For neonate give D_{10} , 0.5-1.0 mg/kg. Thiamine, 100 mg IV, and Narcan, 0.01-0.2 mg/kg.
C. Perform a gastric lavage with activated charcoal, 1.0 g/kg po q 6-8 hours.
D. Provide specific antidotes to toxic drug levels found in screen or based on clinical toxidrome.
E. Consider triple antibiotics, such as ampicillin, gentamicin, or ceftr/Flagyl for suspected sepsis/meningitis.
F. Obtain a trauma/neurosurgeon consultation for a suspected thoraco-abdomen or a closed head trauma.
G. Consider benzodiazepines, Dilantin, or phenobarbital for seizures.
H. **Disposition:** Admit patients with suspected prolonged detoxification, infection, trauma, intractable, or those seizing for the first time.

2. Acute Transverse Myelitis:

Acute transverse myelitis is an inflammation of a segment of the spinal cord, usually thoracic, resulting in loss of function inferior to the lesion.

2.1 Clinical Evaluation:

A. **History/Signs:** Radicular or back pain is followed by bilateral feet paresthesias. These signs are succeeded by ascending sensory loss and weakness. The time from onset to paralysis is a few days to 12 days.

B. **DDX:** MS, acute epidural abscess, spinal mass, and ICH.

C. **Work-up:** Perform an LP looking for elevated protein and xanthochromia. Obtain appropriate tests to rule out differential diagnosis items.

2.2 RX:

A. Support ABCs, IV, O_2, and monitor.

B. **Disposition:** Admit.

3. Amyotrophic Lateral Sclerosis:

A progressive, fatal disease of unknown etiology marked by the destruction of motor cells in the anterior gray horns of the spinal cord and degeneration of pyramidal tracts. Rare sensory changes are also exhibited.

3.1 Clinical Evaluation:

A. **Symptoms:** Weakness, atrophy, and initial muscle fasciculations of hands and arms are followed by spastic paralysis of limbs.

B. **Signs:** Consistent with the progression cited above.

C. **DDX:** Cervical spondylosis, plasma cell dyscrasias, lead intoxication, spinal muscular atrophy, primary lateral sclerosis, spinal multiple sclerosis, and tropical spastic paraparesis.

D. **Work-up:** Perform an electromyography and a muscle biopsy.

3.2 RX:

A. Support ABCs, IV, O_2, and monitor.

B. Treat for complications of immobility, such as pneumonia, urosepsis, and respiratory problems.

C. **Disposition:** Admit.

4. Cerebrovascular Accident:

Cerebral ischemia/infarction is caused by an occlusive syndrome from the thrombus, the emboli (ulcerated arterial plaques, cardiac mural thrombi, endocarditis, fat emboli of fractures, dysbaric injury), or from a hemorrhage (aneurysm, AV malformation, HTN, blood dyscrasia, neoplasm, infection, and anticoagulants).

4.1 Clinical Evaluation:

A. **Symptoms:** Associated risks of HTN, atherosclerosis, coronary artery disease, diabetes, hypercholesterolemia, smoking, and gout. Many have TIAs- 70% of the patients with such episodes proceed to cerebrovascular accident within 2 years. Symptoms of TIA or cerebrovascular accident are sudden. Clinical improvement over hours is the rule with TIAs, ± incomplete improvement over weeks to months with embolic/thrombotic CVAs, and little improvement with hemorrhagic stroke.

B. **Signs:** Vessel bruit suggests > 70% stenosis. Presence is associated with high risk embolism. However, absence does **not** rule out ulcerated plaque. Exam findings are coincident with vascular/parenchymal distribution affected. Occlusive syndromes include the following:

Middle cerebral artery: Contralateral hemiplegia where the upper extremity weakness > lower extremity, hemianesthesia and homonymous hemianopsia. Contralateral conjugate gaze is affected. Aphasia with dominant hemispheric involvement is displayed.

Anterior cerebral artery: Contralateral extremity weakness, lower > upper, gait apraxia, abulia, and incontinence.
Posterior cerebral artery: Contralateral homonymous hemianopsia, hemiparesis, hemisensory, ipsilateral CN III, and memory loss.
Vertebrobasilar artery: Ipsilateral CN, cerebellar ataxia, contralateral hemiplegia, and hemisensory loss. N/V, nystagmus, vertigo, and tinnitus/hearing loss.
Basilar artery: Quadriplegia, upward gaze/"locked-in" syndrome.
Cerebellar: Ataxia, especially with vermis infarct, vertigo, tinnitus, N/V, and nystagmus.
Lacunar: Lipohyalinotic, cystic infarcts off penetrating cerebral arterioles within internal capsule. Specific syndromes include midpons- dysarthria/clumsy hand, pons/internal capsule- ataxia, leg paresis or pure motor hemiplegia, and thalamus- pure sensory syndrome.
Transient global amnesia: Amygdaloid/hippocampus infarcts, commonly in patients > 60 years, that last minutes to hours with complete resolution. Patient's somatic/speech, cognition and long-term memory are intact during and after an episode, but the patient has no knowledge of event. Hemorrhagic events include subarachnoid and intracerebral. (Refer also the "Intracranial Hemorrhage" section.)
Other intracranial hemorrhages include: Pontine- pinpoint pupils, decerebration, and coma. Thalamic- contralateral hemiparesis, hemianesthesia, and dysconjugate gaze. Putamen- similar to middle cerebral artery syndrome but with much depressed level of consciousness. Cerebellar- ataxia, dizziness, and nausea/vomiting.

C. **DDX:** Trauma- concussion, epidural/subdural hematoma, cerebral contusion (coup/contrecoup), neoplasm, infection, abscess, metabolic abnormalities (ex: hyponatremia), and toxidromes (ex: narcotics, phenothiazines, cyclic antidepressants, cholinesterase inhibitors/pesticides, and pilocarpine), postictal.
D. **Work-up:** Order CBC, oximetry or ABG, CBC, SMA-7, calcium, magnesium, ammonia, culture of blood, urine, ± CSF (negative head CT) for fever, a head CT and c-spines for clinical suspicion. Consider noninvasive cervical vascular Doppler to search for plaques.

4.2 RX:

A. Support airway, IV, O_2, and monitor.
B. Provide ICP management.
C. Consider heparinization for patients with history and clinical evidence of TIA. Heparinization should also be considered for patients with smaller infarcts due to embolization, normal mental status and little deficit; precise decision point for treatment is controversial so consider early consultation.
D. Consider antihypertensive therapy and control of intracranial pressure. (Refer to "Intracranial Hemorrhage").
E. Obtain a neurology/neurosurgery consultation for possible angiography and/or surgical intervention. Also consult for possible use of thrombolytic agents.
F. If you decide on thrombolytic therapy obtain a neurology consult, perform an NIH stroke scale, review inclusion and exclusion criteria, and obtain consent. The drug of choice is t-PA 0.9 mg/kg (max dose of 90 mg), 10% as a bolus dose, and the remainder given over 60 minutes.
G. **Disposition:** Admit.

5. Headache:

Brain parenchyma, dura, pia and arachnoid have no pain fibers. Headaches are due to tension, inflammation, and swelling of pain sensitive tissues, such as skin, muscle, sinuses, vessels, and somatic/visceral nerves. Headache types include the following.

A. **Vascular:**

Migraines are induced by environmental changes, emotional stress, sleep deprivation, hunger, and thirst, which leads to arterial vasoconstriction. Hypoxia is a result of a parenchymal distribution that develops into a specific aura. Examples are: 1) MCA- contralateral hemiparesis, and hemisensory changes, and 2) Vertebrobasilar- scotoma, ataxia, N/V, LOC. Occipital cortex- scintillations, uni/bilateral scotoma, and field cuts. Eventually vasodilation and reperfusion occur which thereby cause the release of pain mediators, such as histamine,

serotonin, prostaglandins, and SRSA. A severe throbbing pain is produced that is initially localized but may become global with associated ocular pain, nausea, and vomiting.
Subtypes of migraines include ophthalmoplegic, unilateral frontal HA associated with ipsilateral CN III palsy, ± CN IV, and CN VI loss. Hemiplegic focal/global pain is associated with unilateral weakness, and sensory loss. Such deficits may persist even after resolution of pain. Although these subtypes are exhibited most commonly in young adults, an intracranial pathology must be ruled out, such as aneurysms, tumors, emboli- TIA, and cerebrovascular accidents. Typical patients are young females in their 30s who complain of progressively painful unilateral to global HA associated with photophobia, and N/V are common. Correlation with menses and family history.
Cluster headaches are accompanied by the sudden onset, severe, burning, boring pain on one side of face. Other symptoms include ipsilateral rhinorrhea, congestion, and ± ipsilateral Horner's syndrome. The afflicted patient is typically a young adult in his/her 30s.
A subarachnoid hemorrhage occurs from bleeding originating from a leaking berry/saccular aneurysm or a AV malformation. It is also commonly associated with a trauma. The associated pain is usually sudden, like a "thunder-clap", and global because blood tracks underneath the arachnoid surrounding the cerebrum causing pressure and inflammation.

B. **Vasculitis** (temporal/cranial arteritis): Granulomatous inflammatory changes involving carotid branches. The patient is usually female, > 40, with complaints of unilateral HA, facial pain, ± jaw/tongue pain, and unilateral eye pain ± vision changes. The exam may a reveal a tender, pulseless temporal artery. Symptoms worsen with arterial compression. If a temporal artery is involved, there is a very high risk that a retinal artery is also involved which may lead to blindness. Do not misdiagnose this as a migraine! ESR is usually > 50.

C. **Tension:** Muscular strain, spasm from repetitive head motion or prolonged positioning. This headache is associated with "stress". Pain may extend globally, similar to a halo around the head, and extend down into the neck, shoulders, and back.

D. **Intraparenchymal mass** (tumor, abscess): HA is insidious in the onset but progressively worsens. The pain is dull, throbbing and is usually unilateral. It is most severe upon awakening. Associated symptoms may include n/v, ataxia, visual changes, LOC, tinnitus/hearing loss, uni/bilateral CN, and distal somatic findings based on lesion location.

E. **Ocular:** Local, global pain, ± vision changes, retinal changes, hyphema, periorbital/conjunctival swelling, erythema, and discharge. Etiologies include trauma, iritis, infection, glaucoma, and corneal abrasion. (Refer to the "HEAD & NECK" section).

5.1 Clinical Evaluation:

A. **DDX:** Refer to the above. Consider also meningitis, encephalitis, subdural/epidural hematoma, skull fracture, sinusitis, tooth abscess, TMJ syndrome, otitis media, external otitis, parotitis, and high altitude sickness.

B. **Work-up:** Customize evaluation for each presentation and include your index of suspicion fro a dangerous cause. Consider CBC, SMA-7, calcium, magnesium, ESR, septic workup for fever. Also, consider head CT, MRI and noninvasive vascular Doppler evaluation.

5.2 RX:

A. **Treat the different stages of Migraines as follows:**

Aural stage: Ergotamines po/PR/inhaler- Cafergot, 1-2 mg po ASAP, maximum of 5 mg/attack, 10 mg/week and 1 suppository ASAP and in 1 hour prn, **or** NSAIDS- especially naproxen, 500-1000 mg po ASAP, repeat in 12 hours prn, **or** Midrin 2 capsules po ASAP, followed by 1 po q hour to maximum 5/day or 10/week, **or** sumatriptan (Imitrex) 6 mg sc, may repeat in 1 hour.

Acute stage: Metoclopramide, 10 mg po/IM/IV, **or** chlorpromazine, 0.1 mg/kg IV q 15 minutes **or** 25 mg IM single dose, **or** dihydroergotamine, 0.5-1.0 mg IV ± chlorpromazine, **or** meperidine, 25-50 mg IM with hydroxyzine, 25 mg po/IM, **or** methylprednisolone, 60-120 mg IV, **or** sumatriptan (Imitrex) 6 mg sc, may repeat in 1 hour. Consider ketorolac, 60 mg IM (contraindication late in pregnancy, history of PUDz).

Prevention: Avoid alcohol, caffeine, chocolate, OCPs, tyramines, and stress. Consider verapamil, 80 mg po tid/qid, or amitriptyline, 50-75 mg po q day, or Phenytoin, 200-400 mg po q day, or ergotamine, 1 mg po bid, no more than 10 tabs/week.

B. **Treat Clusters as follows:**
Oxygen, 7-15 L/minute. Ergotamines po/PR/IV. (Refer also to the "Migraine" section). Consider trying intranasal viscous lidocaine.
Prevention: Avoid alcohol, nitrates, and histamines. Consider verapamil, 80 mg po tid/qid, or amitriptyline, 50-75 mg po q day, or lithium carbonate, 300 mg po tid.

C. **Arteritis:** Treat with prednisone, 80-120 mg po q day with 2 week taper. Prescribe NSAIDS for pain relief.

D. **Subarachnoid hemorrhage:** Refer to the relevant section shown above.

E. **Tension:** Prescribe NSAIDS, massage, and stress management.

F. **Ocular:** Refer to the "ENT" section.

G. **Space-occupying lesion:** Support airway, IV, O_2, and monitor. Implement seizure prophylactic measures, BP management, and ± ICP monitoring.

H. **Disposition**: Admit the patient for a work-up if there is concern of intracranial pathology or if there is no clinical improvement from ED intervention. If the patient is to be discharged, arrange an appropriate follow-up. Provide strict instructions to return for progressive symptoms.

6. Intracranial Hemorrhage (ICH):

Intracranial Hemorrhage may occur with trauma, such as in subdural and epidural hematomas, or may occur spontaneously. Spontaneous ICH is the cause of about 10% of all cerebrovascular accidents. Hypertensive Hemorrhage is most commonly caused from small penetrating arteries located within the MCA and within the basal ganglia. Subarachnoid hemorrhage is typically associated with a ruptured aneurysm. AV malformations are the sources of some of these aneurysms. A one month mortality rate is 50%. (Refer also to the "Cerebrovascular Accident" section presented above as well as the "Subdural" and "Epidural Hematomas" sections described within the Trauma chapter).

6.1 Clinical Evaluation:

A. **Symptoms:** Trauma, HTN, previous known history of aneurysm or AVM, inducing stress. Sudden onset of worst HA of life or previous "sentinel" HAs suggest SAH. Obtain a history of antithrombotic or thrombolytic meds, and cocaine use.

B. **Signs:** ABC, neuro exam evaluating for focal deficits, change in mental status, and frequent or continuous reassessment. Check gag. BP often is very high. Cheyne-Stokes respirations with elevated ICP may occur with pinpoint pupils and a pontine hemorrhage.

Grading scale for SAH:

Grade I: Change in mental status, focal deficit, mild HA, and meningismus.
Grade II: Mild change in mental status, some focal deficit, severe HA, and meningismus.
Grade III: Major change in mental status or major focal deficit.
Grade IV: Semicomatose or comatose.

C. **DDX:** Non-hemorrhagic cerebrovascular accident, change in mental status, recurrence of symptoms of previous cerebrovascular accident brought about by another new insult, including infection, metabolic abnormality, meningitis, encephalitis, metabolic derangement, brain tumor, or abscess.

D. **Work-up:** Order non-contrast brain CT, pulse oximetry or ABG, CBC, SMA-7, PT, PTT, and CXR. Obtain a neurosurgical consultation for angiography and possible surgery.

6.2 RX:

A. Support airway, including ICP management, IV, O_2, and monitor. Consider arterial BP monitoring.

B. BP management: Titrate to S/D BP 160-200/100-110 (don't overdo it, patients with baseline HTN and cerebral edema need perfusion pressure). Administer nitroprusside, 0.5 μg/kg/minute up to 10 μ/kg/minute, **or** hydralazine, 10-20 mg IV q 30 minutes, **or** Labetalol, 20 mg IV q 10 minutes up to 300 mg.

C. For evidence of elevated ICP or impending herniation, RSI for intubation with care of ICP.

D. Hyperventilate with goal of a pCO_2 of 25-30 mm Hg, elevate HOB to 30 degrees, and consider mannitol, 1 g/kg.
E. Manage seizure. Consider possible prophylaxis with phenytoin load of 15-20 mg/kg IV at a maximum rate of 50 mg/minute.
F. SAH: Consider nimodipine for grade I & II to decrease possible incidence of vasospasm and other calcium-channel mediated benefits. Obtain a neurosurgical consultation.
G. **Disposition:** Admit to ICU unless the patient is clearly stable.

7. Landry-Guillain-Barré:

An acute idiopathic polyneuritis characterized by progressive motor weakness usually starting distally in the legs and occasionally in arms. The motor weakness ascends to involve trunk, upper extremities, and cranial and respiratory muscles. Onset occurs over several days and recovery may require months.

7.1 Clinical Evaluation:

A. **Symptoms:** Progressive motor weakness, some sensory loss, and autonomic disturbance.
B. **Signs:** Decreased or absent DTRs, weakness as above, examine for a tick.
C. **DDX:** Tick paralysis, poliomyelitis, hypokalemia, periodic paralysis, acute transverse myelitis, radiculopathies, myopathy includes polymyositis, neurotoxins include botulism, tetanus, and diphtheria.
D. Myasthenia gravis: Usually presents with bulbar involvement.
E. Botulism: Usually presents with bulbar involvement; respiratory compromise follows as paralysis descends.
F. Polymyositis: Affects proximal muscles more, tender muscles, and elevated CK.
G. Polymyalgia rheumatica: Proximal muscle pain without weakness.
H. **Work-up:** Perform acute evaluation only in the ED. Consider obtaining CBC, SMA-7, calcium, magnesium, and appropriate imaging. The work-up may include LP. A few cells with elevated protein may be found from days to weeks into the disease course. Nerve conduction studies and other evaluation of respiratory function are inpatient concerns.

7.2 RX:

A. Support ABCs, IV, O_2, and monitor.
B. Plasmapheresis inpatient.
C. **Disposition:** Admit for further neurological evaluation and treatment. Consider outpatient management only for a patient who is currently safe, reliable, and has transportation to return to the ED if the condition worsens. Obtain a consultation with the primary physician or a neurologist before discharging the patient.

8. Myasthenia Gravis:

Condition involves the autoimmune acetylcholine receptor destruction and poor neurotransmission resulting in weakness. There are two types of myasthenic crises as described below.

Myasthenic: Usually occurs in a undiagnosed patient with severe weakness resulting from a functional lack of acetylcholine. Administer edrophonium (Tensilon), 2 mg IV, followed by 8 mg IV slow, will improve symptoms.

Cholinergic: Displayed in patients undergoing treatment for myasthenia with excess acetylcholine esterase (anticholinesterase). Severe muscle weakness occurs. Edrophonium increases symptoms! Examine for muscarinic symptom-SLUDGE. Administer atropine, 1 mg IV and prn, for bradycardia, low BP, wheezing/rales, or SLUDGE.

Myasthenia gravis classifications include the following.

Localized: Non-progressive, and limited to ocular weakness (diplopia and ptosis.) The prognosis is good.

Generalized: Both cranial and skeletal muscle weakness without sensory loss. The prognosis is also good.
Acute Onset: Systemic involvement with poor response to therapy. The prognosis is poor.
Gradual Progression: Onset of symptoms appear over several years. The prognosis is poor.
Generalized Disease: Muscle atrophy beginning several months post onset. Variable prognosis.

8.1 Clinical Evaluation:

A. **Symptoms:** Complaints of muscle weakness, worsened by prolonged activity, and improved with rest. Most common symptoms begin with ocular ptosis, diplopia, and blurred vision.
B. **Signs:** Ocular weakness- ptosis, extraocular weakness, diplopia, blurriness, and facial, oral and distal extremity weakness with depressed DTRs. Examine for respiratory difficulty.
C. **DDX:** Eaton-Lambert Syndrome (symptoms improve with repetitive exercise!), botulism, Guillain Barre, tick paralysis, familial periodic paralysis (seen with normal, high or low K^+), chronic fatigue syndrome, oculopharyngeal dystrophy, polymyositis, MS, and sleep paralysis.
D. **Work-up:** Typically occurs outside ED; "double blind" Tensilon test- increases acetylcholine and improves symptoms. Electromyogram is a gold standard. Determine ± serologies for acetylcholine receptors.

8.2 RX:

A. Treat with edrophonium, 2 mg IV then 8 mg IV slow. Clinical improvement, myasthenic crisis. If symptoms worsen, consider cholinergic crisis.
B. **Disposition:** Admit.

9. Seizures:

Primary epilepsy, idiopathic, onset occurs before the age of 20. Secondary epilepsy, symptomatic, is caused by parenchymal abnormality, including aneurysm, AVM, tumor cyst, abscess, contusion, hematoma, or an old scar. Status epilepticus describes seizures persisting longer than 20 minutes **or** repetitive events without lucid intervals. Untreated status is associated with a 20% mortality rate.

9.1 Clinical Evaluation:

A. **Symptoms:**

Generalized/grand mal: Witnessed LOC with generalized activity.
Minor/petit mal(absence): Prolonged unresponsive staring without LOC, +/- focal muscular activity.
Focal: Repetitive motor activity without LOC.
Temporal lobe: Hallucinations (visual, auditory, and olfactory), memory loss, and/or bizarre behavior which may progress to focal-generalized motor activity.
Todd's paralysis: Focal weakness/paralysis after seizure lasting up to several days.
Febrile: Generalized activity associated with rapidly rising fever, continuing for several minutes. Exhibited in the 3 months to the 5 years age group. There is no increased risk for permanent seizure disorder, mental retardation, cerebral palsy, or death.
Infantile spasm: Myoclonic jerking and spasm, especially flexion/extension of neck or back. Displayed by 3-9 month olds. Associated with severe mental retardation.

B. **Signs:** ABCs. Examine for trauma, including head/facial abrasions, contusions, lacs, tongue, buccal lacs, neck deformity, and urine/stool incontinence. Is patient seizing? Is patient awake? Look for eye deviation and focal/generalized tonic/clonic activity.
C. **DDX:** Drug intoxication/withdrawal, hypoglycemia, hyper/hyponatremia, hypocalcemia, pyridoxine deficiency, infection, breath-holding spells, TIA/cerebrovascular accident, syncope, cataplexy, narcolepsy, myoclonia, and pseudo-seizures, i.e., watch for purposeful movement during episode.
D. **Work-up:** Initiate O_2 saturation and Dexi-stick stat. Order CBC and SMA-7. Consider calcium, magnesium, toxicology screen (serum/urine), serum osm., anticonvulsant levels, serum, urine and csf culture for fever. Obtain CXR to rule out aspiration, head CT/MRI, and EEG. Eliminate the possibility of trauma as the etiology or an episode prn by obtaining an X-ray/CT evaluation, etc.

9.2 RX:

A. **Adults:** Support airway, IV, O_2, and monitor. Dexi-stick or start D_{50}, Narcan, 2-4 mg, and thiamine, 100 mg IV. For pregnant patients, begin $MgSO_4$, 4-6 g load, followed by 1-2 g/hour IV. Consider pyridoxine, 5 g of a 5-10% solution IV, for suspected INH toxicity. Prescribe diazepam, 5 mg/minute IV q 5 minutes to 30 mg, **or** lorazepam, 0.1 mg/kg IV, to suppress activity. If there is no response, start phenytoin, 15-20 mg IV load at 50 mg/minute, **or** after benzo suppression. Consider phenobarbital, 15-20 mg/kg IV at 50 mg/minute, repeated twice for seizures that are unresponsive to benzos **or** Dilantin. For status epilepticus unresponsive even to phenobarbital, consider Lidocaine, 2-4 mg/minute IV, **or** a Valium drip, 1 mg/kg/hour IV, **or** pentobarbital drip, 5 mg/kg load with 1-3 mg/hour IV, **or** a generalized anesthesia, including halothane.

B. **Peds:** Support airway, IV, O_2, and monitor. Dexi-stick **or** start D_{25}, 2-4 cc/kg, and Narcan, 0.01-0.1 mg/kg IV. For neonates, administer pyridoxine, 50-100 mg, slow infusion, and calcium gluconate, 4 cc/kg IV. Prescribe diazepam, 0.2-0.3 mg/kg IV at 1 mg/minute to 10 mg maximum. Consider phenobarbital, 15-20 mg/kg IV at 25 mg/minute if there is no response or after benzo suppression. Consider phenytoin, 15-20 mg/kg IV at 50 mg/minutes, for seizures unresponsive to phenobarbital infusion.

Pearls of phenytoin: Contraindicated in second to third degree heart block.

Infuse Dilantin, no faster than 50 mg/minute, to reduce risk of hypotension and heart block.

Prescribe Isoniazid, chloramphenicol to raise serum phenytoin levels. Lower phenobarbital and alcohol levels.

Phenytoin toxicity, levels > 20 μg/m, is associated with following symptoms. 1) Nausea/vomiting and lateral nystagmus, > 20 μg/mL, 2) lateral, vertical nystagmus, and ataxia, > 30 μg/mL, 3) lethargy, dysarthria, confusion, and seizures, > 40 μg/mL, and 4) Bradycardia, heart block, idioventricular rhythm, and asystole, > 70 μg/mL

C. **Disposition:** Admit all status epilepticus patients. Discharge individuals with first-time seizures, negative primary work-up, and no additional activity during 6 hours of observation. Ensure that these patients obtain a neurology follow-up in 24-48 hours after being discharged. Provide instructions to return for any aura or activity. Discharge patients with known seizure disorders not related to drug intoxication or withdrawal pending therapeutic anticonvulsant levels. Observe patients with a question of drug intoxication/withdrawal as etiology for seizures for a minimum of 6 hours. There are no data currently available that supports a shorter length of stay.

Inclusion criteria for rt-PA Administration:

- Ischemic stroke.
- Patient presentation within 3 hours of symptom onset (some studies show a benefit within 6 hours of symptom onset).
- Clearly define time of symptom onset.
- CT scan negative for hemorrhage.

Exclusion criteria:

- Substantial edema, mass effect or midline shift on CT scan.
- Intracranial surgery in past 3 months.
- Intracranial neoplasm.
- AV malformation or aneurysm.
- Uncontrolled hypertension >190 mm Hg systolic and > 100 mm Hg diastolic.
- Subarachnoïd hemorrhage or hx of ICH.
- Major surgery in the past 2 weeks.
- Platelet count <75,000.
- GI bleed in the past 3 weeks.
- Known bleeding diathesis and prolonged PT and PTT.
- Heparin use within the last 48 hours.

Administer: rt-PA 0.9 mg/kh, 10% as a bolus with the remainder given over 60 minutes (maximum dose of 90 mg).

OBSTETRICS

1. Ectopic Pregnancy:

Ectopic pregnancy is the implantation of a fertilized ovum outside the endometrium. This implantation typically occurs in the lateral two thirds of the Fallopian tube. The fertilized ovum can also implant in an ovary or the abdominal cavity. The risk factors associated with ectopic pregnancies include tubal abnormalities, scarring from PID, tubal ligation, IUDs, recent abortion (< 2 weeks), and future ectopic pregnancies.

1.1 Clinical Evaluation:

A. **Symptoms:** Amenorrhea, abdominal pain, followed by vaginal bleeding. Positive pregnancy test commonly occurs 2-4 weeks after last menstrual cycle.

B. **Signs:** Diffuse or localized abdominal pain, and pallor. Shoulder pain can be present from diaphragmatic irritation. Pelvic tenderness is displayed. Hemorrhagic shock can be exhibited if a rupture occurs.

C. **DDX:** PID, threatened abortion, corpus luteal cyst, and dysfunctional uterine bleeding.

D. **Work-up:** Order quantitative βHCG, serial values, q 48 hours, may 'plateau', non-exponential rise in value. Consider CBC, T&C, U/A, and a pregnancy test. Perform a pelvic US. Consider culdocentesis if US is not available. Aspiration of non-clotting blood with hematocrit > 15% represents a positive finding. A clear tap is negative. A dry tap is non-diagnostic.

1.2 RX:

A. For shock, start IV, O_2, and place on monitor. For Trendelenburg, consider blood transfusion and a STAT referral for laparotomy.

B. Discharge reliable patients with serial quantitative βHCGs and who are within the time range of 2-5 weeks in which a pregnancy test may be positive but a US does not yet indicate an IUP. If βHCG decreases, perform a D&C and evaluate products of uterine extraction for chorionic villi. If there is no villi, perform a laparoscopy to locate ectopic. If serial βHCGs plateau or do not increase exponentially, consider laparoscopy.

C. **Disposition:** Admit patients for positive culdocentesis, shock, unreliable follow up, or when there is no intrauterine pregnancy with a βHCG above 6000.

2. Emergency Delivery:

2.1 Clinical Evaluation:

A. **Symptoms:** True labor: Regular uterine contractions with increasing intensity and decreasing intervals. First stage results in cervical dilation and effacement. It continues for 6-8 hours in the multiparous patient and for 8-12 hours in the primiparous patient. The second stage of labor begins with complete cervical dilation and ends with the delivery of the infant. This stage lasts for several minutes to 2 hours. Pain in uterine fundus radiates over the uterus into the lower back. "Bloody show" consists of a bloody mucous discharge representing expulsion of the cervical mucus plug and indicates ongoing labor. Spontaneous rupture of membranes also verifies active labor.

B. **Signs:** If vaginal bleeding, not just a "bloody show", is present, avoid a pelvic exam but perform an ultrasound to assess for placenta previa. Otherwise, perform a sterile speculum exam to confirm ruptured membranes by inspecting vaginal secretions for ferning and for turning Nitrazine paper blue. Check the fetal heart tones with Doppler. Expect FHT 120-160 with variation. Monitor continuously, if available, or q 15 minutes in stage 1, q 5 minutes in stage 2, and for 30 seconds after contractions. If prolonged bradycardia or tachycardia occurs after contractions, fetal distress is present. Determine position, presentation (portion of fetus in birth canal), lie (longitudinal vs. transverse) of fetus and stage of labor. Check for cord prolapse, cervical effacement, cervical dilation (10 cm is complete) and station (relationship of fetal part to ischial spines). A delivery in the second stage presents as crowning, pressure on rectum with urge to defecate, and an uncontrolled bearing down movements of mother.

2.2 RX:

A. For a premature delivery, consider transferring the patient to an institution with Obstetrics and Neonatal facilities.
B. For fetal distress, position mother on left side. Start IV, O_2, and place the patient on a monitor. Arrange for immediate delivery.
C. For cord prolapse, exert manual pressure through vagina to lift presenting part away from cord. Place patient in knee-chest or deep Trendelenburg position. Use tocolytic agents to stop labor, such as magnesium sulfate, 4-6 g IV, **or** terbutaline, 0.25 sq, **or** ritodrine, 0.1 mg/minute IV.
D. Above all, don't drop the baby!
E. Position mother on stretcher with thighs abducted, knees flexed and feet on stretcher with buttocks raised on bed pan. If time permits, cleanse and drape perineum. Control delivery of head with one hand on the occipital area and one hand supporting the mother's perineum. The baby's chin can be lifted from posterior position. After delivering the baby's head, suction oral cavity with bulb syringe. If cord is wrapped around the baby's neck, loosen and slip over head or cut. The head will rotate to one side and then the shoulders are delivered next. Grasp head and exert gentle pressure downward until anterior shoulder appears beneath the pubic symphysis. Lift head upward to aid posterior shoulder delivery. If shoulders are impacted perform episiotomy, anesthetize area with lidocaine and cut from perineum avoiding the anal sphincter. After shoulders are delivered, support head with one hand and prepare to catch body and legs with other hand.
F. Hold the baby horizontal to introitus and suction mouth and nose. Cut umbilical cord after clamping twice. Send cord blood for infant serology and Rh. Place a sterile cord clamp or tie around cord 1-3 cm distal to navel. Place neonate on warm blankets in heated isolette. Take 1 and 5 minute Apgar scores.
G. Apply pressure above pubic symphysis and minimal traction on cord to deliver placenta. A placental delivery is recognized by a sudden gush of blood and by an umbilical cord protrusion. Excessive traction results in uterine inversion. Check placenta for completeness. Gently massage the uterus and administer oxytocin, 20 units to IV bag. Inspect and repair lacerations of cervix or vagina with a 3.0 chromic catgut. Repair episiotomy.
H. For birth with thick meconium, intubate baby and suction under direct laryngoscopy.

3. First Trimester Hemorrhage:

First trimester bleeding can result from an ectopic pregnancy, a normal pregnancy, or an abortion. Spontaneous abortion (AB) is common. An abortion can be idiopathic or it can be caused by drugs, infection, radiation, or chromosomal defects. AB is defined as the termination of pregnancy before 20 weeks when the fetus is < 500 g. Normal pregnancies can also exhibit implantation bleeding.

3.1 Clinical Evaluation:

A. **Symptoms:** Refer to the above discussion.
B. **Signs:**

Threatened AB: os closed, mild cramping and bleeding, no passage of fetal tissue, viable fetus. Twenty percent abort.
Inevitable AB: os dilated and effaced, cramps and moderate bleeding.
Complete AB: Uterine contents expelled, cervix closed, and slight cramping or bleeding.
Incomplete AB: Clots and tissue in cervical os, os open, cramps and bleeding are severe.
Missed AB: Uterus fails to expel fetus for 2 months, os closed, fetal heart tones are absent, and pregnancy test is negative.

C. **DDX:** Carcinoma, polyps, cervicitis, and molar pregnancy.
D. **Work-up:** Check for fetal heart tones with Doppler, and US pelvis prn. Send products of conception to lab. Order CBC, quantitative βHCG, type and screen, and SMA-7.

3.2 RX:

A. Start IV, O_2, and monitor. Position mother on left side. For a threatened AB, discharge the patient if she is stable and there is no vaginal bleeding. Instruct her to avoid strenuous activity for 1 day and to return to the ED if fever, increased bleeding, or abdominal pain occur.

B. For incomplete or inevitable AB, consider D&C or IV Pitocin, 20 units in 1 L of NS.

C. For Rh negative, administer 50 Mg Rh immunoglobulin.

D. **Disposition:** Discharge a patient with missed abortion. However, ensure that a close follow up is arranged because most will abort spontaneously. Admit patients who are hemodynamically unstable or diagnosed as an incomplete AB for Ob/Gyn management and usually a D&C. Also admit patients with serious conditions, such as missed AB with coagulopathy, an ectopic pregnancy, a threatened AB with continued pain, and cramps/bleeding.

4. Gestational Hypertension:

Gestational hypertension is a blood pressure of 140/90 in the second half of pregnancy. Blood pressure returns to normal after delivery with no signs of proteinuria or edema. Preeclampsia is hypertension > 140/90 that is displayed at 20 weeks with edema and proteinuria. This condition is common in primigravidas. Eclampsia is seizures or coma exhibited by a patient diagnosed with preeclampsia in the third trimester or postpartum. Chronic hypertension is characterized by a blood pressure of > 140/90 and occurs before pregnancy and persists after delivery. Risk factors for preeclampsia are family history, plural gestation, diabetes, and heart or renal disease.

4.1 Clinical Evaluation:

A. **Symptoms:** Edema, headache, visual disturbances, mental status changes, abdominal pain, and seizures.

B. **Signs:** Papilledema, abdominal tenderness, and ankle clonus of hyperreflexia. Tremulousness may indicate impending eclampsia. Check fetal heart tones by Doppler. Perform a bimanual to examine for cervical dilation.

C. **DDX:** Chronic hypertension and seizures after 2 weeks may indicate CNS pathology, meningitis, or intracranial bleeding.

D. **Work-up:** Order U/A, SMA-7, CBC, transaminases, and 24 hour urine sample for protein and T&C.

4.2 RX:

A. For gestational HTN, observe for 6 hours. Discharge patient if BP is < 90 diastolic with follow up.

B. For mild preeclampsia without proteinuria, instruct patient to decrease activity. Discharge with a close follow up.

C. For preeclampsia with proteinuria, hospitalize for bed rest. Check 24 hour urine for protein.

D. Hospitalize patients with severe preeclampsia and a pregnancy > 36 weeks. Position patient on left side, maintain urine output, and start magnesium sulfate, 2-4 g IV load, followed by magnesium sulfate maintenance, 1 g/hour drip. Control BP with hydralazine, 5-10 mg IV q 20 minutes with goal of lowering the BP to < 90 diastolic. If refractory, use labetalol or nitroprusside.

E. Deliver baby when the following conditions are evident: Altered mental status, coagulopathy, increase in serum creatinine, uncontrolled HTN, decreased fetal movements or distress.

F. For eclampsia with seizures, use magnesium sulfate, 2-4 g over 5-10 minutes IV **or** 1 g/hour continuous infusion. For resistant seizures, administer diazepam, 5 mg IV, repeat q 5 minutes up to 15-20 mg. If seizures continue, administer phenobarbital, 200 mg IV, and treat hypertension.

G. Treat chronic hypertension with methyldopa, hydralazine, or labetalol.

H. Definitive treatment of eclampsia is delivery. However, control seizures and BP first. Complications of hypertension in pregnancy are intracranial bleeding, papilledema, pancreatitis, renal failure, liver failure, pulmonary edema, and coagulopathy.

5. Hyperemesis Gravidarum:

5.1 Clinical Evaluation:

A. **Symptoms:** N&V in first trimester.
B. **Signs:** Orthostatic hypotension, decreased skin turgor, tachycardia, and thirst.
C. **DDX:** Cholecystitis, gastroenteritis, pyelonephritis, PUD, reflux esophagitis or appendicitis.
D. **Work-up:** Order U/A, CBC, and SMA-7.

5.2 RX:

A. Administer IVF and Compazine in ED. Discharge the patient with instructions to consume frequent small meals.
B. **Disposition:** Admit patients with severe dehydration, acidosis, or ketosis.

6. Post Abortion Sepsis:

6.1 Clinical Evaluation:

A. **Signs and Symptoms:** Three to seven days post abortion- fever, excessive bleeding, uterine tenderness, and purulent bloody discharge. Risk factors are advanced gestational age and untreated pelvic infections.
B. **Work-up:** Order CBC, SMA-7, U/A, and blood and U/A cultures.

6.2 RX:

A. Start IV, O_2, and monitor.
B. Initiate an IV antibiotic regime, including clindamycin, 900 mg IV q 9 hours, plus gentamicin, 2 mg/kg IV load, followed by 1.5 mg/kg q 8 hours, **or** Cefoxitin, 2 g IV q 8 hours, plus, doxycycline, 100 mg IV q 12 hours.
C. **Disposition:** Admit.

7. Post Partum Hemorrhage:

In post partum hemorrhage, the maternal blood loss > 500 mL after delivery. This loss of blood may be immediate, < 24 hours, or delayed, 7-14 days, after delivery. Immediate hemorrhage is caused by uterine atony which, in turn, is a result of a ruptured uterus. Delayed hemorrhage involves the retention of placental tissue or endoparametritis. There is a potential for profound shock with post partum hemorrhage. Risk factors are a prolonged or rapid labor, high parity, large or multiple fetuses, and lacerations to the vagina or cervix.

7.1 Clinical Evaluation:

A. **Symptoms:** An immediate hemorrhage is accompanied by steady and brisk bleeding. A delayed hemorrhage is associated with sudden, painless bleeding preceded by foul smelling lochia.
B. **Signs:** Soft, boggy uterus or uterine inversion
C. **DDX:** Endometritis.
D. **Work-up:** Order CBC, PT, PTT, fibrinogen, T&C, and US.

7.2 RX:

A. Start IV, O_2, and monitor.
B. Start a transfusion for shock and a FFP for DIC.
C. For immediate hemorrhage, massage uterus and administer oxytocin, 20-40 μg/L at 200-500 mL/hour.
D. For persistent bleeding, administer Methergine, 0.2 mg IM, **or** inject 0.5 mg of prostaglandin F into uterus. Repair lacerations.
E. Perform vaginal packing for multiple small lacerations.
F. For refractory immediate hemorrhage, transfer patient to surgery to ligate uterine artery or hysterectomy.

G. For delayed hemorrhage when the bleeding has stopped, discharge the patient home with a prescription of ergonovine, 0.2 mg po q 6-12 hours.
H. **Disposition:** Admit patients with severe bleeding and large amounts of retained products for a D&C.

8. Retained Product of Conception:

8.1 Clinical Evaluation:
A. **Symptoms:** Occurs typically after abortions with local anesthesia. Approximately one week after the abortion, the patient presents with cramping, heavy bleeding, and fever.
B. **Signs:** Vaginal blood, products of conception, and uterine tenderness.

8.2 RX:
A. Perform a D&C and start IV antibiotic regime which includes clindamycin, 900 mg IV q 9 hours, plus gentamicin, 2 mg/kg IV load, followed by 1.5 mg/kg q 8 hours, **or** Cefoxitin, 2 g IV q 8 hours, plus doxycycline, 100 mg IV q 12 hours.
B. **Disposition:** Admit.

9. Third Trimester Hemorrhage:

9.1 Clinical Evaluation:
A. **Symptoms:**
Placenta previa: Placental implantation in lower uterus adjacent to or over the os. Presentation is painless, bright red vaginal bleeding after 28 weeks. Risk factors include multiple surgeries and multiple pregnancies.
Abruptio placenta: Premature separation of the placenta from the uterine wall. Presentation is painful, dark red bleeding (80%), and abdominal pain. Risk factors are eclampsia, diabetes, renal disease, hypertension, and abdominal trauma.
B. **Signs:** Avoid vaginal or speculum exams. Abdominal palpation for fundal height, contractions, or tenderness of uterus. Previa is soft and non-tender. Abruptio has a firm and irritable uterus.
C. **DDX:** Normal labor, uterine rupture, vasa previa, and bloody show.
D. **Work-up:** Order Pelvic US, CBC, PT, PTT, fibrinogen, SMA-7, and T&C. Monitor fetal heart tones by Doppler. DIC present 20% with abruptions. A US can detect or rule out placenta previa, but does not reliably detect an abruption.

9.2 RX:
A. Obtain an obstetrics consultation STAT.
B. Start IV, O_2, and monitor.
C. Position patient on left side, transfuse early, implement FFP for DIC, and MAST.
D. **Disposition:** For unstable patients, admit to OR and ensure that an obstetrician is available to perform an exam and a possible C-section. Admit the patient to the Obstetrics unit. Instruct bedrest and a close follow up for stable patients with abruption carrying an immature fetus. This condition may be managed expectantly if bleeding is slight.

ORTHOPEDICS

1. Carpal Tunnel Syndrome:

1.1 Clinical Evaluation:

A. **Symptoms:** More common in women than in men. Complaints include tingling, numbness, burning, paresthesias along distribution of median nerve, and cold sensitivity. Symptoms often awaken patient but may be relieved by shaking or lowering the hand. Symptoms may increase with repetitive hand motion.

B. **Signs:** Decreased two-point discrimination and light touch. Positive Phalen's test in which flexing of the wrists for 30 seconds reproduces symptoms. Tinel's sign is positive if tapping on the wrist over the median nerve causes tingling sensation in the hand. Weakness of median nerve innervated muscles may also be present.

C. **Work-up:** Obtain a wrist X-ray to exam for calcific deposits, callus, or osteophytes. Perform a c-spine if cervical radiculopathy is considered. In some cases, chemistry, thyroid function, sedimentation rate, rheumatoid factor, and antinuclear antibody tests should also be considered.

1.2 RX:

A. Apply wrists splints, administer NSAIDs, and instruct patient to discontinue repetitive motion.

B. **Disposition:** Refer to a hand surgeon.

2. Compartment Syndromes:

Limited space, with increased tissue pressure, produces decreased tissue circulation which results in an abnormal neuromuscular function.

2.1 Clinical Evaluation:

A. **Symptoms:** Pain is usually severe and constant. Hypoesthesia with tingling and numbness may be present.

B. **Signs:** Tenderness, swelling, and increased pain with passive muscle movement.

C. **Work-up:** Measure compartment pressures, i.e., 0-10 mm Hg is usually normal. Capillary blood flow is compromised at about 20 mm Hg. Nerves and muscles are at risk when pressures greater than 30-40 mm Hg are produced.

2.2 RX:

Obtain an immediate surgical consultation with elevated compartment pressures. A fasciotomy, which involves a longitudinal skin incision, should be performed in the operating suite.

3. Fractures:

Diagnosis, treatment, and disposition of patients with fractures.

3.1 Clinical Evaluation:

A. **Symptoms:** Age of patient, mechanism, pain site and character, and changes in sensation.

B. **Signs:** Neurovascular exam, swelling, deformity, and evidence of integument disruption.

C. **Work-up:**

Plain films: X-ray pain site and joint above and below.

Radionuclide bone scanning: Detects occult and stress fractures as well as osteomyelitis that is not present radiographically. Fracture must be at least 72 hours old.

CT: Confirms suspicious fractures and defines alignment, fragmentation, or displacement.

MRI: Used to diagnose lesions of bones, ligaments, cartilage, menisci, and disks.

D. **Description:** Exam and X-ray findings should describe and include the following:

Anatomical location: Proximal, middle, and distal.

Position: Valgus-described part angled away from midline. Varus-described part angled toward midline.

Apposition: Contact between fracture surfaces, apposed, displaced, or distracted.

Alignment: Along longitudinal axis, deviation is angulation and should be measured.

Open versus closed.

Fracture line direction: Transverse, spiral, or oblique.

Avulsion present: Bone fragment pulled away from its normal position by ligament or muscle.

Articular involvement: Percentage of articular surface involvement.

Pathologic: Fracture which occurs through bone that is not normal.

Stress: Repeated low-intensity trauma.

Complete versus incomplete: Complete-disruption of both cortices; incomplete-disruption of one cortex.

Impaction: Depression or compression.

Comminuted: More than two fragments.

E. **Fractures In Children:**

Greenstick: Incomplete, angulated fractures of long bones.

Torus: Buckling or wrinkling of the cortex.

Classification (Salter-Harris): I- Involves slip of the zone of provisional calcification. II- Similar to type I with fracture extension into metaphysis. III- Involves slip of the growth plate plus a fracture through the epiphysis and involves the articular surface. IV- Similar to type III with involvement of metaphyseal fracture. V- Crush injuries of the metaphyseal plate. III-V may result in growth problems.

F. **Fracture Complications:**

Hemorrhage: Radius and ulna, 150-250 mL, humerus, 250 mL, tibia and fibula, 500 mL, femur, 1 L, and pelvis, 1.5-3 L.

Nerve: Shoulder dislocation-axillary, elbow-medial (supracondylar) and ulnar, sacral-cauda equina, hip dislocation-femoral, acetabulum-sciatic, femoral shaft- peroneal, knee dislocation-peroneal or tibial, and lateral tibial plateau-peroneal.

Compartment syndrome: Pain with passive stretching, with active flexing against resistance, or with compartment pressure.

Vascular: First rib and clavicle fractures are associated with vascular bleeding. Knee fractures and dislocation are associated with popliteal artery injury.

Avascular Necrosis tends to occur in comminuted fractures of bones with poor blood supply, such as capitate, scaphoid, and femoral head.

Fat Embolism commonly follows long bone fractures, tibia, fibula, and hip. Symptoms may include tachypnea, dyspnea, tachycardia, pulmonary edema, restlessness, confusion, petechial rash, fever, jaundice, retinal changes, and renal involvement. Fat may be found in the urine.

Immobilization Complications: Pneumonia, UTI, ulcers, muscle atrophy, GI hemorrhage, DVT, pulmonary embolism, and psychological disorders.

Cast Problems: Patients often present with pain, local irritation, swelling, and numbness. Bivalve cast and inspect. If bivalve does not relieve symptoms, consider compartment syndrome.

3.2 RX:

A. For open fractures, obtain culture and start antibiotics. Irrigate with saline solution and cover with Betadine-soaked sponges. Treat with tetanus immunoglobulin for large crush wounds. Obtain immediate orthopedic consultation.

B. For closed fractures, splint or immobilize all fractures or suspected fractures. Obtain an orthopedic consultation.

C. Non-displaced fractures may not be apparent on initial radiographs. If fracture is clinically suspected, splint and repeat films in 7 days or perform a more definitive test, such as a CT or a bone scan.

4. Hand Infections:

Soft-tissue infections have a high risk of morbidity and mortality. Meleney's gangrene, a progressive bacterial synergistic, is a spreading infection of the subcutaneous tissue commonly caused by *Staphylococcus*. Necrotizing fasciitis spreads even more quickly and is typically caused by *E. coli*. Bites caused by cats or dogs often become infected with *Pasteurella multocida*. Wounds are especially dangerous in patients that are immunosuppressed. Fungal hand infections are also common, especially in gardeners infected with *Sporothrix schenckii*.

4.1 Clinical Evaluation:

A. **Symptoms:** Trauma is usually a puncture, cut, bite, or crush injury.

B. **Signs:** Examine for crepitus, erythema, vesicle formation, change in skin color, pain with passive or active movement, and pus.

C. **Work-up:** X-ray to eliminate possibility of a foreign body or air in tissue or joint.

4.2 RX:

A. Irrigate with high pressure saline, allow wound to remain open, dress wound, splint in position of function, and start appropriate antibiotics.

B. **Disposition:** Admit patient with signs of serious hand infection. Obtain an immediate consultation of hand surgeon.

5. Hand Injuries:

5.1 Clinical Evaluation:

A. **Symptoms:** Age, occupation, dominant hand, mechanism of injury, and clean or contaminated environment.

B. **Signs:** Location, bone exposure, neurovascular status, including color, pallor, cyanosis, and capillary refill. Perform an Allen's test to evaluate radial and ulnar arteries, a motor and sensory nerve evaluation, and a tendon evaluation.

5.2 RX:

A. For a flexor tendon, refer to a hand surgeon.

B. For an extensor tendon, repair by EP, if so trained, with close follow-up.

C. For amputations, clean amputated part to remove gross debris and then wrap the part in a moist saline towel or sponge and place it in a plastic container. Place the container on ice, if possible. Refer to a hand surgeon immediately.

D. A Boutonniere Deformity is a sudden forced flexion of the proximal interphalangeal joint disrupting the central slip of the extensor tendon. Splint the proximal interphalangeal joint in extension for 6-8 weeks.

E. A Mallet Finger is the flexion of the distal interphalangeal joint which ruptures the extensor tendon at the base of the distal phalanx. Splint the distal interphalangeal and proximal interphalangeal joints in extension for 6 weeks. If avulsion of the bone occurs, splint in hyperextension. Consult a hand surgeon immediately if bony avulsion involves 1/3 or more of the joint.

F. For a subungual hematoma, make a hole over the center of the hematoma by using either an electric cautery or a heated paper clip.

G. A Ganglion Cyst is a benign tumor-like swelling which generally occurs on the volar-radial aspect and dorsum of the wrist. Lesions are filled with a jelly-like substance. Surgical removal may be required if pain, tenderness, or weakness is present.

H. A DeQuervain's Tenosynovitis occurs in the abductor pollicis longus and extensor pollicis brevis. This condition is usually associated with repetitive motion. Perform a Finkelstein's test by placing the thumb in the palm and then deviating the wrist in an ulna direction. If pain is produced, treat with rest and splinting. Hand surgeons may inject steroids or perform a release.

6. Hip Fractures and Dislocations:

6.1 Clinical Evaluation:

A. **Symptoms:** Trauma, falls, and motor vehicle accident.

B. **Signs:** Gentle palpation. Auscultate symphysis pubis while tapping patella, dullness suggests fracture (Wood's sign). Evaluate distal neurovascular status.

Femoral Neck Fractures: Extremity slightly shortened, externally rotated, and abducted.
Intertrochanteric Fractures: Extremity shortened and markedly externally rotated.
Anterior dislocations: Extremity abducted and externally rotated.

C. Posterior dislocations: Extremity is shortened, internally rotated, and adducted.

D. **Work-up:** Obtain plain films of the pelvis and hips. Order CT, bone scans, and vascular studies for further evaluation. Order trauma labs.

6.2 RX:

A. Refer the patient immediately to an orthopedic surgical consultation. Treat hemorrhage.

B. **Disposition:** Admit.

7. Joint Dislocations:

Subluxation is the disruption of joint with continued proximal and distal approximation of the articulating surfaces. Dislocation is the disruption of joint with complete loss of articulation. Rapid treatment is important to prevent injury to nerves and blood vessels, as well as to avoid the onset of avascular necrosis of the bone.

7.1 Clinical Evaluation:

A. **Symptoms:** May be minor or major trauma. Complaints of pain with movement.

B. **Signs:** Deformity. Detailed neurovascular exam.

C. **Work-up:** Obtain X-rays.

7.2 RX:

A. Reduce after X-ray evaluation. Reduce immediately if there is evidence of a neurovascular compromise. Obtain postreduction films to document reduction and rule out the possibility of a fracture. Splint. Always refer to an orthopedic surgeon.

Distal Interphalangeal Joint: Splint in full extension for 4 weeks.
Finger or Thumb Proximal Interphalangeal Joint: Splint 15 degrees of flexion for 4 weeks.
Finger and Thumb Metacarpophalangeal Joints: Splint 40-50 degrees of flexion for 4 weeks.
Wrist: Usually requires urgent ORIF.

Radial Head Subluxation (Nursemaid's Elbow): Children age 1-4 with radial head subluxed through annular ligament with sudden traction, treat with simultaneous traction and supination, click confirms reduction, and do not splint.
Elbow: Associated with Median N., Ulnar N., and Brachial A. injury. After reduction, position splint for a posterior dislocation in 120 degrees of flexion and anterior dislocation in 90 degrees of flexion.
Shoulder: Anterior is most common. High risk of Axillary N. injury. Reduce and sling for 2-3 weeks. Posterior is rare.
Hip: Occurs with large forces. High incidence of avascular necrosis of the femoral head. Often requires operative reduction. After reduction treat with traction.
Knee: Associated with Popliteal a. and Peroneal N. injury. If a suspicion of arterial injury arises, obtain an arteriography. After reduction, splint 20 degrees of flexion.
Patella: Associated with osteochondral fracture. After reduction, splint in a knee immobilizer for 3-4 weeks.
Ankle: Almost always associated with fracture and ORIF to repair. Position in a cast 6 weeks.

B. **Disposition:** Admit most hip, knee, and ankle dislocations after obtaining a consultation.

8. Knee Soft-Tissue Injuries:

8.1 Clinical Evaluation:

A. **Symptoms:** Mechanism, position of injury, abnormal bending, force applied, and sounds heard (popping suggests anterior cruciate tear, ripping or click suggests meniscus tear).

B. **Signs:** Swelling suggests fracture or ligament disruption, deformity, straight-leg raises, and palpation. Varus and valgus stress for collateral ligament tears. Anterior drawer test for anterior cruciate tears consists of gentle forward traction of the flexed knee specifically examining for laxity. Examine for meniscal tears by performing the Apley and McMurray tests. Apley compression test consists of first positioning the patient to lie prone with the knee flexed 90 degrees. The examiner applies downward pressure on the posterior thigh with one hand while applying downward pressure on the plantar surface of the foot and rotating the lower leg. Pain occurs on the affected side. McMurray test consists of positioning the patient to lie supine and hyperflexing the knee. One hand applies pressure on the distal anterior thigh while the other applies caudal pressure on the plantar surface of the foot while rotating the lower leg. Pain or clicking is a positive test.

C. **Work-up:** Obtain an X-ray. Consider tapping large effusions after consulting with an orthopedic surgeon.

8.2 RX:

A. After eliminating the possibility of a fracture and dislocation, treat soft tissue injuries by applying ice to the injury for 20 minutes several times. Instruct the patient to elevate the injury to use crutches, and to immobilize the knee as possible.

B. **Disposition:** Refer the patient to an orthopedic surgeon for further evaluation and for a possible arthrography and arthroscopy.

9. Low Back Complaints:

Low back pain is a very common complaint. Causes may include trauma, neoplasms, congenital disorders, degenerative disease, metabolic disorders, infections, metabolic disorders, inflammatory disorders, vascular disorders, psychosocial disorders, and visceral inflammation.

9.1 Clinical Evaluation:

A. **Symptoms:** Location, duration, frequency, and radiation of pain. Assess bowel and bladder function, neurologic symptoms, and weakness.

B. **Signs:** Neurologic deficits, deformity, tenderness, range of motion, straight leg raises, gait, reflexes, muscle strength, sensory/motor, and rectal tone/sensation.

C. **Work-up:** Order plain films. Consider CT, MRI, and bone scan to rule out focal lesions or unexplained symptoms. Obtain a myelogram or MRI if cord compression is considered.

9.2 RX:

A. For fractures, immobilize on back board. Refer to an orthopedic or neurosurgical specialist.

B. For disk herniation, rupture, extrusion with out neurologic involvement, initiate analgesics, NSAIDS, muscle relaxants. Instruct the patient to +/- bedrest and physical therapy. Obtain an orthopedic consult.

C. Instruct patients with a disk herniation, rupture, extrusion with neurologic involvement or acute cauda equina syndrome, and bladder/rectal dysfunction to rest in bed. Obtain an immediate neurology/neurosurgery/orthopedic surgery consult.

D. For osteomyelitis, discitis, and paraspinal abscess disk space narrowing usually is present 10-14 days after symptoms. Admit the patient, obtain an immediate consultation, and start IV antibiotics.

E. For neoplasia, obtain a bone scan and a myelogram. Admit patient, in most cases, and refer to oncology/radiation oncologist and neurosurgeon.

10. Pelvic Fractures:

Pelvic fractures usually occur from falls or high speed blunt trauma. These types of fractures may cause severe hemorrhage. Pelvic fractures are associated with pelvic organ injury, i.e., especially the bladder.

10.1 Clinical Evaluation:

A. **Symptoms:** Trauma and pelvic pain.

B. **Signs:** Evaluate for shock. Gently palpate pelvis for pain sites. Perform pelvic and rectal if not contraindicated. Evaluate neurovascular status. There is a high mortality with severe fractures; therefore, immediate intervention is required after assessment.

C. **Work-up:** Obtain X-rays. CT should be considered. Order trauma labs. If urethral bleeding, boggy prostate, or scrotal hematoma is present, perform am urethrogram before Foley insertion. Obtain a cystogram to determine bladder integrity.

10.2 RX:

A. Treat for hemorrhage and shock. Mast trousers should be considered. Consult trauma, orthopedic, and urologic surgeons. Placement of external fixator or other operative management may be required.

B. Classifications:

Fracture I: Fracture individual bones without break in continuity of the ring. Stable. Treat with bedrest.

Fracture II: Single break in the pelvic ring. Stable. Twenty five percent of these types of fractures are associated with tissue injury, visceral injury, genitourinary injury, and bleeding.

Fracture III: Double break in pelvic ring. Unstable. Associated with soft tissue, visceral, genitourinary injury, and major hemorrhage.

Fracture IV: Fracture of the acetabulum. Associated with nerve injury.

11. Sprains:

1st degree: Minor tear ligamentous fibers with mild hemorrhage and swelling. Stress joint produces pain but no abnormal joint motion.
2nd degree: Partial ligament tear. Moderate hemorrhage, swelling, tenderness, pain, and loss of function.
3rd degree: Complete ligament tear with loss of joint stability.

11.1 Clinical Evaluation:

A. **Symptoms:** Abnormal or exaggerated force on joint. Often hear a pop or snap. History should include position and forces applied.
B. **Signs:** Evaluate for swelling, hemorrhage, point tenderness, function, and joint stability.
C. **Work-up:** In most cases, include plain films to eliminate possibility of fracture.

11.2 RX:

Treat sprain with ice, elevation, and analgesia. Instruct patient to avoid weight bearing and to immobilize the injury as much as possible. Refer to an orthopedic specialist prn.

12. Strains:

1st degree: Minor tearing of musculotendinous unit with spasm, swelling, tenderness, and mild loss of function.
2nd degree: More tearing without complete disruption. Swelling, muscle spasm, ecchymosis, and loss of strength.
3rd degree: Complete disruption of muscle or tendon often with avulsion fracture.

12.1 Clinical Evaluation:

A. **Symptoms:** Pulled muscle usually is caused by a rapid acceleration or use of excessive force.
B. **Signs:** Local tenderness, swelling, spasm, ecchymosis, and loss of function.

12.2 RX:

A. Instruct the patient to rest, apply ice to the strain, and elevate/immobilize the injured part. Also inform the patient that passive stretching during early post injury may impede healing, and result in calcium or fibrosis in the injured muscle. Obtain an orthopedic consultation. Prescribe NSAIDS.
B. **Disposition:** Discharge as an outpatient with therapy follow-up.

PEDIATRICS

1. Resuscitation:

An overwhelming majority of cardiorespiratory compromise is due to hypoxia. Bradycardia leading to asystole from hypoxemia causes the majority of cardiac dysrhythmias. V-tachycardia/V-fibrillation are actually rare but when there is such an occurrence, it is commonly associated with cardiac anomaly. PSVT is typically the result of WPW. Other causes requiring resuscitation include prematurity, birth trauma, congenital and other medical problems, trauma, environmental injury, acute infection, toxic ingestion, and seizures.

1.1 Clinical Evaluation:

A. **Symptoms:** Attempt to obtain a vestige of history from EMS or caretaker while initiating ABCs.

B. **Signs:** Assess airway, breathing, and circulation.

C. **Work-up:** Determine appropriate laboratory and X-ray evaluation after stabilization. Pulse oximetry or ABG may be useful during resuscitation. Refer also to algorithms in reference section.

Newborn Resuscitation (Delivery): Hold neonate in slight Trendelenburg, suction nares and oropharynx. Clamp and cut cord, move to radiant warmer, dry and stimulate patient, suction again. If spontaneous respiration is present but is not clearly adequate, provide 100% O_2.

Assist ventilation with bag-valve-mask for pulse < 100, apnea, and persistent cyanosis, at a rate of 40-60/minute.

Intubate for meconium aspiration (and suction with DeLee trap) and difficulties with bag-valve-mask ventilation, persistent apnea, or cyanosis.

Initiate chest compressions for pulse < 60 or persistent pulse < 80 after performing the steps described above at a rate of 120/minutes and a depth of 1/2-3/4 inch.

Intervene pharmacologically for pulse < 80 after conducting the steps cited above. Obtain access via the umbilical vein (single, larger vessel) using -5.0 Fr umbilical venous catheter. Epinephrine, 1:10,000, 0.1 mg/mL, 0.01-0.1 mg/kg; $NaHCO_3$, 1 mEq/kg; and consider naloxone, 0.01 mg/kg.

Pediatric Resuscitation:

AGE	Kg	Pulse	BP	ET	ET length	Blade	NG
Preemie	< 2	140	55	3.0	6+kg	0	5
Term	3	125	65	3.5	6+kg	1	6
6 months	7	120	90	3.5	11	1	8
1 year	1	120	96	4.0	11	1	10
3 years	15	110	100	4.5	13	2	10
5 years	18	100	100	5.0	14	2	12
6 years	20	100	100	5.5	15	2	12
8 years	25	90	105	6.0 c	17	2	14
12 years	40	85-90	115	6.5 c	19	3	18

Airway: 1) ET tube size- (16+age)/4 or table above, 2) < 1 year- back blows and chest thrusts for FB, Heimlich, 3) > 1 year- back blows, chest thrusts, and Heimlich for FB, 4) Intubation < 6 years- Increase succinylcholine to 2 mg/kg, consider atropine 0.01 mg/kg if using succ., especially in peds < 3 years, and 5) Intubation < 8 years- use uncuffed tube.

1.2 RX:

A. **Common Drug Doses:**

Epinephrine, 0.01 mg/kg 1:10,000 IV or IO.
Epinephrine, 0.1 mg/kg 1:1000 ET.
Atropine, 0.02 mg/kg, (minimum 0.1 mg, maximum 0.5 mg child, 1.0 mg adolescent).
Lidocaine, 1 mg/kg, repeat up to 3 mg/kg.
Amiodarone 5 mg/kg IV
Naloxone, 0.01 mg/kg.
$NaHCO_3^-$, 1 mEq/kg of 8.4% solution IV or IO.
$NaHCO_3^-$, 0.5 mEq/mL solution for neonates.
Diazepam, 0.2 mg/kg q 2-5 minutes to 10 mg maximum (titrate 0.5 mg units), 0.5 mg/kg rectal dose.
Phenobarbital, 15-20 mg/kg slow IV or IM, may -repeat q 20 minutes to 30 mg/kg maximum.
Dobutamine, 5-15 μg/kg/minute.
Dopamine, 2-20 μg/kg/minute for pressor, 0.5-2 μg/kg/minute increases renal and splanchnic blood flow.
Epinephrine, 0.1-1.0 μg/kg/minute.
Isoproterenol, 0.1-1.0 μg/kg/minute.
Lidocaine, 20-50 μg/kg/minute.
NAVEL drugs can go down the ET tube, such as lidocaine, atropine, Naloxone, epinephrine, and Valium or Versed.
The algorithms, cited below, all consist of ABCs which include intubation, CPR as appropriate, O_2, reassessments after each step, and venous or intraosseous access.

B. **Asystole:**

Hyperventilate.
Check 2 leads.
Administer epinephrine, 0.01 mg/kg of 1:10,000 IV/IO.
Administer epinephrine, 0.1 mg/kg of 1:1000 IV/IO q 3-5 minutes.

C. **Bradycardia:**

Administer atropine, 0.02 mg/kg, minimum 0.1 mg, maximum 0.5 mg for child, 1.0 mg for adolescent. Repeat one time.
Start epinephrine, 0.01 mg/kg of 1:10,000 IV/IO q 3-5 minutes, or 0.1 mg/kg 1:1000 ET if IV/IO not available.
Consider pacing.

D. **PEA:**

Hyperventilate.
Seek and treat cause, including hypoxia, hypovolemia, tension pneumothorax, cardiac tamponade, hypothermia, or acidosis.
Start epinephrine, 0.01 mg/kg of 1:10,000 IV/IO, or 0.1 mg/kg 1:1000 ET, if IV/IO is not available.
Administer epinephrine, 0.1 mg/kg of 1:1000 IV/IO/ET q 3-5 minutes.
Atropine 0.02 mg/kg IV with a minimum dose of 0.1 mg q 5-10 minutes to a max dose of 1.0 mg.

E. **SVT:**

For unstable, synchronized shock, 0.5-1 J/kg.
Synchronized shock, 2 J/kg.

Synchronized shock, 4 J/kg, repeat after each drug round.
Start adenosine, 0.1 mg/kg rapid IV, double dose and try again up to two more times.
Administer verapamil, 0.1-0.3 mg/kg up to 5 mg. However, do not use for those < 1-2 years.
For stable, vagal maneuvers (ice on face, simulated dive reflex).
Prescribe adenosine, 0.1 mg/kg rapid IV, double dose and try again up to two more times.
Prescribe digoxin or β-blocker.
Administer verapamil, 0.1-0.3 mg/kg up to 5 mg. Do not use for those < 1-2 years.

F. **V-fibrillation/pulseless V-tachycardia:**

Shock, 2 J/kg.
Shock, 4 J/kg.
Shock, 4 J/kg.
Start epinephrine, 0.01 mg/kg of 1:10,000 IV/IO, or 0.1 mg/kg 1:1000 ET if IV/IO is not available.
Administer lidocaine, 1 mg/kg IV/IO or amiodarone 5 mg/kg IV/IO.
Shock, 4 J/kg 30-60 s after each med.
Administer epinephrine, 0.1 mg/kg of 1:1000 IV/IO/ET q 3-5 minutes.
Administer lidocaine, 1 mg/kg IV/IO.

G. **V-tachycardia, stable:**

Start lidocaine, 1 mg/kg IV or amiodarone 5 mg/kg.
Give phenytoin, 2-4 mg/kg IV over 5 minutes, **or** procainamide, 2-6 mg/kg slowly.

2. Analgesia / Sedation:

Pain management and the appropriate use of sedation are part of the art of emergency medicine. Use of medications carries inherent risks that must be understood and weighed when deliberating over the prescribing meds and dosing. Adequate patient monitoring should be in place as appropriate for each situation as well as the equipment and personnel that are necessary for airway management. Some of the meds that are used in practice include the following, (Annal EM 23:2, 241, 1994). Check contraindications before usage:

Medication	Route	Dose (mg/kg)	Max Dose (mg)	Cautions
Analgesics				
ASA	PO/PR	10-15	975	Flu, PUDz, viral illness
Ibuprofen	PO	5-10	800	PUD
Acetaminophen	PO/PR	10-15	1000	
Sedative Analgesics				Respiratory depression
Morphine	IV/IM/PO	0.1-0.2	10	
Meperidine	IV/IM	1.0-2.0	100	
Fentanyl	IV/IM	0.001-0.005	0.05	
Codeine	PO	1.0	60	
Hydrocodone	PO	0.2	7.5	
Sedatives				Respiratory Depression
Midazolam	IV/IM PR/IN	0.01-0.8 0.3-0.7	4	
Diazepam	IV PR	0.05-0.2 0.5	10	
Chloral	PO	50-100	1,000	Liver disease
Hydrate				
Pentobarbital	IV/IM	2.0-5.0	200	
Thiopental	IV	3.0-5.0	500	Hypotension
Etomidate	IV	0.2-0.5		N, V
Other				
Ketamine	IV IM PO	1.0 3.0-5.0 6.0-10.0	100 50 50	Laryngospasm, V, dysphoric reactions
Nitrous Oxide	Inhaled	30-50%	50%	

3. Apnea:

Apnea is no spontaneous respirations > 20 s. Sudden Infant Death Syndrome (SIDS) is the leading cause of death in first 1-12 months of life. Incidence of males to females deaths is 2:1. Apnea occurs at a higher rate in the winter months and in the early morning hours. Other risks include prematurity, low birth weight, IUGR (growth retardation), bronchopulmonary dysplasia, mothers who smoke, and IV drug abusers. Apparent Life Threatening Event (ALTE, or near-miss SIDS) is associated with apnea spells, cyanosis, listlessness, or LOC with complete resolution.

3.1 Clinical Evaluation:

A. **Symptoms:** Infant found unconscious, unresponsive, ± cyanosis, and apneic. Patient aroused spontaneously, via tactile stimulation (ALTE) or remains unresponsive despite CPR (SIDS). There is no history of trauma, ± history of recent URI, and gastroenteritis.

B. **Signs:** Unconscious, unresponsive, apneic, ± cyanotic, and no vitals or asystole on monitor if SIDS.

C. **DDX:** Seizure, hypoglycemia, sepsis/meningitis, cardiomyopathy, and botulism.

D. **Work-up:** Determine O_2 saturation or ABG, CBC, SMA-7, and ECG. Order septic work-up to include blood, urine, csf and stool culture. Obtain a head CT ± I. Consider inpatient Holter, pneumogram, and ± swallowing study.

3.2 RX:

A. Support ABCs, including IV, O_2, monitor, and PALS.

B. **Disposition:** Admit for monitoring and work-up if there is any question of ALTE and apneic episode.

4. Bronchiolitis:

The majority of cases of bronchiolitis occur within the first 2 years. RSV is the most common cause among infants followed by parainfluenza virus. Mycoplasma pneumoniae typically causes bronchiolitis among school-aged children. Epidemics usually occur as a result of RSV. Most pediatric patients that die from bronchiolitis are < 6 months old.

4.1 Clinical Evaluation:

A. **Symptoms:** Poor appetite, apparent dyspnea, coryza, and rhinitis.

B. **Signs:** Tachypnea, chest hyperexpansion, wheezing, and anxiety. Retractions and grunting are late signs.

C. **DDX:** Asthma, pneumonia, other debilitating respiratory or cardiac illness, cystic fibrosis, and FB aspiration.

D. **Work-up:** Pulse oximetry, consider ABG and CXR. Look for peribronchiolar cuffing which appears as small white circles, especially near the periphery, elevated and flattened diaphragms associated with air trapping/hyperinflation, and rib angle flattening also associated with trapping on the CXR.

4.2 RX:

A. Antibiotics are not useful unless a secondary infection is evident. Bronchodilators are helpful. Consider ribavirin for RSV when verified or if patient is very ill. Rehydrate IV prn.

B. **Disposition:** Admit patients who are younger, have other underlying disease, are immune compromised, and who appear severely ill. Follow up within 1 day for those discharged from the ED.

5. Dehydration:

5.1 Clinical Evaluation:

A. **Symptoms:** Associated with F, N, V, D, and decreased po intake from any cause.

B. **Signs:** Percentage dehydrated:

	5%	10%	15%
Tachycardia	-	+	+
Orthostatic	-	±	+
Dry mucous membranes	±	+	+
Poor skin turgor	-	±	+
BUN	Normal	Increasing	**Increasing**
UO	±	Decreasing	**Decreasing**
S.g. urine	1.020	1.030	1.035

C. **Work-up:** Order CBC, SMA-7, U/A, and other appropriate evaluations for underlying problem.

5.2 RX:

Treat with NS, 20 mg/kg IV bolus for severe dehydration, repeat prn.

6. Fever, Bacteremia, and Sepsis:

Managing patients of < 3 years who have a fever but no clear source of the cause is challenging. Controversy exists and optimal management is unknown. Always perform a thorough examination to find the cause of the fever by obtaining the history of the patient and performing appropriate lab exams/tests, i.e., especially U/A.

Fever: T > 38.0 °C (100.4 °F) rectal.

Toxic: Decreased consciousness, poor or absent eye contact, does not interface with environment, septic or cyanotic appearance, and lowered perfusion or ventilation. Risk of serious bacterial infection in peds < 90 days who meet toxic criteria is 17.3%.

Low-risk criteria: Previously healthy patients who contracted a bacterial source. WBC are 5,000-15,000, bands are < 1,500, U/A is normal, < 5 WBC/hpf in diarrhea when condition is present. Risk of serious infection in peds < 90 days who meet low-risk criteria is 1.4%.

6.1 Clinical Evaluation:

A. **Symptoms:** Fever with or without V, D, and signs of toxicity. Determine duration and magnitude of fever and other symptoms. Determine recent po intake as accurately as possible. UO or diaper changes required.

B. **Signs:** Perform a thorough pulmonary exam to seek source of fever and gauge degree of dehydration. Examine skin for signs or rash or petechia that could be associated with meningococcal sepsis.

C. **DDX:** Septic appearing infants may be suffering from infectious causes, i.e., bacterial sepsis, meningitis, UTI, congenital syphilis, or viral infection. Non-infectious causes of septic appearance include gastroenteritis with dehydration, congenital heart disease, PAT, myocardial infarction, pericarditis and myocarditis, congenital adrenal hyperplasia, hypoglycemia, Reye's syndrome, anemia or methemoglobinemia, pyloric stenosis, intussusception, child abuse, or other metabolic derangement.

D. **Work-up:** Controversial. Consider CBC, SMA-7, LP, UA, CXR, and blood & urine culture. Several algorithms exist; however, conservative algorithms include:

0-28 days: Complete work-up as above, ± CXR, admit with or without parenteral antibiotic pending culture results. Usually administer if patient does not meet low-risk criteria cited above. (Controversial: Rate of serious bacterial infection in patients < 28 days meeting low- risk criteria approximately 1%.)

28-90 days: If patient appears toxic (as above), admit, and obtain U/A, blood and urine culture, LP, and administer a parenteral antibiotic.

28-90 days: Non-toxic appearance, choice A- U/A, blood and urine culture, LP, ceftriaxone, 50 mg/kg IM up to 1 g. Discharge patient home with follow up in 1 day.

Choice B: Obtain urine culture. Discharge patient home without antibiotic but with close observation and follow up within 1 day.

3 months-3 years: If patient has a toxic appearance, admit, perform a sepsis workup, and administer a parenteral antibiotic.

3 months-3 years: For non-toxic appearing patients, use temperature as the decision point. If the T > 39 °C, obtain a urine culture for males < 6 months and for females < 2 years. Order stool cultures, if blood or mucus is in stool or if there are 35 WBC/hpf. CXR for respiratory symptoms or findings, blood culture (some recommend only if WBC > 15,000), and empiric antibiotic (some recommend only if WBC > 15,000). Discharge with follow up in 1-2 days. If patient is non-toxic and T < 39.0 °C, no lab work-up is required. Discharge with acetaminophen, follow up 1-2 days, and advise parents to return with the child if symptoms worsen or fever persists > 2 days.

6.2 RX:

A. Implement algorithms as cited above. For all patients, perform ABCs, IV, O_2, and monitor if appropriate. Administer NS, 20 mg/kg IV for dehydration, repeat prn. Prescribe antipyretics, such as acetaminophen, 15 mg/kg, **or** ibuprofen, 10 mg/kg, when patients > 1 year do not respond to acetaminophen.

B. **Disposition:** Admit, unless patient is nontoxic in appearance, and arrange a close follow-up.

7. Laryngotracheobronchitis (Croup):

Etiologies include parainfluenza 1, 2, 3, respiratory syncytial virus, influenza A, and rhinovirus. Spasmodic croup is associated with personal or family history of allergies and with multiple bouts of croup.

7.1 Clinical Evaluation:

A. **Symptoms:** A few days of viral prodrome often precedes gradual onset of characteristic barking, "seal" like cough. Inspiratory stridor can progress to respiratory distress. For many patients, particularly those with spasmodic croup, changes in temperature or breathing humidified air can cause significant, rapid improvement. Peak incidence occurs at age 2. A variable fever may be displayed.

B. **Signs:** Cough as above, may not appear toxic.

C. **DDX:** Croup must be differentiated from epiglottitis. The latter is characterized by a slightly older age group, rapid onset, absence of cough, muffled voice, ill or toxic appearance, anxious, and sitting up and drooling. Other croup differential diagnoses include tracheitis, FB, tracheal stenosis, and diphtheria.

D. **Work-up:** Perform CXR, AP neck to check for "steeple" sign, and lateral if there is a concern about possible epiglottitis. Consider CBC, ABG, blood C&S, U/A, and C&S. Obtain urine antigen screen, nasopharyngeal washings for direct fluorescent antibody (RSV, adenovirus, parainfluenza, influenza virus, and Chlamydia) and viral cultures.

7.2 RX:

A. Use a non-threatening approach by allowing child to remain in parent's arms. Treat symptomatic patients with humidified O_2 by blow-by or by 40-60% by mask. Maintain O_2 saturation at > 92%. For stridor at rest, retractions, and tachypnea, initiate treatment with racemic epinephrine, 2.25% solution, 0.05 mL/kg/dose, or a 0.5 mL/dose nebulized in 4 mL NS, repeat q 1-6 hours. Some authors recommend dexamethasone (Decadron), 0.25-0.5 mg/kg IV/IM q 6 hours. Patients with serious respiratory compromise should be intubated by using an ET tube 0.5-1.0 mm smaller than predicted (usual size (16+age)/4).

B. **Disposition:** Admit all patients requiring treatment with racemic epinephrine or steroids with the exception of patients observed in the ED that appear well > 6 hours after such treatment. The latter patients may be discharged. Consider admission for patients who do not have quick access to an ED. Patients responding well to conservative treatment in the ED may be discharged with instructions for using a vaporizer or, alternatively, producing steam by turning on the shower in a closed bathroom. Instruct parents to return with the child if symptoms worsen.

8. Orbital / Periorbital Cellulitis:

Infection of orbital/periorbital structures is more common in children than in adults. A common cause is extension of sinusitis (ethmoid). Other causes include URI and otitis media with effusion. Ninety percent of blood cultures indicate the presence of *H. influenzae* and *S. pneumoniae.* However, *H. influenzae* is more common in peds.

8.1 Clinical Evaluation:

A. **Symptoms:** Lid swelling, pain, usually in one eye, that persists over a day or two. Often, there is a history of URI and/or sinus infection.

B. **Signs:** Fever. Periorbital erythema, edema, warmth, tenderness of one or both lids, and closure of palpebral fissure can also be displayed. Mucopurulent discharge is evident along with orbital chemosis, proptosis, tenderness, ophthalmoplegia, pupillary sluggishness or paralysis, and decreased visual acuity. Tenderness/pain with EOMs is present.

C. **DDX:** Orbital (more serious) vs periorbital cellulitis, allergy, trauma, orbital abscess, subperiosteal abscess, cavernous sinus thrombosis, neoplasm, and thyrotoxicosis.

D. **Work-up:** Order CBC, chemistries, blood cultures (most negative), and CT of orbit (differentiates orbital from periorbital).

8.2 RX:

A. Treat adults and children over 5 years with nafcillin, 150 mg/kg/day q 6 hours, or those with a penicillin allergy with vancomycin, 40 mg/kg/day q 6 hours).

B. For children under 5 years, administer cefuroxime, 75 mg/kg/day q 8 hours.

C. Obtain an immediate ophthalmologic consultation.

D. **Disposition:** Admit children and all but mildest adult cases.

9. Pertussis:

Bordetella pertussis is the usual cause of "Whooping Cough”. Immunization is not life-long. However, the disease is most common in patients < 5 years and is most dangerous in those < 1 years.

9.1 Clinical Evaluation:

A. **Symptoms:** Catarrhal stage- F, URI symptoms, and conjunctivitis.

Paroxysmal stage: Coughing, increasing in frequency and severity with characteristic inspiratory "whoop" after a series of coughs. Severe congestion in obligate nasal breathers (< 4-6 months), and choking or apnea can complicate disease and require management.

Convalescent stage: Improvement.

B. **Signs:** Subconjunctival hemorrhages, engorged conjunctivae, facial petechia and epistaxis are signs of increased venous pressure during coughing. Any of these signs, along with post-tussive emesis, suggests pertussis.

C. **DDX:** Viral URI, bronchiolitis, laryngotracheobronchitis, reactive airway disease, and FB.

D. **Work-up:** CBC with leukocytosis of > 20,000 is common. CXR findings include emphysema, atelectasis, and perihilar infiltrates.

9.2 RX:

A. Treat with erythromycin, 12.5 mg/kg qid. Treat household members and close contacts.

B. **Disposition:** Consider admission primarily for patients < 1 year and those presenting complications.

10. Retropharyngeal Abscess:

Retropharyngeal abscess is most common in children < 3. Abscess formation occurs between the retropharyngeal fascial planes (alar fascia), the prevertebral fascia and the vertebral bodies. Potential exists for mechanical airway obstruction, abscess extension inferiorly to mediastinum and/or pericardium. There is a high morbidity/mortality if the condition is not treated. Usually mixed mouth flora, anaerobic infection, *Staphylococcus aureus* and *H. influenzae* are often implicated as the causative origins. The disease is contracted primarily through tissue inoculation via retropharyngeal trauma, such as surgery, dental work, falling onto popsicle/lollipop stick, etc. Other etiologies include otitis media, parotitis, and retropharyngeal adenopathy from naso-pharyngitis.

10.1 Clinical Evaluation:

A. **Symptoms:** Sore throat, progressive sensation of mass in throat, dysphagia, ± difficulty breathing, ± fever, ± toxic appearing, ± cough, and pleuritic chest pain. Inquire about recent trauma to mouth or pharynx.

B. **Signs:** Hyponasal voice, muffled voice, noisy breathing, toxic appearance, dehydration, stiff and painful neck. Redness or swelling to the neck with tenderness to palpation. Pharyngeal wall may appear erythematous, boggy, and displaced toward the uvula.

C. **DDX:** Pharyngitis, foreign body, epiglottitis, croup, tonsillar abscess, submandibular abscess, Ludwig's angina, Diptheria, and vascular anomaly.

D. **Work-up:** Order CBC, SMA-7, and throat, blood and urine cultures for fever. Soft tissue neck films may reveal prevertebral soft tissue swelling, ± AFL, normal trachea, and epiglottis. Consider CT if needed.

10.2 RX:

A. Support ABCs. Maintain equipment for emergency management of the airway, including cricothyroidotomy set. Monitor the patient carefully for respiratory distress. Obtain otolaryngologic consultation for surgical I&D. Administer IV antibiotics, including nafcillin, 100-150 mg/kg/day q 4 hours IV, plus metronidazole, 35-50 mg/kg/day tid IV, **or** clindamycin, 15-40 mg/kg/day q 6-8 hours IV, plus a cephalosporin.

B. **Disposition:** Admit, either to intensive care or directly to the OR.

PSYCHIATRY

1. Anorexia Nervosa:

1.1 Clinical Evaluation:

A. **Symptoms:** Refusal to maintain body weight over a minimum normal weight, profound weight loss, disturbed body image, preoccupation with losing weight, excessive dieting and exercise, and absence of menses.

B. **Signs:** Bradycardia, hypothermia, pedal or pretibial edema, brittle hair and nails, petechiae or purpura, peripheral neuropathy, paresthesias of the fingers and toes, diminished deep tendon reflexes, and impaired gross motor coordination.

C. **DDX:** Schizophrenia, depressive illness, hysterics, borderline personality disorders, superior mesenteric artery syndrome, inflammatory bowel disease, chronic hepatitis, Addison's disease, diabetes, hyperthyroidism, hyperemesis gravidarum, tuberculosis, and malignancy.

D. **Work-up:** Consider CBC, electrolytes, BUN, creatinine, liver function studies, glucose, magnesium, lipase, and ECG.

1.2 RX:

A. Start aggressive replacement with isotonic saline, thiamine, multivitamins, and magnesium.

B. Consider admission with a psychiatric and internal medicine consultant.

C. **Disposition:** Hospitalization is suggested for the following: Weight loss > 30% over 3 months, severe metabolic disturbance, depression severe enough to be at risk for suicide, severe bingeing and purging, failure to maintain outpatient weight contract, psychosis, family crisis. It may be necessary to confront patient and family denial. Suggest the initiation of therapy (individual, family, and pharmacotherapy), and complex differential diagnosis.

2. Bulimia Nervosa:

2.1 Clinical Evaluation:

A. **Symptoms:** Eating binges, self-induced vomiting, or diarrhea secondary to laxative abuse, preoccupation with diet and exercise, and disturbed body image. Symptoms of esophagitis.

B. **Signs:** Normal weight, parotid and submandibular swelling, scars and abrasions on the knuckles and hands, unexplained amenorrhea, and extensive loss of dental enamel.

C. **DDX:** Primary affective or schizophrenic disorder.

D. **Work-up:** Obtain electrolytes, CBC, lipase, liver function studies. Determine BUN and creatinine, and glucose level.

2.2 RX:

A. Initiate aggressive replacement with isotonic saline, thiamine, multivitamins, and magnesium. A period of 48 hours in an inpatient setting is important in order to determine the extent and severity of illness and its complications.

B. **Disposition:**

Admit to an "Eating Disorders" unit if possible and obtain a psychiatric and internal medicine evaluation should.

Hospitalization is suggested for the following: Weight loss > 30% over 3 months, severe metabolic disturbance, depression severe enough to be at risk for suicide, severe bingeing and purging, failure to maintain outpatient weight contract, psychosis, family crisis. It may be necessary to confront the patient and the family members. Suggest the initiation of therapy.

3. Conversion Disorder:

3.1 Clinical Evaluation:

A. **Symptoms:** The most typical conversion symptoms involve loss of neurologic functions, such as blindness, aphonia, seizures, paralysis, hemianesthesia, tunnel vision, unresponsiveness, and amnesia. An attitude of relative unconcern despite the seriousness of the symptoms that may be present (La Belle indifference) along with vomiting and symptoms of pregnancy.

B. **Signs:** Inconsistent and incomplete sensory loss of one leg with preservation of deep tendon reflexes and antigravity muscle activity. Slowness of motion, inconsistencies in physical signs during unresponsiveness may be present. Non-organically unresponsive patients always demonstrate both the fast and slow component of nystagmus on oculovestibular stimulation. Inconsistencies in blindness and cogwheel response on manual muscle testing are evident.

C. **DDX:** Conversion disorder must be distinguished from organic illness, malingering, and Munchausen's syndrome, as well as from somatization disorders and hypochondriasis.

3.2 RX:

A. Patients with conversion disorders must be handled delicately, deftly, and with a great deal of respect. The patient should be told that although the symptoms are bothersome, they do not appear to be manifestations of a serious illness. Simultaneously, the physician can probe for underlying psychosocial conflicts that may lead to the appearance of symptoms.

B. **Disposition:**

Request a neurologic consultant to assist in differentiating organic from nonorganic.

Many patients with conversion disorders experience resolution of their physical symptoms during their ED stay but others require admission to the hospital.

If the diagnosis of conversion disorder is uncertain and if presenting symptoms could signify dangerous illness, hospital admission is warranted.

Even when the diagnosis of conversion disorder is clear, patients with persistent manifestations and those who cannot manage on their own require inpatient care.

4. Depression and Suicide:

4.1 Clinical Evaluation:

A. **Symptoms:** Vague, ill-defined somatic symptoms, pain in a wide variety of anatomic sites, nervous symptoms, such as increased tension and feelings of anxiety, self- inflicted wounds, drug overdoses, and falls from heights. Symptoms of depression include a diminished sense of self-esteem and general physical and mental well being, including loss of interest in or employment of pleasurable activities, loss of energy, poor appetite, sleep disturbances, decreased attention span and concentration ability, decreased effectiveness or productivity at school, work, or home, episodes of tearfulness or crying, irritability or excessive anger, pessimistic attitude toward the future, and recurrent thoughts of death or suicide.

B. **Signs:** Detailed neurologic workup, including extensive mental status examination.

C. **Work-up:** Consider thyroid studies, CBC, SMA-7, and liver function studies as well as ammonia levels where indicated. Chemical and mechanical restraint may be necessary. Obtain a psychiatric consultation.

4.2 RX:

A. A potentially suicidal patient generally requires admission to an inpatient psychiatric unit. Do not consider discharge from ED unless the following conditions have been met.

The patient has been evaluated and deemed actively nonsuicidal or at risk to self or others.

Short-term outpatient follow-up can be arranged.

The patient agrees to return to the ED immediately if further self-destructive urges arise.
A positive, supportive environment of family or friends is available into which the patient can be released. Transfer of patient who is suicidal requires formal "commitment" of patient so personnel have authority to restrain patient prn.

5. Management of the Difficult Patient:

A high index of suspicion of an organic cause must be maintained in order to reach an accurate diagnosis in the difficult-to-manage patient. The acutely psychotic patient may harm himself/herself, or others to avoid some imagined or projected threat. These types of patients may also pose danger simply because he/she is confused.

5.1 Clinical Evaluation:

A. **Symptoms:** Onset of abnormal behavior, psychiatric history, and history of violent behavior or assault. Ask about medication specifically pain pills, nerve pills, sleeping pills, and any other pills that the patient may have been using recently.

B. **Signs:** If the patient is confused, his wallet, purse, or pocket should be searched for medication, identification, and physician appointment cards. The patient's muscle tone and overall state of attention may indicate that he is posed for fight or flight. Speech may be loud or profane, indicating impending loss of control. Motor activity, such as restlessness or pacing, especially if it is escalating, is another clue.

C. **DDX:** Drug or alcohol withdrawal, hypoglycemia, meningitis or encephalitis, hypertensive encephalopathy, intracranial hemorrhage, subdural or epidural hematoma, thyrotoxicosis, porphyria, and hemorrhagic shock.

D. **Work-up:** The workup is extensive and may require a CT scan, ECG, CXR, electrolytes, CBC, blood cultures, liver function studies with ammonia, alcohol level, and a screen for drugs of abuse.

5.2 RX:

A. Physical restraints may be required for protection of the patient and staff. Chemical restraint such as a neuroleptic drug may be necessary to decrease agitation, such as:

Haloperidol, 5-10 mg IM q 30 minutes up to a 40 mg maximum, **or** chlorpromazine (Thorazine), 100 mg IM, **or** trifluoperazine (Stelazine), 10 mg IM, **or** thiothixene (Navane), 10 mg IM.

Consider prophylactic administration of an anti-Parkinson drug, such as benztropine, 2 mg IM.
When physical restraint is necessary, each staff member must physically cease and/or control movements in one of the patient's extremity. The patient is brought to the ground backwards while protecting the head. The legs are restrained at the knees. The patient's arms are crossed over the head to control head movement. After physical control is established, the patient can be moved to a seclusion room. A suitable number of staff members must be available to lift the patient in the recumbent position with his/her arms pinned to the sides.

B. **Disposition:** Agitated or violent patients who require the use of restraints or medication should be considered for evaluation by a psychiatric consultant and for admission to an inpatient facility. Even after behavioral control is achieved, long term treatment may be necessary and more complete medical assessment is often required as well.

6. Panic Disorder:

6.1 Clinical Evaluation:

A. **Symptoms:** Sudden extreme surge of anxiety, dread, palpitations, tachycardia, shortness of breath, chest tightness, dizziness, sweating, and tremulousness.

B. **Signs:** Typically there are no specific physical findings other than tachycardia and tachypnea.

C. **DDX:** Thyrotoxicosis, carcinoid syndrome, hypoglycemia, pheochromocytoma, migraine, myocardial infarction, cardiac arrhythmia, schizophrenia, depressive disorders, somatoform disorders, phobic disorders, post-traumatic stress disorder, drug withdrawal, complex-partial seizures, and alcohol withdrawal.

D. **Work-up:** Order ECG, CXR, thyroid profile, glucose level, and electrolyte profile.

6.2 RX:

A. Benzodiazepines are generally considered the first line of treatment because they are safe and have a relatively rapid onset of action. Other helpful drugs are sedating antihistamines, diphenhydramine (Benadryl) and hydroxyzine (Vistaril and Atarax).

B. **Disposition:** When diagnosis is certain, psychiatric consultation is indicated. If the patient has responded to emergency intervention and family support is available, consultation can be accomplished on an outpatient basis. Consider inpatient care for all patients who do not respond to supportive measures in the ED or those who are a suicide risk.

PULMONARY

AIRWAY MANAGEMENT & INTUBATION

There is no single guideline for managing the airway. Differences in clinical presentation and condition, patient anatomy, situation, and physician and institution practices mandate that airway management be individually customized. The following are some suggestions; however, obtain consultation with appropriate specialists as clinically indicated.

1. Orotracheal Intubation:

A. ETT Size (interior diameter):
   Women: 7.0-9.0 mm.
   Men: 7.5-10.0 mm.
   Peds: (Age + 16)/4 mm.

B. Prepare all equipment, including suction, O_2, bag-valve- mask, ET tubes, cricothyroidotomy or needle-jet equipment, CO_2 indicator, laryngoscope, and pulse oximeter.

C. If sedation and/or paralysis is required, prepare all meds, including those required for a rapid sequence induction, if so planned. These may include:
   Fentanyl (Sublimaze), 50 μg increments IV (2-3 mg/kg).
   Midazolam (Versed), 1 mg IV every 2-3 minutes, maximum 0.1-0.15 mg/kg.
   Vecuronium, 0.015 mg/kg priming dose (at 1 mg adult) and 0.15 mg/kg paralytic dose (at 7-10 mg).
   Atropine, 0.01 mg/kg with more available for peds < 3 years.
   Lidocaine, 1.0-1.5 mg/kg;
   Pentothal, 4 mg/kg IV;
   Succinylcholine, 1 mg/kg. There is a risk for vomiting and aspiration; therefore, apply cricoid cartilage pressure as soon as the patient is unable to protect airway (Sellick maneuver).
   Considerable expertise is required for use of paralyzing agents and rapid sequence intubation.

D. Position patient's head in a "sniffing" position with head flexed at neck and extended. If necessary, elevate head with a small pillow or towel.

E. Preoxygenate by allowing patient to breathe 100% oxygen. Avoid unnecessary gastric filling by minimizing assisted bag-valve-mask ventilation.

F. Hold laryngoscope handle with left hand. Insert along right side of mouth to the base of tongue and push tongue to left. Advance to the vallecula (superior to epiglottis, if using curved blade) and lift anteriorly. If a straight blade is used, place it beneath the epiglottis and lift anteriorly.

G. Intubate until cuff disappears behind vocal cords. If unsuccessful after 30 seconds, stop and resume bag-valve-mask ventilation before re-attempting.

H. Inflate cuff with syringe and attach the tube to an Ambu bag or ventilator.

I. Confirm ET tube location by checking for equal bilateral breath sounds, no gastric air, CO_2 monitor or syringe test and CXR. If any questions arise about proper ETT location, repeat laryngoscopy with tube in place to ensure it is endotracheal. Secure tube with tape and note centimeter mark at the mouth. Suction oropharynx and trachea.

2. Nasotracheal Intubation:

Nasotracheal intubation may be the preferred method if prolonged intubation is anticipated (increased patient comfort). Intubation can be facilitated if patient is awake and breathing spontaneously.Use of a tube with directional tip control ("ringed", Endotrol) may also help.

A. ETT Size (interior diameter):
   Women: 6.0-7.0 mm tube.
   Men: 7.5-9.0 mm tube.

B. Spray nasal passage with vasoconstrictor spray, such as cocaine 4%, 4 cc , **or** phenylephrine 0.25% (Neo-Synephrine), 2 cc, unless contraindicated. Apply topical anesthesia with viscous lidocaine 2% or topical spray. If sedation is required, administer fentanyl, 1 μg/kg, **or** midazolam, 0.05-0.1 mg/kg, titrate.

C. Position patient. Intubation may be performed with patient sitting up. Place tube into nasal passage and guide it into nasopharynx. Monitor progress by listening for air movement and observing fogging of the tube. As the tube enters oropharynx, gradually guide the tube downward. If the sounds stop, withdraw the tube 1-2 cm until breath sounds are heard again. Reposition the tube, and if necessary, extend the head and advance. If difficulty is encountered, perform laryngoscopy under direct visualization or use Magill forceps.

D. Successful intubation occurs when the tube passes through the cords. A cough may occur and breath sounds will reach a maximum intensity if the tube is correctly positioned. Confirm placement of tube as cited in the "Orotracheal Intubation" section.

PULMONARY CASES

1. Asthma:

1.1 Clinical Evaluation:

A. **Symptoms:** Prior known history, recent exposure to trigger, and aggravated wheezing and dyspnea.

B. **Signs:** Anxious, tachypneic, wheezing, accessory muscle use, cough, and cyanosis. Be alert of patients moving very little air that they are not wheezing and those that are tiring from respiratory effort.

C. **DDX:** Pneumonia, bronchitis, croup, bronchiolitis, COPD, congestive heart failure, pulmonary embolism, allergic reaction, and upper airway obstruction.

D. **Work-up:** Peak flow measurements mandatory. Pulse oximetry and/or ABG may be useful in patients with severe symptoms. Order CXR and labs prn.

1.2 RX:

A. Maintain O_2 saturation > 90% with supplemental oxygen. Monitor peak flow rates before and after bronchodilator treatments.

B. Treatment may include:

   Albuterol (Ventolin), 2.5 mg, in 3 mL of saline q 20 minutes.

   Epinephrine, 0.3-0.5 mL of 1:1000 sq given q 20 minutes for 3. Determine relative contraindications in ages > 40 years and do not administer to patients with known coronary artery disease, if it can be prevented.

   Terbutaline, 0.25 mg sq q 30 minutes up to x 3. This drug is preferred over epinephrine for pregnant patients.

   Steroids, such as methylprednisolone (Solu-Medrol), 60-120 mg IV (optimal dosing is unknown), **or** prednisone, 40-60 mg po. Some recent research suggest oral glucocorticoids may be as effective and as fast-acting as IV administration.

Magnesium sulfate, 2 g IV over 20 minutes, may be transiently useful.

Heliox (80% Helium + 20% O_2) via face mask is also effective.

C. **Disposition:** Asthmatic patients should not have to stay longer than 4 hours in the ED. During that time, a decision to admit or discharge has to be made. A decision to admit a patient is based primarily on clinical impression and peak flow measurements. Admit patients showing no improvement, tiring from work of breathing (objectively measured by rising CO_2), exhibiting low peak flows, and displaying other complications, such as pneumonia or ischemia. Patients returning to the ED after a recent previous visit should also be admitted. There is a low threshold to admit pregnant asthmatics. All asthmatics discharged from the ED should have their medications carefully checked, be given adequate prescriptions, and be advised to seek medical attention as an outpatient within the week.

2. Aspiration Pneumonia:

2.1 Clinical Evaluation:

A. **Symptoms:** Risk factors include debilitation, cerebrovascular accident, CP, seizures, alcoholic, use of depressant drugs, dyspnea, and chest pain.

B. **Signs:** Copious foul-smelling purulent sputum, cough, fever and hypothermia, rales, and egophony.

C. **Work-up:** Order CXR, CBC, sputum for Gram's stain, C&S, pulse oximetry, and ABG with A-a gradient. Obtain other labs as pertinent for history.

2.2 RX:

A. Manage airway and maintain adequate oxygenation with supplemental O_2. Rehydrate. Administer clindamycin (Cleocin), 600 mg IV q 8 hours, and gentamicin, 1-1.5 mg/kg IV or 5-7 mg1kg q 24 hours, or ampicillin/Sulbactam (Unasyn), 1.5-3 g IV q 6 hours, or ticarcillin/clavulanate (Timentin), 3.1 g IV q 6-8 hours.

B. **Disposition:** Admit.

3. COPD / Bronchitis:

Treatable component of COPD is caused by tracheo-bronchial inflammation and mucous production leading to chronic, productive cough. Pathology implicated in its etiology include previous infection, cigarettes, and environmental pollutants which increase secretions and impair mucociliary response. Although most episodes have viral etiology, superimposed and chronic bacterial infections contribute to inflammation and chronic obstruction.

3.1 Clinical Evaluation:

A. **Symptoms:** Stages are as follows.

Morning/smoker's cough, no respiratory difficulty.

Periodic exacerbations of copious, purulent sputum, a "chest cold", with little dyspnea or disability.

Chronic cough, DOE, and disability. Severe, heightened symptoms with "colds". Clinical evidence suggestive of central cyanosis and chronic hypoxia/hypercarbia, early right heart failure.

Progressive disability, DOE with minimal exertion. Chronic respiratory difficulties of cough paroxysms and wheezing. Work up reveals cor pulmonale.

End stage. Incapacitation, O_2 dependence, chronic dyspnea at rest, chronic respiratory failure, and refractory cor pulmonale.

B. **Signs:** ± obese, ± central cyanosis, pursed lip breathing, loose rales, rhonchi, and diffuse wheezes.

S4 suggests low RV compliance, S3 RV failure and systolic murmur may suggest tricuspid insufficiency. Sputum may reveal mixed bag of bugs.

C. **DDX:** Pneumonia, atelectasis, asthma, congestive heart failure, cardiogenic shock, ARDS, pulmonary embolism, foreign body, aspiration pneumonitis, and tumor.

D. **Work-up:** ABG more reliable than FEV1. pCO_2 indicates adequacy of ventilation, pO_2 the degree of hypoxia. Ex: 80-100, stage A; 60-80, stage B; < 60, stage C. pH and HCO_3 values indicate the degree of respiratory and renal compensation. CXR verifies ± atelectasis, edema, infiltrate (rarely hyperexpanded) and ± cardiomegaly. FEV1 low (establish < 60 to > 300) is useful for baseline comparison prior to exacerbation and as an indicator of clinical response to treatment.

3.2 RX:

A. Support airway, IV, O_2, and monitor. Increase O_2 by 1-2 L/minute prn.

B. Prescribe bronchodilators, such as β-adrenergics (albuterol, 0.5 cc of 0.5%, metaproterenol, 0.3 cc of 0.5%). Anticholinergics, including glycopyrrolate neb or ipratropium bromide MDI may emerge to play a role in acute ED management.

C. Treat with steroids, including prednisone, 40-60 mg po initial dose, **or** methylprednisolone, 60-125 mg IV (or equivalent) q 6 hours for acute flare. Taper doses of outpatient prednisone over 5-7 days beginning at 40-60 mg.

D. Administer antibiotics although data are unclear of their efficacy.

For inpatients, treat with ampicillin, 1 g IV q 6 hours, **or** 250-500 mg po q 6-8 hours, **or** TMP/SMX (Septra, Bactrim D), 160/800 mg po bid, **or** ampicillin/sulbactam (Unasyn), 1.5 g IV q 6 hours, **or** cefuroxime, 1.5 g IV q 8 hours.

For outpatients, prescribe doxycycline, 100 mg po q 12 hours for 10 days, erythromycin, 333 mg po q 8 hours for 10 days, TMP/SMX day q 12 hours for 10 days. Cephalosporin 1, ciprofloxacin, or Augmentin are no longer effective.

E. **Disposition:** Admit patients with acute exacerbation or little clinical improvement with treatment. Consider outpatient follow-up if respiratory status, FEV, and patient 'road tests' improve.

4. Hemoptysis:

Inflammatory (bronchitis, bronchiectasis, lung abscess, pneumonia, and TB). Neoplastic, cardiovascular (AV malformation, congestive heart failure, pulmonary embolism, pulmonary hypertension, mitral stenosis), and congenital (cystic fibrosis). Immunologic, extrapulmonary (thrombocytopenia, coagulopathy, and trauma).

4.1 Clinical Evaluation:

A. **Signs:** Quantify the bleeding as massive (600 mL/24-48 hours or a rate of > 100 mL/hour), or submassive. Seek history of pulmonary embolism associated with coagulopathy.

B. **Work-up:** T&C 4-6 units PRBCs. Pulse oximetry, ABG, CBC, platelets, SMA-7, and PT/PTT. Sputum gram stain, C&S, AFB, parasites and fungal, and cytology. CXR and ECG. Consider nasopharyngoscopy to rule out upper airway source, a VQ scan, and a contrast CT scan.

4.2 RX:

A. Manage airway. Obtain immediate thoracic surgical consultation for massive hemoptysis. Keep patient in lateral decubitus and Trendelenburg positions. Quantify all sputum and blood, suction prn. Transfuse and manage coagulopathy as indicated. Consider empiric antibiotics if infection may be contributing to hemoptysis.

B. **Disposition:** Transfer patient with massive bleeding to ICU and refer to a surgeon. Bronchitis is usually managed as an outpatient. Discharge only those patients who are reliable and stable. Arrange an appropriate follow-up.

5. Pleural Effusion:

There are many causes for pleural effusion, including acute aortic dissection, esophageal rupture, pulmonary embolism, congestive heart failure, pulmonary infection, tumor, sarcoid, cirrhosis, pancreatitis, nephrotic syndrome, and myxedema.

5.1 Clinical Evaluation:

A. **Symptoms:** Occasionally asymptomatic, weight loss, fever, orthopnea, edema, cough, dyspnea, and chest pain.

B. **Signs:** Decreased breath sounds with dullness to percussion.

C. **DDX:** Pneumonia or other infiltrate, tumor, and herniated diaphragm with viscera in thorax.

D. **Work-up:** CXR, pulse oximetry, ABG, CBC, SMA-7, LFTs, amylase, lipase, protein, PT, ECG, and thoracentesis. Pleural fluid:

Tube 1: LDH, protein, amylase, lipase triglyceride, and glucose (10 mL).
Tube 2: Gram stain, C&S, AFB, fungal C&S, and wet mount (20-60 mg heparinized).
Tube 3: Cell count and differential (5-10 mL of EDTA).

5.2 RX:

A. Manage airway and maintain adequate oxygenation with supplemental O_2. Consider thoracentesis for diagnostic or therapeutic purposes.

B. **Disposition:** If a thoracentesis is performed in the ED, consider admission. Patients with an effusion not evacuated may require admission, depending on the severity of their symptoms, underlying diagnosis, and response to treatment.

RESPIRATORY FAILURE and VENTILATOR MANAGEMENT

Potential indications for ventilatory support: Patient appears in severe respiratory distress. Patient can't state their name due to respiratory distress, impending respiratory failure, and uncorrectable hypoxia by ABG or pulse oximetry. Decision in ED is primarily based on clinical impression.
Sample initial orders: FiO_2 = 100%, PEEP = 3-5 cm H_2O, assist control 8-14 breaths/minute, tidal volume = 800 mL (10-15 mL/kg ideal body weight), set rate so that minute ventilation (VE) is approximately 10 L/minute.
If patient is "fighting" ventilator despite appropriate sensitivity, flow rate settings, and tidal volume, consider IMV or SIMV mode, or add sedation with or without paralysis (exclude complications or other causes of agitation).
Never use paralytic agents without concurrent analgesia/sedation.

RADIOGRAPHIC EVALUATION OF COMMON INTERVENTION PEARLS

1. Central Intravenous Lines:

Central venous catheters should be located well above the right atrium in the superior Venn cava. Rule out pneumothorax by ensuring that the lung markings extend completely to the rib cages on both sides. An upright, expiratory X-ray may be helpful. Examine for a hydropericardium ("water bottle" sign, mediastinal widening). Pulmonary artery catheters should be positioned centrally and posteriorly and must not be more than 3-5 cm from midline.

2. Endotracheal Tubes:

After insertion, verify that the tube is located 3 cm below the vocal cords and 2-4 cm above the carina. The tip of the tube should be at the level of the aortic arch.

3. Tracheostomy:

Ensure, by CXR, that the tube is located half the distance from the stoma to the carina. The tube should be parallel to the long axis of the trachea. The tube should also be approximately 2/3 of width of trachea and the cuff must not cause bulging of the trachea walls. Check for subcutaneous air in the neck tissue and for mediastinal widening secondary to air leakage.

4. Nasogastric Tubes:

Verify that tube is located in the stomach and not coiled in the esophagus or in trachea. The tip of the tube should not be near the gastroesophageal junction.

5. Chest Tubes:

A chest tube for pneumothorax drainage should be superior and nearly level to the third intercostal space. To drain a free flowing pulmonary effusion, position the tube inferior-posteriorly at or about the level of the eighth intercostal space. Verify that the proximal side port of the tube is within the chest cavity.

6. Mechanical Ventilator:

After initiation, obtain CXR to eliminate the possibility of pneumothorax, subcutaneous emphysema, pneumomediastinum, or subpleural air cysts. Infiltrates may diminish or disappear due to increased aeration of the affected lung lobe.

RHEUMATOLOGIC / ALLERGIC

1. Anaphylaxis:

Anaphylaxis is a life-threatening allergic reaction that occurs in sensitized persons causing the release of histamine, prostaglandins, and kallikrein from mast cells and basophils. Mediators illicit massive vasodilation and capillary leakage that results in hypotension, urticaria, and angioedema of the skin, upper airway, and GI tract. Most common antigens are penicillin and bee/wasp stings. Laryngeal edema may obstruct upper airway obstruction and, if untreated, can result in the death of the patient. Urticaria is edema of superficial dermis and appears as red wheals. Angioedema is edema of deep dermis. A patient with the latter condition exhibits swelling of the mucous membranes that is prominent in face, lips, and pharynx.

1.1 Clinical Evaluation:

A. **Symptoms:** Antibiotics, NSAIDS, aspirin, iodinated contrast media, Hymenoptera stings, and seafood. Onset is < 1 hour after exposure. Early symptoms are itching, a warm feeling, chest tightness, and a lump in the throat. Dizziness, secondary to hypotension, occurs after a prolonged period of exposure.

B. **Signs:** Tachycardia, arrhythmia, and hypotension. Angioedema, stridor, wheezing, decreased breath sounds, and urticaria.

C. **DDX:** Hereditary angioedema, viral or bacterial infection, scombroid fish poisoning, reaction to monosodium glutamate, and carcinoid syndrome.

1.2 RX:

A. For mild cases, treat with diphenhydramine (Benadryl), 50 mg po and severe IV.

B. For severe cases, treat as follows.
   Methylprednisolone (Solu-Medrol), 60-125 mg IV push (Peds, 1 mg/kg).
   Zantac, 50 mg IV.
   Epinephrine (1:1000 solution), 0.3 cc sq (Peds, 0.001 mg/kg).
   Epinephrine (1:1000 solution), 0.4 cc may be given sublingually.

C. In life-threatening situations, give epinephrine, 0.3-0.5 mg of 1:10,000 solution IV.

D. For persistent shock, administer 1 mg in 250 cc D_5W and infuse at 2 μg/minute-IV RL wide open.

E. For persistent hypotension, treat with MAST suit and dopamine infusion.

F. If patient with mild allergic reaction responds rapidly and completely, observe in ED for 3 hours. Admit all moderate or severe cases for observation.

G. **Disposition:** Admit all unstable patients to ICU.

2. The Hot Joint:

Causes of monoarticular arthritis include trauma, crystal-induced and non-crystal induced inflammation, immunologic disorders, degenerative joint disease, and infection. The organism that typically induces this infection is *Gonococcus*, followed by *Staphylococcus*, *Streptococcus*, *Pseudomonas* (IV drug abusers), and *Salmonella* (sicklers). The timely diagnosis of septic arthritis is the most important consideration in the ED.

2.1 Clinical Evaluation:

A. **Symptoms:** Viral syndrome, pharyngitis, trauma, fever, vaginal, urethral discharge, rash, alcohol, IV drug abuse, previous episodes, major diseases, and meds.

B. **Signs:** Fever, tachycardia, tophi, pharyngitis, rales, murmur, and abdominal organomegaly or tenderness. Affected joint-hot, edematous, red, tender, and decreased ROM. First MP, ankle (gout), knee (pseudogout, infectious), and sternoclavicular joint (IV drug abuse).

C. **DDX:** Cellulitis, bursitis, gout, pseudogout, septic arthritis, trauma, osteoarthritis, rheumatoid arthritis, collagen vascular disease, and coagulopathy.

D. **Work-up:** Order CBC, SMA-7, ESR, joint X-ray, and blood C&S.

Arthrocentesis: Synovial fluid analysis for appearance, viscosity, cell count with differential, glucose level, presence of crystals, Gram stain, and C&S. Normal synovial fluid is clear yellow, viscous, WBC < 200/μL, and glucose >50% of serum glucose.

Hemorrhagic (trauma, coagulopathy) has bloody appearance.

Inflammatory (osteo/rheumatoid, psoriatic) has opaque appearance, low viscosity, glucose 90-100%, rheumatoid may show > 75, and cell count 2000-50,000 WBC/μL.

Crystal-induced (gout, pseudogout) shows inflammatory response plus urate crystals of gout or positively birefringent calcium pyrophosphate crystals of pseudogout.

Infection has opaque turbid appearance, low viscosity, glucose < 40, and cell count > 50,000. Gram stain is positive in 75% of infectious arthritis.

2.2 RX:

A. Therapeutic arthrocentesis for tense joint effusion.

B. For hemorrhagic patients, splint and elevate the affected area. Advise patient not to place weight on the area. Treat for analgesia and apply appropriate therapy for bleeding disorder.

C. For inflammation, treat with indomethacin (Indocin), 25 mg q 6 hours prn, or aspirin.

D. For crystal-induced cases, administer indomethacin 50 mg qid for 2 days, followed by 25 mg qid prn, **or** colchicine, 2 mg IV (diluted in 20 cc NS injected slowly), **or** 0.6 mg po q 2 hours until symptoms subside or nausea/diarrhea occurs.

E. Treat infectious cases as follows.

For gram-positive infections, administer nafcillin, 1 g IV q 6 hours.

For gram-negative rod infections, treat with gentamicin, 5-7 mg/kg/day, + carbenicillin, 500 mg/kg/day IV.

For *H. influenzae*, give ampicillin, 200 mg/kg/day, + chloramphenicol, 50 mg/kg/day IV.

For *Gonococcus* infections, prescribe pen G, 10 million units/day IV.

F. **Disposition:** Admit all patients with infectious causes. Discharge all others.

TOXICOLOGY

1. General:

Toxicity results from the ingestion of a toxic substance or from an overdose of prescription or non-prescription drugs.

1.1 Clinical Evaluation:

A. **Symptoms:** History is extremely important. Obtain information from patient, friends, relatives, and EMS. Drug bottles should be brought to ED. Time of ingestion, quantity of drugs consumed, the occurrence of vomiting, psychiatric history, previous similar episodes, drug and alcohol abuse, and change in mental status before and after ingestion must be determined.

B. **Signs**:

Change in mental status: Loss of consciousness (Glasgow coma scale), confusion/delirium (cocaine, narcotics, and PCP), and mania (PCP).
Vital signs: Temperature, hyperthermia (atropine), tachycardia (cyclic antidepressants, and cocaine), bradycardia (narcotics and organophosphates), hyperventilation (aspirin and acidosis), and bradypnea (narcotics).
Skin for redness: (CO and anticholinergics), track marks.
HEENT: Signs of trauma, pupil size, equality and light reaction (narcotics, barbiturates- miosis, cocaine- mydriasis), fundi, visual acuity, and nystagmus (PCP).
Neuromuscular: Dystonic reaction (phenothiazines).

C. **Work-up:** Depends on presentation. Consider CBC, SMA-7, toxicology screen, or ASA/acetaminophen/alcohol levels. Specific drug levels, ABG, osmolality, CXR, CO, KUB, and U/A may also be useful.

1.2 RX:

A. Support airway, IV, O_2, and monitor.

B. Treat patients with decreased level of consciousness with opioid antagonist naloxone (Narcan), 2 mg IV, thiamine, 100 mg IV, glucose 1 amp D_{50} IV.

C. Prevent absorption by using activated charcoal, 1 g/kg po or a NG tube. (Do not use with caustics, hydrocarbons, lithium, or iron.) Repeat doses q 2-4 hours in some cases. Gastric lavage may be performed if ingestion occurred within the 1 hour or if indicated otherwise. Intubation should be performed first if there is a decreased level of consciousness and no gag reflex.

D. After ethanol therapy, perform immediate dialysis with methanol and ethylene glycol, salicylate level 100 mg% or greater, lithium level > 3.5 mg%.

E. **Disposition:** Admit for all but benign ingestions. Recommend psychiatric consultation as indicated.

2. Acetaminophen:

Acetaminophen is metabolized in the liver. A small dosage of the drug is metabolized via the cytochrome P-450 oxidase system to a final toxic metabolite. This metabolite is detoxified by glutathione and excreted in urine. In the case of an overdose of acetaminophen, glutathione is depleted and the toxic metabolite accumulates in liver. Hepatic necrosis is thereby induced.

Phase I (to 24 hours): Anorexia, nausea, and vomiting.
Phase II (24-72 hours): Abdominal pain.
Phase III (3-5 days): Jaundice, hypoglycemia, coagulopathy, and encephalopathy.
Phase IV (1 week): Resolution if Phase III is not lethal.

2.1 Clinical Evaluation:

A. **Symptoms:** Identification of drug, time of ingestion, medical and psychiatric illnesses, and current meds. Nausea, vomiting, abdominal pain, diaphoresis, malaise, and jaundice (sometimes asymptomatic).

B. **Signs:** Change in mental status, scleral icterus, hepatomegaly, RUQ tenderness, pallor, diaphoresis, and jaundice.

C. **DDX:** Liver disease, including alcoholic and viral hepatitis, gall-bladder and biliary tract disease, and amanita mushroom poisoning.

D. **Work-up:** Order CBC, SMA-7, PT, PTT, LFTs, toxicology screen, and serum acetaminophen level. A nomogram is valid at 4 hours.

2.2 RX:

A. Support airway, IV, O_2, and monitor. Administer naloxone, thiamine, glucose, and charcoal (refer to the "General" section). Consider gastric lavage if presentation within 1 hour of ingestion.

B. Toxicity by nomogram, > 150 µg/mL at 4 hours, requires administration of glutathione-substitute N-acetylcysteine (Mucomyst and NAC). Standard loading dose is 140 mg/kg diluted with soda or juice, followed by 70 mg/kg q 4 hours for 17 doses. Consider 48 hours IV NAC (not yet FDA approved) at the same doses and frequency or a higher load with charcoal, 235 mg/kg.

C. **Disposition:** Admit all patients requiring NAC. Refer to a psychiatric consultation.

3. Alcohols:

Methanol (wood alcohol) is found in antifreeze, paint solvents, canned fuels (Sterno), gasoline additives and home heating fuels. It is metabolized in the liver to formic acid. **Ethylene glycol** is a component of detergents, paints, antifreeze and coolants. This alcohol is metabolized to glycolic and oxalic acids. Both methanol and ethylene glycol produce profound anion gap acidosis. **Isopropyl alcohol** (rubbing alcohol) is metabolized to acetone but does not cause acidosis. (Refer to the "Endocrine/Alcoholic Ketoacidosis" section for a discussion on ethanol.)

3.1 Clinical Evaluation:

A. **Symptoms:** Symptoms of isopropyl alcohol ingestion are similar to acute ethanol intoxication. CNS depression, nausea, and vomiting are exhibited. Symptoms of nausea, vomiting, abdominal pain, and blurred or change in vision occur 1 to 2 days after ingestion of methanol. Symptoms of ethylene glycol toxicity are displayed 1 to 12 hours after ingestion and include slurred speech and lethargy. Within 12 hours, cardiac and respiratory symptoms occurs, including palpitations and SOB. If patient survives this stage, renal failure transpires at about 48 hours as a result of intratubular deposition of oxalate crystals.

B. **Signs:**

Decreased level of consciousness (methanol, ethylene glycol, and isopropyl alcohol).

Vitals: Tachycardia, hypertension (ethylene glycol), and hyperventilation (compensatory from metabolic acidosis - methanol or ethylene glycol).

Photophobia, mydriasis, hyperemia of optic disk, papilledema (methanol), and nystagmus (ethylene glycol).

Rales and arrhythmias (ethylene glycol).

Abdomen: Diffuse tenderness (methanol and isopropyl alcohol).

Neuro: Ataxia, myoclonus (ethylene glycol), confusion, and seizures (methanol and ethylene glycol).

C. **DDX:** Differential of change in mental status: TIPS-AEIOU (Refer to "Sedative/Hypnotics" and "Change in Mental status" within the Neurology section).

D. **Work-up:** Order CBC, SMA-7, ABG, U/A, serum osmolality, toxicology screen, serum methanol and ethylene glycol (if available), CXR, and ECG (as needed). (Refer also to "Anion Gap Metabolic Acidosis" section.) Serum acetaminophen and salicylate level.

3.2 RX:

A. Support airway, IV, O_2, and monitor. Administer naloxone, thiamine, and glucose (refer to the "General" section).
B. Use a symptomatic treatment for isopropyl alcohol poisoning.
C. If ingestion of methanol/ethylene glycol occurred within 1 hour, perform a gastric lavage (minimal absorption to charcoal). Start a HCO_3^- IV to correct acidosis, up to 400 mEq may be required, and an IV ethanol with a 10% loading dose of 10 mL/kg, followed by maintenance infusion of 1.5 mL/kg/hour to achieve a level of 100 mg/dL, which should competitively block conversion to toxic metabolites. Alternative treatment with 4-methylpyrazole (Fomepizole) load 15 mg/kg slow IV over 30 min followed by 10 mg/kg IV q 12 hours for 4 doses.
D. Consider hemodialysis if there is no improvement with bicarbonate and ethanol, if the serum level of either substances > 50 mg/dL, or if there is visual impairment (methanol).
E. **Disposition:**

Observe and then discharge individuals poisoned by ethanol or isopropyl alcohol if there is no clinical evidence of intoxication. Admit patients exhibiting respiratory depression or decreased levels of consciousness.
Admit all patients poisoned with methanol/ethylene glycol to the ICU as needed. Obtain renal and ophthalmologic consultations as required.
Refer to a psychiatric consultation as appropriate.

4. Anion Gap Metabolic Acidosis:

Normal anion gap = Na - (HCO_3 + Cl) (8-12 mEq/L).
Discussion obtained from Emergency Medicine Pearls of Wisdom, 4th ED. Causes: A MUDPILE CAT.

A = alcohol,

M = methanol,
U = uremia,
D = DKA,
P = paraldehyde,
I = iron and isoniazid,
L = lactic acidosis,
E = ethylene glycol,

C = carbon monoxide,
A = aspirin,
T = toluene.

History and physical exam of the patient greatly assist in narrowing this list down. Also, a large anion gap, > 35 mEq/L, is usually caused by ethylene glycol, methanol. or lactic acidosis. Smaller anion gap, 16-22 mEq/L, may be due to uremia. However, uremia must be in an advanced stage to induce a larger anion gap.

The "osmolar gap" can also serve as an aid in diagnosing the onset of an anion gap acidosis. Osmolar gap is the difference between the measured osmolality and the calculated osmolarity. Osmolar gap is determined by using the following relationship.

Measured osmolality - calculated osmolarity = osmolar gap.
(Normal = 275 - 285 mOsm/l and normal gap <10 mOsm/l)

$$CalculatedOsmol(mOsm/l) = 2(Na) + \frac{glucose}{18} + \frac{BUN}{2.8}$$

Different substances contribute variably to the osmolar gap as shown in this Table:

Substance	mg/dL to increase serum osmol 1 mOsm/L	# mOsm/L increase due to each mg/dL
Methanol	2.6	0.38
Ethanol	4.3	0.23
Ethylene glycol	5.0	0.20
Acetone	5.5	0.18
Isopropyl alcohol	5.9	0.17
Salicylate	14.0	0.07

Thus, smaller amounts of methanol result in greater increases in osmolality. Large amounts of salicylate will eventually increase the osmolar gap. Note also that the contribution of alcohol to the osmolar gap may be calculated. This value can be useful when a mixed alcohol ingestion is suspected.

4.1 Clinical Evaluation:

A. Methanol: Visual disturbances and headache common. High anion and osmolar gap.
B. Uremia: Advanced before it causes an anion gap.
C. Diabetic ketoacidosis: Usually exhibits both hyperglycemia and glucosuria.
D. Alcoholic ketoacidosis (AKA): Often displays a lower blood sugar and mild or absent glucosuria.
E. Salicylates: High levels are required to contribute to gap.
F. Lactic acidosis: Check serum level. There is a broad differential.
G. Ethylene glycol: Calcium oxalate or hippurate crystals are produced in urine. High anion and osmolar gap.

5. Anticholinergics:

A wide variety of prescription and non-prescription drugs have anticholinergic properties. Some of these drugs include antidepressants, antiemetics, antihistamines, antiparkinson meds, major tranquilizers, antispasmodics, ophthalmoplegics, over-the-counter cough and cold meds, and sleep aids. Parasympathetic blockade creates clinical picture of:

Hot as hades.
Blind as a bat.
Dry as a bone.
Red as a beet.
Mad as a hatter.

5.1 Clinical Evaluation:

A. **Symptoms:** Identify drug, time of ingestion, medical and psychiatric illnesses, and current meds. Symptoms of toxicity are dry mouth, fever, blurred vision, and confusion.
B. **Signs:** Level of consciousness/change in mental status. Examine for hyperthermia, tachycardia, hypertension, mydriasis, poor visual acuity, flushed and dry face, decreased bowel sounds, disorientation, and confusion.
C. **DDX:** CNS infection, dehydration, psychiatric disorder, and sepsis.

D. **Work-up:** Order CBC, SMA-7, ABG, CXR, ECG, and toxicology screen.

5.2 RX:

A. Support airway, IV, O_2, and monitor. Administer naloxone, thiamine, glucose, and charcoal (refer to the "General" section).
B. Perform conservative and supportive therapy in ED.
C. For uncontrollable agitation/unstable, LIFE THREATENING arrhythmias, treat with physostigmine (reversible inhibitor of acetylcholinesterase), 1 mg over 2 minutes q 30 minutes as needed. However, this drug is very dangerous, use is controversial, avoid if possible.
D. **Disposition:** Observe patient in the ED until condition resolves. Admit for severe symptoms or complications. Obtain a psychiatric consultation as appropriate.

6. Antipsychotics:

Antipsychotic (neuroleptic) drugs block dopaminergic, adrenergic, and muscarinic and histaminic receptors. Dopamine blockade modifies behavior and can cause dystonic reactions. α-Adrenergic blockade produces the onset of vasodilation (orthostatic hypotension). Antipsychotics have anticholinergic properties (refer to the "Anticholinergics" section). Common phenothiazines are chlorpromazine (Thorazine), fluphenazine (Prolixin), prochlorperazine (Compazine), thioridazine (Mellaril), and trifluoperazine (Stelazine). Some typical butyrophenones consist of haloperidol (Haldol) and droperidol (Inapsine).

6.1 Clinical Evaluation:

A. **Symptoms:** Symptoms, such as nervousness, stiff neck, and pacing, are usually side effects of the prescribed drug. Determine dosage, frequency, other meds and psychiatric history.
B. **Signs:** Level of consciousness is usually not affected except in severe overdoses. Hyperthermia, tachycardia, orthostatic hypotension, dystonias, including torticollis, involuntary movements, spasms, and akathisia.
C. **DDX:** Malignant hyperthermia, heatstroke, extrapyramidal reaction, hyperthyroidism, and infectious disease.
D. **Work-up:** Order CBC, SMA-7, ECG, and CXR.

6.2 RX:

A. Support airway, IV, O_2, and monitor. Administer naloxone, thiamine, glucose, and charcoal (refer to the "General" section).
B. Hypotension: RL or NS IV.
C. For dystonias, prescribe diphenhydramine (Benadryl), 50 mg IM, or benztropine (Cogentin), 2 mg IM. May repeat as needed.
D. **Disposition:** Unless otherwise indicated, discharge with psychiatric follow-up.

7. β-Blockers / Calcium Channel Blockers:

β-blockers obstruct adrenergic receptors which, in turn, can produce the condition of hypoglycemia. **Calcium channel blockers** obstruct calcium in slow channels of myocardium, depress SA and AV nodes, and inhibit calcium-dependent insulin release which results in hyperglycemia. Toxicities are similar in both, including bradycardia, depression of myocardial contractility, and hypotension. CNS effects are secondary to hypoperfusion. Common β-blockers are metoprolol (Lopressor) and atenolol (Tenormin), which are cardioselective, as well as labetalol (Normodyne and Trandate), nadolol (Corgard), propranolol (Inderal), and esmolol/timolol (Blocadren). Prevalent calcium channel blockers include diltiazem (Cardizem), nifedipine (Procardia), verapamil (Calan and Isoptin), and nicardipine (Cardene).

7.1 Clinical Evaluation:

A. **Symptoms:** Identification of drug, time of ingestion, medical and psychiatric illnesses, and current meds. Chest pain, lethargy, nausea, and vomiting.

B. **Signs:** Mental status is usually not decreased. Seek bradycardia, hypotension, bradyarrhythmias, and rales (pulmonary edema).

C. **DDX:** Digoxin, cholinergic agents (organophosphate insecticides), cyclic antidepressants, α-methyldopa, anaphylaxis, cardiogenic shock, and sepsis.

D. **Work-up:** Order CBC, SMA-7, ABG, CXR, ECG, toxicology screen, serum acetaminophen ans salicylate level.

7.2 RX:

A. Support airway, IV, O_2, and monitor. Administer naloxone, thiamine, glucose, and charcoal (refer also to the "General" section).

B. For calcium blocker bradycardia/hypotension, treat with RL or NS IV, calcium gluconate 3 g slow IV push up to 5 g. Pacemaker as needed.

C. For β-blocker bradycardia/hypotension, administer RL or NS IV, atropine, 0.5-1 mg IV, glucagon (stimulates membrane receptors, cardiac contractility, heart rate, and BP) 5 mg IV, followed by infusion of 1 mg per hour.

D. **Disposition:** Discharge patients with mild toxicity after 4-6 hours with or without a psychiatric consultation as necessary. For more severe case, admit to the ICU unit and obtain a psychiatric consultation.

8. Carbon Monoxide:

Carbon monoxide is a colorless, odorless gas with an affinity for hemoglobin which is 240 times that of O_2. Toxic exposure occurs with smoke inhalation during fire and from improperly vented exhausts originating from stoves, furnaces, and automobiles. Toxic exposures induce hypoxia because of a decrease in carrying capacity of hemoglobin for O_2. Half-lives are 6 hours on room air, 1.5 hours on 100% O_2, and 0.5 hours 100% O_2 HBO.

8.1 Clinical Evaluation:

A. **Symptoms:** Occupational exposure, home and business heaters, and suicide attempt. Early symptoms (CO-Hb level - 10-20%): Mild headache and dyspnea on exertion and angina.

20-30%: Moderate headache, dyspnea, nausea, and dizziness.
30-40%: Severe headache, vomiting, fatigue, and poor judgment.
40-50%: Confusion, syncope, tachypnea, and tachycardia.
50-60%: Syncope, seizures, and coma.
> 60%: Convulsions, respiratory failure, arrhythmias, and death.

B. **Signs:**

Level of consciousness. Tachycardia, tachypnea, cyanosis vs red color (rare), if involved in fire, soot around nose, lips, mouth, and stridor (see Smoke Inhalation).
Lungs: Rales or rhonchi.
MSE: Confusion and poor judgment.

C. **DDX:** Differential of change in mental status: TIPS-AEIOU.

D. **Work-up:** Obtain CBC, ABG, CXR, ECG, and CO-Hb (carboxyhemoglobin) level.

8.2 RX:

A. Support airway, IV, O_2, and monitor.

B. Ensure that all patients receive 100% oxygen by using a tight-fitting, non-rebreather mask or by a endotracheal tube.

C. **Disposition:**

Admit all patients with CO-Hb levels of 25-30%, with cardiac, pulmonary or neurologic disease, and with anemia.

Transport patients who are unconscious, seizing, have CO-Hb levels > 40% (many recommend HBO for level of 35%), and those who are in respiratory failure to a hyperbaric oxygen (HBO) chamber. Also treat pregnant females and infants with hyperbaric oxygen.

Refer to a psychiatric consult as appropriate.

9. Caustics:

The major caustic (corrosive) materials are acids and alkalis. Acids, such as hydrochloric, sulfuric, and nitric, are a component(s) in toilet bowel cleaners, battery acid, drain cleaners, and industrial cleaners. Ingestion of an acid results in coagulation necrosis and burns to the distal stomach, duodenum, and jejunum. Alkalies (lye), including sodium hydroxide, potassium hydroxide and ammonium hydroxide, are found in paint removers, drain and pipe cleaners, toilet bowl cleaners, dish washing liquids, bleaches, laundry detergents, disinfectants, and oven, tile, wall, and floor cleaners. Direct exposure of bases causes liquefaction necrosis and burns with tissue penetration. There is a high risk of perforation in esophagus and stomach when an alkali is ingested. Household ammonia or bleach (sodium hypochlorite) are usually not caustic except in large amounts.

9.1 Clinical Evaluation:

A. **Symptoms:** Time, type, concentration and amount of corrosive. Symptoms include drooling, throat pain, chest pain, vomiting, abdominal pain, hematemesis, hoarseness, and shortness of breath.

B. **Signs:**

Level of consciousness.

Vitals: Fever (alkali) and hypotension (perforation).

HEENT: Soapy mucosal lesions (alkali), white/grey-white necrotic areas (acid), dysphagia, aphonia, stridor, and dyspnea.

Abdomen: Rigidity (perforation and peritonitis).

Rectal: Hemoccult.

C. **DDX:** FB ingestion, iron ingestion, esophagitis, gastritis, peptic ulcer disease, esophageal varices, Mallory-Weiss syndrome, Boerhaave's syndrome, perforated viscus, epiglottitis, croup, retropharyngeal abscess, and malignancy.

D. **Work-up:** Obtain CBC, SMA-7, coagulation studies, U/A, ABG, type and cross, toxicology screen, CXR, abdominal series, and lateral soft-tissue of neck.

9.2 RX:

A. Support airway, IV, O_2, and monitor. Administer naloxone, thiamine, and glucose. Charcoal is not indicated; instead, use a small amount of diluent, such as milk or water. Prescribe NPO/opioid analgesics for pain control. Initiate immediate surgical intervention if GI hemorrhage or perforation. (Use of steroids for alkali ingestion is controversial).

B. **Disposition:** Admit patients to the ICU and obtain an immediate gastroenterology an otolaryngology consult. Refer to a psychiatric specialist as appropriate.

10. Cocaine:

Cocaine affects the central and peripheral sympathetic system stimulating primarily the CNS and cardiovascular systems. Hyperthermia is induced from the combined effects of increased motor and metabolic activity, vasoconstriction, and hypothalamic stimulation. Routes of administration are oral, inhalation, and intravenous. IV heroin/cocaine ("speedballing") drug use is common.

10.1 Clinical Evaluation:

A. **Symptoms:** Route, amount, and time of ingestion, medical and psychiatric illnesses, and current meds. History of IV drug use, complications, and hospitalizations. Palpitations, chest pain, and nervousness.

B. **Signs:** Agitation, altered level of consciousness, and lethargy (heroin). Examine for hyperthermia, tachycardia, tachypnea, hypertension, dilated pupils, rales, track marks, restlessness, paranoia, and hallucinations.

C. **DDX:** Anticholinergic agents, sympathomimetics, hallucinogens, pheochromocytoma, hypoglycemia, drug withdrawal, thyrotoxicosis, malignant hypertension, MAO reaction, and psychiatric illness. Differential of change in mental status: TIPS-AEIOU.

D. **Work-up:** Order CBC, SMA-7, ± oximetry or ABG, ECG, and toxicology screen.

10.2 RX:

A. Support airway, IV, O_2, and monitor. Administer naloxone, thiamine, glucose, and charcoal for oral ingestions (refer also to the "General" section).

B. Order diazepam, 2.5 to 5 mg IV prn agitation. Assist in stopping chest pain and hypertension. Avoid β-blockers alone. (Refer to "Myocardial Infarction" and "Thrombolysis" sections for chest pain and for indications of an acute myocardial infarction.)

C. **Disposition:** Observe the patient in the ED for 3 to 6 hours and discharge mild cases. Admit individuals with sustained chest pain, altered vitals, and ECG changes. Obtain a psychiatric consultation as appropriate.

11. Cyclic Antidepressants:

Tricyclic antidepressants are the #1 cause of ingestion-related deaths and account for one-half of ICU admissions for drug toxicity. Primary mechanism of toxicity is the blockade of norepinephrine re-uptake resulting in an anticholinergic effect, a quinidine-like effect, and an α-adrenergic blockade effect. Tricyclic antidepressants affect primarily the cardiovascular and central nervous systems. Common tricyclics are imipramine (Tofranil), amitriptyline (Elavil), nortriptyline (Pamelor), and doxepin (Sinequan). Newer unicyclic and bicyclic agents, such as fluoxetine (Prozac), trazodone (Desyrel), bupropion (Wellbutrin), block serotonin and dopamine re-uptake and have less affect on the CNS and cardiovascular systems. The main toxic effects of an overdose are cardiac arrhythmias/heart blocks, hypotension, and decreased level of consciousness. **Twenty five percent of the patients that die from TCA are responsive upon initial presentation.**

11.1 Clinical Evaluation:

A. **Symptoms:** Identification of drug, time of ingestion, medical and psychiatric illnesses, and current meds. Palpitations, dry mouth, slurred speech, and drowsiness.

B. **Signs:**

Level of consciousness (monitor very frequently or constantly).
Vitals: Hyperthermia, tachycardia, bradycardia, irregular rhythm, and hypotension (monitor every 15 minutes).
HEENT: Mydriasis, dry mouth, and flushed face.
Heart: Abnormal rate and rhythm.
Abdomen: Decreased bowel sounds.
Neuro: Hyperreflexia and myoclonus.
MSE: Disorientation.

C. **DDX:** Hypoxia, metabolic abnormalities, cardiac disease, β-blockers, propoxyphene, quinidine, procainamide, phenothiazines, anticholinergics, cocaine, amphetamines, and withdrawal from sedative-hypnotic drugs. Differential of change in mental status: TIPS-AEIOU.

D. **Work-up:** Order CBC, SMA-7, ABG, ECG (arrhythmias, blocks, widened QRS), serum acetaminophen and salicylate level, and toxicology screen. QRS > 100 ms has a specificity of 75% and a sensitivity of 60% for serious complications. A normal ECG will not rule out a serious overdose.

11.2 RX:

A. Initiate aggressive airway management with very low threshold for intubation. Start IV, O_2, and place on monitor.
B. Administer naloxone, thiamine, glucose, and charcoal (refer to the "General" section). A nondepolarizing agent, such as vecuronium, is preferred. Succinylcholine, a depolarizing agent, causes more vagal effects and therefore should be avoided.
C. Basis of treatment is alkaline diuresis to reduce sodium channel blockade and increase plasma protein binding and excretion. Either hyperventilate patient and/or provide 2 mEq/kg bicarbonate IV initially with subsequent doses to maintain arterial pH of 7.5.
D. Treat hypotension with IV NS, bicarbonate (as above), epinephrine, norepinephrine, or phenylephrine. Dobutamine is contraindicated.
E. Most patients with seizures do not need treatment because the episodes tend to be brief. Diazepam, 5-10 mg IV, has been used but its efficacy is questionable. Phenytoin is effective in treating conduction defects and seizures but it will not eliminate myoclonic jerks. Alkalinize with IV sodium bicarbonate, 1-5 mEq/kg.
F. **Disposition:** Admit to ICU for all but the most benign ingestions. Asymptomatic patients may be discharged after 6 hours observation with a psychiatric consultation.

12. Digoxin:

Therapeutic serum digoxin levels are 0.5 to 2.0 ng/mL. Toxicity is usually produced from dosing anomalies and exaggerating therapeutic effect (bradycardia and AV blocks).

12.1 Clinical Evaluation:

A. **Symptoms:** Time of ingestion, quantity consumed, frequency and dosage of chronic therapy, other meds, and previous illnesses.
   Acute toxicity: Weakness and slow heart rate with skipped beats.
   Chronic toxicity: Confusion, depression, fatigue, headache, weakness, disturbances of color vision, and skipped beats.

B. **Signs:**
   Level of consciousness.
   Vitals: Bradycardia and hypotension.
   HEENT: Scotoma.
   Heart: Bradyarrhythmias.
   Neurology: Confusion, muscle weakness, and paresthesias.

C. **DDX:** Myocardial infarction, cardiac disease with arrhythmia, hyperkalemia, hypokalemia, glaucoma, cyclic antidepressant, β-blocker, and calcium-channel blocker.
D. **Work-up:** Order CBC, SMA-7 (hyperkalemia- acute, hypokalemia- chronic), ECG (most common arrhythmia is PVC's, PAT with block pathognomonic), and serum digoxin level.

12.2 RX:

A. Support airway, IV, O_2, and monitor. Administer naloxone, thiamine, glucose, and charcoal (refer to the "General" section).
B. For treatment of bradyarrhythmias, refer to the "Cardiovascular" and "Bradycardia" sections.
C. For acute ingestion, life-threatening dysrhythmias, coma or hyperkalemia, administer 10 vials of digoxin-specific Fab fragments (Digibind) given IV over 30 minutes. For chronic toxicity, body

load = serum concentration x 5.6 x patient's weight (kg)/1000. Example: 4 ng/mL x 5.6 x 70 kg/1000 = 1.57 mg. This number is divided by 0.6 for the total number of vials required for neutralization, or 3 vials.

D. **Disposition:** Admit to monitored bed if patient is symptomatic or to ICU if he/she is unstable.

13. Hallucinogens:

Hallucinogens produce sensory misperceptions and mood changes from the stimulation and/or distortion of multiple receptor sites in CNS. Common hallucinogens are phencyclidine (PCP, "angel dust"), lysergic acid diethylamide (LSD, "acid"), peyote, mescaline, and tetrahydrocannabinol (?9-THC, marijuana). PCP causes dissociative anesthesia.

13.1 Clinical Evaluation:

A. **Symptoms:** Identification of drug, time of ingestion, medical and psychiatric illnesses, and current meds. Mood swings and bizarre behavior may be exhibited.

B. **Signs:**

Level of consciousness is not usually affected.
Vitals: Hyperthermia, tachycardia, tachypnea, and hypertension.
HEENT: Pupil size and reactivity, vertical nystagmus (PCP).
Skin: Diaphoresis (PCP) and track marks.
Neuro: Sensory loss, hyperreflexia, dystonia, ataxia, and analgesia (PCP).
Mental status: Hallucinations/delusions.

C. **DDX:** Differential of change in mental status: TIPS-AEIOU and cocaine.

D. **Work-up:** Order CBC, SMA-7, oximetry or ABG, U/A (including myoglobin - PCP), and toxicology screen.

13.2 RX:

A. Support airway, IV, O_2, and monitor. Administer naloxone, thiamine, glucose, and charcoal (refer also to the "General" section).

B. Decrease environmental stimulation, i.e., dim the lights or quiet the room.

C. Restrain patient by using physical and pharmacologic means, including haloperidol, mg IM q 30 minutes prn.

D. For hypertension, sedate with haloperidol as above, or use diazepam, 5 mg IV prn.

E. Treat rhabdomyolysis with vigorous solute diuresis on an inpatient basis.

F. **Disposition:** Observe mild cases for several hours and discharge. Admit patients with unstable vitals and mental status to the ICU as indicated. Refer to a psychiatrist as appropriate.

14. Insecticides:

Organophosphate and carbamate insecticides are inhibitors of acetylcholinesterase which result in varying degrees of acetylcholine accumulation at muscarinic, nicotinic, and CNS cholinergic synapses. Common agents include Chlorothion, parathion, diazinon, and malathion. Carbamates are reversible and less toxic. Poisoning typically occurs as result of accidental agricultural exposure. Absorption into the skin, respiratory and GI routes is rapid. Mnemonics are SLUDGE and DUMBELS:

SLUDGE		DUMBELS	
S	= Salivation	**D**	= Diarrhea
L	= Lacrimation	**U**	= Urination
U	= Urination	**M**	= Miosis
D	= Diarrhea	**B**	= Bronchospasm
G	= GI cramps	**E**	= Emesis
E	= Emesis	**L**	= Lacrimation
		S	= Salivation

14.1 Clinical Evaluation:

A. **Symptoms:** Occupational information about possible industrial or agricultural exposure. Amount, time, and route of exposure, as well as identity and type of cholinesterase inhibitor should be determined. Symptoms are headache, dizziness, blurred vision, weakness, tremors, diarrhea, abdominal cramping, wheezing, and incontinence.

B. **Signs:**

Level of consciousness.
Vitals: Bradycardia, tachycardia, and tachypnea.
Breath: Garlic odor.
Skin: Diaphoresis.
HEENT: Miosis and salivation.
Lungs: Wheezes.
Abdominal: Diffuse tenderness and increased bowel sounds.
Neuromuscular: Fasciculations and weakness.

C. **DDX:** Opiates, phencyclidine, phenothiazines, and poisonous mushrooms. Differential of change in mental status: TIPS-AEIOU.

D. **Work-up:** Order CBC, SMA-7, U/A, and ECG. Serum cholinesterase may be sent from the ED.

14.2 RX:

A. Support airway, IV, O_2, and monitor. Administer naloxone, thiamine, glucose, and charcoal for oral ingestions (refer to the "General" section).

B. Remove contaminated clothing and clean skin and hair.

C. To competitively block acetylcholine, use atropine, 2 mg IV q 15 minutes but may require 40 mg or more.

D. To reactivate cholinesterase, use pralidoxime (Protopam, 2-PAM), 2 g IV in 250 cc NS over 60 minutes. Repeat in 2 hours.

E. **Disposition:** Admit the patient to the ICU and obtain a psychiatric consultation as appropriate.

15. Iron:

Iron toxicity is caused by three major items: Ferrous compounds, vitamins with iron, and prenatal vitamins. Most prevalent cause of pediatric poisoning is multivitamins containing iron. In the initial stage, first few hours after ingestion, GI symptoms are exhibited, although hypotension and CNS symptoms may occur. The patient is asymptomatic in the next stage, up to 12 hours, because the iron is absorbed. In the third stage, several hours later, impaired oxidative phosphorylation, hepatic dysfunction, obtundation, hypovolemia with hypotension, metabolic acidosis, and shock may occur. During the fourth stage, days to weeks, gastric outlet or small bowel obstruction transpires. Symptoms may follow after the ingestion of 20 mg/kg of **elemental** iron. Iron poisoning is classified as "severe" when 40 mg/kg of the material is consumed. Percent quantities of **elemental** iron contained within ferrous gluconate, ferrous sulfate, and ferrous fumarate are 11%, 20%, and 33%, respectively.

15.1 Clinical Evaluation:

A. **Symptoms:** The time of ingestion and amount of iron consumed is important. Early symptoms include abdominal pain, nausea, vomiting (occasionally hematemesis), diarrhea (sometimes black and tarry stools), weakness, lethargy, later obtundation, and seizures.

B. **Signs:** Change in mental status, tachycardia, tachypnea, hypotension, pallor, diffuse abdominal tenderness, and increased bowel sounds.

C. **DDX:** Aspirin and other NSAIDS, theophylline, caustics, and isopropyl and ethyl alcohol (differential of anion-gap metabolic acidosis).

D. **Work-up:** Order CBC, SMA-7, anion gap, ABG (anion-gap metabolic acidosis), PT, PTT, serum iron (reliable if within 6 hours), TIBC, and KUB (may show radio-opaque tablets).

15.2 RX:

A. Support airway, IV, O_2, and monitor.
B. Administer naloxone, thiamine, glucose, and perform a gastric lavage (charcoal does not bind iron).
C. Initiate chelation therapy with a symptomatic patient, when the serum iron level is > TIBC, or when the serum iron level is > 350 μg/dL. Start a deferoxamine mesylate (Desferal) intravenous infusion at 15 mg/kg/hour. Do not delay treatment in a symptomatic patient.
D. **Disposition:** Admit patient to the ICU if chelation therapy is required.

16. Lithium:

Lithium is administered as a therapeutic drug for bipolar affective disorder. The optimal serum concentration should be between 0.6-1.25 mEq/L. Mild to moderate toxicity occurs at an intake level of 1.5 to 2.5 mEq/L with 3.5 mEq/L being regarded as life-threatening. Most toxicities are triggered by an infection and/or decreased salt intake in patients that are already taking lithium for medical problems. Dehydration and drug interactions, particularly NSAIDS, methyldopa, and thiazides, are prevalent. Major systems that are affected consist of the GI (early), CNS, and cardiovascular (late).

16.1 Clinical Evaluation:

A. **Symptoms:** History should include drug name, concentration, dosage, time of last ingestion, medical and psychiatric history, and other meds. Nausea, vomiting, diarrhea, tremors, agitation, confusion, and drowsiness are common early symptoms.
B. **Signs:**
Level of consciousness.
Vitals: Bradycardia, arrhythmia, and hypertension.
HEENT: Dysarthria.
Abdominal: Mild diffuse tenderness, particularly LUQ.
Neuromuscular: Tremor, hyperreflexia, fasciculations, and ataxia.
C. **DDX:** Gastroenteritis, labyrinthitis, cerebrovascular insufficiency, seizure disorder, cardiac disease, tricyclic antidepressants, salicylate, theophylline overdose, and change in mental status.
D. **Work-up:** Order CBC, SMA-7, U/A, ECG, and serum lithium level.

16.2 RX:

A. Support airway, IV, O_2, and monitor. Administer naloxone, thiamine, glucose, and perform a gastric lavage (charcoal does not absorb lithium). (Refer to the "General" section).
B. Initiate saline diuresis with NS IV wide open. Sodium exchange enhances lithium excretion.
C. Begin hemodialysis on patients with severe poisoning (> 3.5 mEq/L) experiencing seizures, in a coma, with arrhythmias, or in renal failure.
D. **Disposition:** Admit patients to the ICU, as appropriate, until symptoms resolve or lithium level is therapeutic. Obtain a psychiatric consultation.

17. Narcotics (opioids):

Narcotics stimulate opiate receptors in the CNS system which causes analgesia, euphoria, miosis, and respiratory depression. Some typical narcotics include morphine, codeine, heroin, propoxyphene (Darvon), meperidine (Demerol), and fentanyl (Sublimaze).

17.1 Clinical Evaluation:

A. **Symptoms:** Mode of administration, frequency, and other drugs. Previous complications include hepatitis, pneumonia, AIDs, endocarditis, and hospitalizations. Drowsiness and slurred speech may be displayed.

B. **Signs:**

Decreased level of consciousness (Glasgow Coma Scale).

Vitals: Hypothermia, bradycardia, bradypnea, and hypotension.

Examine for fever, track marks, pupillary miosis (midrange or mydriasis with diphenoxylate, meperidine, and other drugs), rales, murmurs, and other stigmata of endocarditis.

C. **DDX:** Differential of change in mental status: TIPS-AEIOU (refer also to "Sedative/Hypnotics" and "Change in Mental Status" sections).

D. **Work-up:** Order CBC, SMA-7, serum/urine toxicology screens, ABG, CXR, and ECG (as needed).

17.2 RX:

A. Support airway, IV, O_2, and monitor. Administer activated charcoal for oral ingestion.

B. Decreased level of consciousness: After restraints are in place, administer naloxone (Narcan), 2 mg IV (larger doses may be required for diphenoxylate, propoxyphene, pentazocine, and fentanyl). Start naloxone infusion, 1 mg/hour as needed, thiamine, 100 mg IV, and D_{50}, 1 amp IV.

C. **Disposition:** Admit all patients with coma, respiratory depression, persistent naloxone requirement, unstable vital signs, or fever. Refer to a psychiatrist.

18. Petroleum Distillates:

Petroleum distillates (hydrocarbons) include gasoline, kerosene, lighter fluid, mineral oil, turpentine, diesel fuel, motor oil, toluene, xylene, benzene, and carbon tetrachloride. The petroleum distillates most commonly ingested are gasoline, kerosene, lighter fluid, and mineral oil. GI symptoms are almost always exhibited with this type of poisoning. Most frequent adverse effect from petroleum distillates poisoning is chemical pneumonitis from aspiration. The lower the viscosity of the material the more likely aspiration will occur. Some patients, mostly children, present as changes in mental status or loss of consciousness.

18.1 Clinical Evaluation:

A. **Symptoms:** Identity, amount, and concentration of distillate, time of ingestion, symptoms present at time of ingestion, other meds, and past and present medical and psychiatric history. Vomiting almost always follows ingestion and increases the likelihood of aspiration. Coughing and gagging are common.

B. **Signs:** Change in mental status, tachycardia, tachypnea, dusky appearance, oral tenderness, dysphagia, drooling, nasal flaring, stridor, coughing, wheezes, and rales.

C. **DDX:** Corrosive ingestion, infectious gastroenteritis, food poisoning, asthma, allergic reaction, pulmonary infection, and gas inhalation.

D. **Work-up:** Order CBC, SMA-7, ABG, CXR, ECG, and toxicology screen.

18.2 RX:

A. Airway management may need to include early intubation and PEEP. Start IV, O_2, and monitor.

B. Administer naloxone, thiamine, and glucose. The efficacy of charcoal is not known.

C. Treat bronchospasm.

D. Order a psychiatric consultation as appropriate.

E. **Disposition:** Discharge home if the patient is asymptomatic for 6 hours and the second CXR (taken at 2 hours) is normal. Admit for symptomatic patients to the ICU as needed.

19. Phenytoin:

Phenytoin (Dilantin) is an anticonvulsant and type Ib antiarrhythmic. It prevents the spread of abnormal discharges by stabilizing neuronal membranes, inhibiting sodium channels, and decreasing the effective refractory period of myocardium. The majority of toxic cases involving phenytoin are from patient or caregiver dosing errors. At serum levels of 20-40 μg/mL, dizziness, ataxia, tremors, lethargy, nausea, vomiting, slurred speech, diplopia, blurred vision, and nystagmus are prevalent. At 40-90 μg/mL, typical symptoms consist of confusion, psychosis, hallucinations, and decreased level of consciousness. Above 90 μg/mL, the patient goes in a coma and respiratory depression. Cardiac arrhythmias usually occur only after IV (iatrogenic) administration.

19.1 Clinical Evaluation:

A. **Symptoms:** Time, amount, and preparation taken, onset of symptoms, other meds, and present and past illnesses. Early symptoms are dizziness, nausea, vomiting, diplopia, and blurred vision. After a prolonged period of time, confusion and psychotic behavior transpire.
B. **Signs:** Bradycardia, hypotension, mydriasis, nystagmus, bradyarrhythmia, ataxia, tremor, slurred speech, confusion, and hallucinations.
C. **DDX:** Other anticonvulsive meds, sedative-hypnotics, alcohol, DKA, hypoglycemia, Wernicke's encephalopathy, postictal state, and cerebellar lesion/bleed.
D. **Work-up:** Order CBC, SMA-7, U/A, ABG, ECG, serum phenytoin level, and toxicology screen.

19.2 RX:

A. Support airway, IV, O_2, and monitor. Administer naloxone, thiamine, glucose, and charcoal (refer to the "General" section).
B. Treat arrhythmias (refer to the "Cardiovascular" section).
C. Treat seizures with phenobarbital, 15-20 mg/kg IV, repeat as needed.
D. **Disposition:** Admit all symptomatic patients. Place individuals on a monitor when their symptoms are a result of IV phenytoin. Obtain psychiatric consultation as appropriate.

20. Rodenticides:

Rodenticides contain warfarin or superwarfarin and related anticoagulants (Bromadiolone, Coumafene and Pindone). Exposure commonly occurs in children who accidentally ingest rat poison.

20.1 Clinical Evaluation:

A. **Symptoms:** Most patients remain asymptomatic. Occasionally abdominal pain and headache occur. History should include name and chemical identity, amount, concentration of poison, and time of exposure. Past medical and psychiatric history should be obtained.
B. **Signs:** Ecchymoses, hematomas, oral bleeding, abdominal tenderness, and occult bleeding.
C. **DDX:** Coagulopathies.
D. **Work-up:** Order CBC, SMA-7, U/A, PT, and PTT.

20.1 RX:

A. Support airway, IV, O_2, and monitor. Administer naloxone, thiamine, glucose, and charcoal (refer to the "General" section).
B. For a prolonged PT, prescribe phytonadione (Vitamin K and AquaMephyton), 10 mg IM or IV (peds, 0.4 mg/kg). Many prefer test dose and IM to limit anaphylaxis if IV dose is 1 mg/minute. Repeat q 6 hours as needed.
C. Transfuse fresh frozen plasma, 10 units IV, plus packed cells as needed for active bleeding.

D. **Disposition:**

Observe asymptomatic patients for 4-6 hours in ED and then discharge. Patients with ingestions of superwarfarin compounds will require daily checks and follow up for delayed coagulopathies that occur.

Admit patients with prolonged PT.

Admit patients with active bleeding to the ICU.

Refer to a psychiatrist as appropriate.

21. Salicylate / NSAIDS:

Aspirin (acetylsalicylic acid, ASA) and **non-steroidal anti-inflammatory drugs (NSAIDS)** inhibit prostaglandin synthesis. Toxicity with NSAIDS is rare even with massive doses. However, treatment consists of supportive care. Toxic doses of aspirin produce gastric irritation, stimulates respiratory center resulting in hyperventilation and respiratory alkalosis, uncouples oxidative phosphorylation ensuing in fever and anion-gap metabolic acidosis, and mobilizes glycogen stores causing hyperglycemia. However, hypoglycemia is common in children. **Chronic aspirin poisoning** causes lethargy, disorientation, and sometimes acute respiratory distress syndrome (ARDS). The prothrombin time is elevated but salicylate level is usually normal. ASA elimination improves with repeated charcoal, alkaline diuresis, and hemodialysis.

21.1 Clinical Evaluation:

A. **Symptoms:** Identification of drug, time of ingestion, medical and psychiatric illnesses, and current meds. Symptoms of early toxicity are nausea, vomiting, abdominal pain, vertigo, and tinnitus. At 12 to 24 hours fever, diaphoresis, pallor, confusion, disorientation, tachycardia, and tachypnea. After 24 hours cerebral edema, coma, seizures, pulmonary edema, arrhythmias, and bleeding may develop.

B. **Signs:** Level of consciousness. Examine for fever, tachycardia, hyperpnea, hypotension, flushing or pallor, rales, stool for blood, disorientation, and hallucinations.

C. **DDX:** Theophylline toxicity, acute iron poisoning, diabetic ketoacidosis, anxiety, cardiopulmonary disease, cerebrovascular disease, sepsis, alcohol withdrawal, meningitis, COPD, and A MUDPILE CAT.

D. **Work-up:** Order CBC, SMA-7 (anion gap), PT, PTT, U/A, ABG (anion gap metabolic acidosis), toxicology screen, salicylate level (Done nomogram valid at 6 hours in acute ingestion of non-enteric coated) acetaminophen level, ECG, and CXR.

21.2 RX:

A. Support airway, IV, O_2, and monitor closely. Administer naloxone, thiamine, glucose, and charcoal (refer to the "General" section).

B. Rehydrate patient with 1-2 L D_5NS ± 1/2 amp HCO_3^-/L and K^+ 10-20 mEq/L over the first 1-2 hours to make up preexisting deficit. After this, slow IVs to < 500 mL/hour.

C. Start alkaline diuresis for patients exhibiting signs of significant toxicity and acid-base abnormalities.

D. Contraindications are cerebral or pulmonary edema, pH > 7.55, and oliguric renal failure.

E. Start with HCO_3^- , 1/2 amp in initial IV as above and add to IV or provide separately (in 500 cc sterile water) about 2 mEq/kg HCO_3^-, over 2 hours. Titrate to urine pH of > 7.5. Aggressive repletion of potassium will probably be required to achieve alkaline diuresis.

F. Initiate hemodialysis on patients if their salicylate level is > 100 mg, or if they are in a coma, seizing, presenting with cerebral/pulmonary edema, or in renal failure.

G. For prolonged PT in chronic patients, administer phytonadione (Vitamin K and AquaMEPHYTON) 10 mg IM (consider test dose). Provide IV at 1 mg per minute with probable higher risk of anaphylaxis (peds: 0.4 mg/kg). Repeat q 6 hours as needed. Fresh frozen plasma is not indicated.

H. **Disposition:** Admit all symptomatic patients to the ICU as needed. Obtain a psychiatric consultation for acute ingestions.

22. Sedative / Hypnotics:

Sedative/hypnotics stimulate gamma-aminobutyric acid (GABA) and synaptic inhibition in the CNS system. Common **benzodiazepines** are diazepam (Valium), lorazepam (Ativan), chlordiazepoxide (Librium), alprazolam (Xanax), flurazepam (Dalmane), temazepam (Restoril), and triazolam (Halcion). Short-acting **barbiturates** include amobarbital (Amytal), pentobarbital (Nembutal), secobarbital (Seconal), and long-acting barbiturates are anticonvulsants, such as phenobarbital and primidone (Mysoline).

22.1 Clinical Evaluation:

A. **Symptoms:** Identify drug, time of ingestion, medical and psychiatric illnesses, and current meds. Drowsiness and slurred speech may be evident.

B. **Signs:**

General: Level of consciousness (Glasgow Coma Scale).
Vitals: Hypothermia (barbiturates), bradycardia, bradypnea, and hypotension.
HEENT: Miosis, corneal reflex, and neck suppleness.
Lungs: Rales (aspiration pneumonia - barbiturates).
Neuro: Serial coma scale assessments.

C. **DDX:** Causes of coma and decreased level of consciousness is mnemonic TIPS-AEIOU (refer to "Neurology" section):

T = trauma, temperature
I = infection
P = Psychiatric
S = stroke, shock, seizure

A = alcohol
E = endocrine
I = insulin
O = opiates
U = uremia

D. **Work-up:** Order CBC, SMA-7, U/A, toxicology screen, acetaminophen and salicylate level, CXR, ECG, and ABGs.

22.2 RX:

A. Support airway, IV, O_2, and monitor. Administer naloxone, thiamine, glucose, and charcoal (refer also to the "General" section).
B. An antidote to benzodiazepines is flumazenil, a competitive inhibitor of benzodiazepine receptor site. Prescribe at 0.2 mg IV over 30 seconds. May repeat at 1 minute intervals with 0.5 mg doses to a total dose of 3 mg. However, this drug can induce seizures and its use is controversial.
C. For phenobarbital poisoning, begin with multiple doses of activated charcoal, q 6 hours for 6 doses. Excretion is enhanced by urinary alkalinization at 2 mEq/kg to maintain urine pH at 7.5 or greater.
D. Initiate hemodialysis or charcoal hemoperfusion for severe cases.
E. **Disposition:** Admit to the ICU for patients with unstable vitals or a decreased level of consciousness. Obtain a psychiatric consultation.

23. Theophylline:

Majority of toxic cases occur from dosing errors. Normal serum levels are 10-20 μg/mL. Symptoms usually occur at serum levels of > 35 μg/mL.

23.1 Clinical Evaluation:

A. **Symptoms:** Time, overdose quantity, usual intake, and medical history. Initial symptoms are nausea, vomiting, and abdominal pain. After a prolonged period of time, diarrhea and GI bleeding occur. Other symptoms include headache, agitation, tremors, tinnitus, heart palpitations, and seizures.

B. **Signs:**

Level of consciousness (seizure activity).

Vitals: Hyperthermia, tachycardia, and tachypnea.

Heart: Tachyarrhythmias.

Abdomen: Tenderness.

Neuro: Tremors and increased DTRs.

Rectal: Occult blood.

C. **DDX:** Cocaine, amphetamines, anticholinergics, hallucinogens, MAO inhibitors, psychiatric states, drug withdrawal, CNS infection, hypoglycemia, pheochromocytoma, and thyroid storm.

D. **Work-up:** Order CBC, SMA-7, U/A, ABG, ECG, theophylline level, serum amylase/lipase, and CXR.

23.2 RX:

A. Support airway, IV, O_2, and monitor. Administer naloxone, thiamine, glucose, and charcoal q 3 hours (refer to the "General" section).

B. For arrhythmias, use a β-blocker, such as esmolol (Brevibloc) at 500 μg/kg/minute loading dose over 1 minute, followed by 50 μg/kg/minute over 4 minutes.

C. To stop seizures, prescribe diazepam (Valium), 5-10 mg IV titrated.

D. **Disposition:**

Admit patient to a monitored bed if serum theophylline level is > 35 μg/mL or ICU for a level > 50 μg/mL.

Obtain a nephrology consultation for charcoal hemoperfusion or dialysis if seizures are evident, hemodynamically unstable, serum level is 60 μg/mL (chronic) or 80 μg/mL (acute).

TRAUMA

TRAUMA PRINCIPLES

1. Trauma Evaluation:

Evaluation and management of the trauma patient includes a primary survey followed by a detailed secondary survey.

1.1 Primary Survey:

A. **Access ABCs**: Identify and treat life-threatening conditions.
B. Control airway and c-spine by using a chin lift or jaw-thrust maneuver and removing foreign debris. Assume a c-spine fracture and maintain in-line immobilization.
C. Survey breathing and ventilation by evaluating oxygenation. Supplement with bag-valve mask ventilation or intubate as necessary. Insert a chest tube prn.
D. Examine circulation and control of hemorrhage by checking pulse, skin color, capillary refill, and consciousness.
E. Survey disability and neuro status by checking alertness, response to vocal or painful stimuli, or degree of unresponsiveness (AVPU).
F. Expose patient.

1.2 Primary Management:

A. Support airway, and start O_2, two large-caliber IVs, and ECG monitoring. Insert urinary and gastric catheters.
B. Immediately administer thiamine, D_{50}, and Narcan, if there is a change in mental status. Reassess AVPU.
C. Obtain c-spine, chest, and pelvic X-rays.
D. Order labs that include CBC, chem profile, U/A, T&C, and toxicology and alcohol screen.
E. Order ABGs, pregnancy test, and cardiac enzymes prn.

1.3 Secondary Survey:

A. Survey head by examining pupil size, fundi for hemorrhage and papilledema, lens for dislocation, conjunctiva for hemorrhage, and penetration.
B. Check ears for tenderness, CSF leak, hemotympanum, and perforation.
C. For maxillofacial trauma, evaluate and treat when patient is stabilized.
D. Survey cervical/neck by maintaining in-line immobilization, and evaluating for tenderness, deformities, penetrating wounds, JVD, and bruits.
E. Examine chest for breath sounds, deformity, and penetrating wounds. Placement of a chest tube may be necessary. Check rate/rhythm, S1/S2, murmurs, and gallops.
F. Inspect the abdomen for palpations, bowel sounds, masses, guarding, and rebound. Consider DPL.
G. Inspect and palpate for fractures in the pelvis. Perform a genital exam.
H. Survey rectum by evaluating for sphincter tone, blood in lumen, fractures, integrity of wall, and high-riding prostate.
I. Inspect and palpate for fractures and penetrating trauma in the extremities. Evaluate pulses.
J. Check integument for warmth, diaphoresis, and edema.
K. Inspect and palpate for fractures and penetrating trauma in the back.
L. Survey neuro by evaluating focal or lateralizing signs, cranial nerves, muscle/sensory exam, Babinski, and Glasgow Coma Score.

1.4 Secondary Management:

A. Obtain Extremity X-rays.
B. Consider CT head, chest, abdomen, and pelvis.
C. Initiate a IVP, cystourethrogram, chest tube placement, and DPL.
D. Administer crystalloid, 1-2 L to the adult, **or** 20 mL/kg bolus in children, followed by packed red blood cells.

2. Airway Management:

Examine for agitation and cyanosis which suggest hypoxia. Auscultate breath sounds bi-laterally. Gurgling and snoring suggest occlusion of the pharynx. Hoarseness may be induced by laryngeal obstruction. Provide airway, deliver oxygen, and support ventilation. Prevent hypercarbia, especially in the head injured patient. Verbal response indicates a patent airway, intact ventilation, and adequate brain perfusion.

2.1 Management:

A. Chin lift: Place fingers of one hand under the mandible and perform a gentle anterior chin lift. Depress the lower lip to open the patient's mouth with your thumb. Avoid hyperextension of the neck.
B. Jaw thrust: Grasp angles of the lower jaw, one hand on each side, and displace the mandible forward.
C. Suction: Use rigid suction catheter to clear airway.
D. Nasopharyngeal airway: Insert into one nostril to provide passage into the hypopharynx.
E. Oropharyngeal airway: Insert into the mouth behind the tongue.
F. Endotracheal intubation: Used in patients with airway compromise. If any risk of c-spine injury, perform an in-line manual cervical, i.e., immobilization followed by orotracheal intubation. May require rapid sequence induction. Contraindicated if midfacial injuries are present.
G. Nasotracheal intubation: Commonly used if cervical fractures are suspected.
H. Cricothyroidotomy: Skin incision through cricothyroid membrane. Dilate with a hemostat and insert a small endotracheal tube or tracheostomy tube. Avoid in children under 12.
I. Jet insufflation: Needle cricothyroidotomy involves insertion of a large-caliber plastic cannula, #12 or #14-gauge, into the trachea below the level of the obstruction.

TRAUMA CASES

1. Hemorrhagic Shock:

ATLS classification of shock:

	Class I	Class II	Class III	Class IV
Blood Loss (mL, %)	< 750, < 15%	750-1500, 15-30%	1500-2000, 30-40%	> 2000, > 40%
Pulse	< 100	> 100	>120	> 140
BP	Normal	Normal	Decreased	Decreased
Cap Refill	Normal	> 3 s	> 3 s	> 3 s
UO(mL/hour)	> 30	20-30	5-15	< 5
Mental Status	Slight anxiety	Some more anxiety	Anxious & confused	Confused - lethargic
Treatment:	Crystalloid	Crystalloid	Crystalloid & *blood	Crystalloid & *blood

*Transfuse type specific blood (10 minutes prep) or crossmatched blood (1 hour prep). Use Type O negative PRBCs for acute Class III, IV hemorrhage.

2. Spinal Cord Trauma:

Always assume a spinal cord trauma until proven otherwise. Maintain spine immobilization until screening roentgenograms have eliminated the possibility of fractures or dislocations. May "clear" the c-spine clinically in selected patients.

2.1 Clinical Evaluation:

A. **Symptoms:** Mechanism of injury, motor/sensory complaints, and pain.

B. **Signs:**

Avoid moving the patient. Palpate for tenderness and deformity. Complete motor/sensory exam.

Tract dysfunction: Corticospinal - motor problem on same side of body. Test by voluntary muscle contractions or involuntary response to pain. Spinothalamic - pain and temperature problem on opposite side. Test by pin prick or pinch. Posterior - proprioceptive impulses from the same side of the body. Test by position sense of fingers and toes or tuning fork vibration.

Cervical cord injury findings may include flaccid areflexia, especially rectal sphincter, diaphragmatic breathing, priapism, hypotension with bradycardia, ability to flex but not extend the elbow, and pain above but not below the clavicle.

C. **DDX:** Transection: Complete - no sensory or motor function. Incomplete - some function; possibility of partial to complete recovery.

Neurogenic shock: Associated with cervical or high thoracic injury. Impaired sympathetic pathways may result in vasodilation, pooling of blood, and consequent hypotension. Bradycardia may occur.

Spinal shock: Initial shock to cord may make it appear functionless. Flaccidity and loss of reflexes occurs instead of spasticity, hyperactive reflexes, and Babinski signs. Spinal shock may gradually disappear, and spasticity may replace the flaccid state.

D. **Work-up:**

C-spine: Order anteroposterior, oblique cervical, open-mouth odontoid, and cross table lateral views. Swimmer's view may be required for lower cervical vertebrae. ID all 7 cervical vertebrae.

Thoracic: Obtain anteroposterior and lateral films.

Lumbar: Anteroposterior, lateral, and oblique. Examine roentgenograms for anteroposterior diameter of the spinal canal, contour and alignment of the vertebra, bone fragments, linear or comminuted fractures, and soft-tissue swelling. CT scan for definitive evaluation.

2.2 RX:

A. Obtain neurosurgery consultation.

B. Immobilize.

C. Start IV fluids. Hypovolemic shock usually includes tachycardia while neurogenic shock includes bradycardia.

D. Administer steroids.

E. **Disposition:** Admit to ICU.

3. Burns:

Maintain airway, assess breathing, restore intravascular volume, control pain, prevent infection, evaluate extent, and obtain appropriate referral.

3.1 Clinical Evaluation:

A. **Symptoms:** Time and duration of contact, heat source, closed or open space, associated trauma or toxic inhalation.

B. **Signs:** Evidence of inhalation injury, i.e., carbon deposits on the nasal and oral mucosa, and carbonaceous sputum. Depressed consciousness suggests toxic inhalation. Rule out constricting full-thickness burns.

C. **Extent- Rule of 9's:** Adult Body Surface Area- 9% head, 9% each upper extremity, 9% back, 9% buttocks, 9% chest, 9% abdomen, 18% each lower extremity, and 1% perineum. A modified Lund and Browder chart may also be used for peds.

Depth (1st degree): Epidermis only (sunburn), blanching erythema, painful, edematous, indurated, not included in estimation of extent of burn injury.

Superficial and Deep partial thickness (2nd degree): Destruction of epidermis extends to dermis, red or mottled, swelling, blister formation, painful.

Full thickness (3rd degree): Destruction of epidermis and dermis, extension into subcutaneous tissues, muscle, fascia, or bone. Includes nerve fibers, translucent, waxy, mottled, leathery, chaired, painless, pale or white, and does not blanch with pressure.

D. **Work-up:** Order ABGs, CBC, SMA-7, total proteins, albumen/globulin ratio, type and cross for FFP or shelf-stored plasma, carbon monoxide, cyanide, and PT, PTT. U/A, myoglobin, ECG, and CXR.

3.2 RX:

A. Support airway, IV, O_2, and monitor.

B. For airway burns, maintain airway, obtain ABGs, CXR, and carboxyhemoglobin level. If patient is stable, start humidified, 100% high flow oxygen by mask. If the patient unstable, intubate and mechanically ventilate. Consider bronchoscopy. Initiate HBO prn.

C. Start Fluids as described below. Required for more than 20% or more TBSA. Ringer's lactate should be infused through a 16 gauge or larger IV line.

Parkland Formula - 4 mL x body weight(kg) x % of second or third degree burn divided by 24 hours = hourly fluid requirement for first 24 hours.

Administer 50% of total 24 hour requirement over the first 8 hours and final 50% over the next 16 hours. Timing begins at time of injury.

Monitor vital signs and urine output, 30-50 mL/hour in adults, and 1 mL/kg/hour in children weighing less than 30 kg.

Colloids or plasma, 0.5 mL/kg/% burn may be given between 24-32 hours.

D. Treat pain with IV narcotics, such as morphine, 5-10 mg, after circulation is stabilized.

E. Initiate burn care by cleaning affected area with sterile saline. Avoid vigorous scrubbing. Remove charred epithelium, surface debris, and excise ruptured blisters. Apply silver sulfadiazine or gauze impregnated with antibiotic ointment. Do not apply silver sulfadiazine to the face.

F. Consider Td, NG, antacids, and IV H_2 blockers.

G. For tar burns, cool affected area immediately, remove tar with Polysporin, Neosporin, and silver sulfadiazine ointments.

H. **Disposition:**

Discharge patients with partial-thickness burns less than 15% of TBSA in adults and 10% in children.

Admit patients with full-thickness burns greater than 10% TBSA, who are extremes in age, are afflicted with burns involving the face, hands, feet, and those individuals with a complicating medical illness .

Transfer patients to a burn unit with the following conditions: 1) Burns that involve more than 25% TBSA, or 20% in children under 10 and adults over 40, 2) third degree burns involving more than 10% of TBSA and second degree burns that exceed 20% of TBSA, and 3) burns involving the eyes, face, ears, hands, feet, or perineum, and those associated with traumatic injury warrant transfer.

4. Abdominal Trauma:

Blunt trauma typically produces spleen and liver injury. Stab wounds in the abdomen require laparotomy in 1 out of every 4 cases. Serious intra-abdominal injury occurs in 95% of GSWs. A laparotomy is required except in certain cases of tangential penetration. Wounds to the lower chest (nipple line anteriorly and the tip of the scapulae posteriorly) often involve the abdomen.

4.1 Clinical Evaluation:

A. **Symptoms:**

Blunt: Knowledge of direction and amount of forces applied, position at impact, location, seat belt type and usage, damage to windshield, steering column, extrication requirements, and status of other victims.

Penetrating: Size and length of knife. Bullet caliber, mass, expandability, and possibility of fragmentation should be considered.

B. **Signs:** Expose and visualize entire body, log roll, inspect abdomen for contusion, distention, abrasion, laceration, auscultation of bowel sounds, palpate for signs of peritoneal irritation, and focal tenderness. Physical exam may be unreliable, despite absence of clinical signs, CT and DPL should be considered in patients with suspected intra-abdominal injury.

C. **Work-up:** Plain films may detect retroperitoneal or free air, fractures, and abnormal fluid collections. Contrast gastroduodenography may be indicated in a stable patient with suspected pancreaticoduodenal injury. ERCP is recommended if pancreatic ductal injury is suspected in a patient not requiring laparotomy. Contrast enema may be used to diagnose colorectal perforations. Lab studies should include CBC, SMA-7, amylase, lipase, T&C, U/A, and toxicology screen. Insert a Foley and a NG. Appropriate diagnostic options should be considered, including DPL, CT, or immediate laparotomy depending on the clinical circumstances and the personnel available.

4.2 RX:

A. Stabilize the patient by controlling the bleeding with direct pressure and starting large bore IVs. Hypotensive patients should receive 2 L RL in adults and 20 mL/kg in children. If there is no response, administer O^- blood and implement an immediate surgical intervention.

B. Treat coagulopathy with FFP, 1 unit for every 4 units of PRBC. Administer calcium chloride, 0.2 g, 2 mL of 10% solution, IV when PRBCs are transfused at a rate of > 100 mL/minute and a maximum of 1 g of calcium chloride.

C. Patients in profound shock and who are unresponsive to initial fluid resuscitation may require transthoracic aortic clamping followed by laparotomy.

D. Consult a trauma surgeon for anticipated injuries or on the arrival of multiply injured patients.

E. Consider administrating tobramycin or gentamicin, 1.5 mg/kg IV, **and** clindamycin, 600 mg IV, or cefoxitin (Mefoxin), 1 g IV.

F. Initiate Td prophylaxis.

G. Perform the following procedures for blunt abdominal traumas:

Acute Abdomen or **Pneumoperitoneum**: Exploratory laparotomy.

Non-acute abdomen: Consider DPL or CT (Positive- laparotomy, Negative- observe). If reduced pain is a response secondary to drugs, alcohol, head trauma, or hypotension of unknown etiology, consider DPL or CT.

H. Perform the following procedures for penetrating abdominal traumas:

GSW: Requires exploratory lap. Tangential wounds may be assessed by DPL.

Stab: For unstable patients with acute abdomen, signs of peritoneal injury, shock, hypotension, upper or lower GI bleeding, evisceration or pneumoperitoneum, perform a laparotomy. For stable patients with wounds between the fourth intercostal space to the costal margin, fascia involvement, or penetration on local exploration, perform DPL (refer also to "Sections on Chest

Trauma"). For stable patients with no fascia penetration with wound exploration, observe for 24 hours and implement local wound care and antibiotics, if clinically appropriate.

I. Criteria for **Positive Peritoneal Lavage** (for blunt trauma) are 5 mL gross blood, RBC > 100,000 cells/mm^3 (RBC >10,000 for penetrating trauma), WBC > 500 cells/mm^3, food particles, bile, feces or bacteria on Gram's stain. Exit of lavage fluid via a chest tube or bladder catheter. Amylase, 320 IU/L, or alkaline phosphatase, 33 IU.

J. **Disposition:** Victims of multisystem trauma should be hospitalized and observed for 12 to 24 hours despite normal diagnostic studies. After initial stabilization, consider transferring patients to a trauma center.

5. Trauma in Pregnancy:

Treatment priorities for trauma pregnancies are identical to the nonpregnant patient. After the twelfth week of gestation, the uterus rises out of the protection of the pelvis. Injuries incurred include penetration, rupture, and abruptio placenta. Abruption is the number one cause of fetal death after blunt trauma. Hemodynamic changes in pregnancy consist of elevated cardiac output and heart rate. Systolic and diastolic blood pressure is decreased by 5-15 mm Hg. Plasma volume increases and WBC increases. There is no change in respiratory rate although the tidal volume does increase. Fetus can be in shock before mother shows any signs; therefore, resuscitate adequately.

5.1 Clinical Evaluation:

A. **Symptoms:** Refer to the "Abdominal Trauma" section.

B. **Signs:** Expose and visualize entire body, log roll, inspect abdomen for contusion, distention, abrasion, laceration, auscultation of bowel sounds, palpate for signs of peritoneal irritation, and focal tenderness. A physical exam may be unreliable despite the absence of clinical signs. Complete a pelvic exam. Consider deferring if blood is present at introitus, and there is an obvious pelvic fracture.

C. **Work-up:** Stat ultrasound and obstetrical consultation. Order fetal heart tones and tocographic monitoring. If DPL is indicated, use open technique above uterus. Perform a Kleihauer-Betke assay to assess amount of fetomaternal hemorrhage. Dose appropriately with Rh immune globulin for a Rh$^-$ mother.

5.2 RX:

A. Unless spinal trauma is suspected, tilt patient to her left side to prevent uterine compression of the vena cava.

B. Perform a trauma workup and evaluation as previously discussed.

C. **Disposition:** Consider observation with cardiotocodynamometry for 4 hours.

6. Aortic Disruption:

Occurrence is prevalent at the level of the ligamentum arteriosum. There is a 90% mortality at the accident scene. Survivors usually have a contained hematoma.

6.1 Clinical Evaluation:

A. **Symptoms:** Maintain a very high index of suspicion especially in setting of decelerating injury.

B. **Signs:** Palpable first or second rib fractures, chest wall tenderness or bruises.

C. **Work-up:** CXR- tracheal deviation to the right, fractures of the first or second ribs, widened mediastinum, obliteration of the aortic knob, presence of a pleural cap, depression of the left main stem bronchus, obliteration of the space between the pulmonary artery and the aorta, elevation and rightward shift of the right main stem bronchus, and deviation of the esophagus to the right. Obtain a CT chest or arteriogram with surgical consultation.

6.2 RX:

A. Support ABCs, IV, O_2, and monitor.

B. **Disposition:** Refer to a STAT cardiothoracic surgeon STAT. Perform a thoracotomy prn.

7. Pericardial Tamponade:

7.1 Clinical Evaluation:

A. **Symptoms:** Most common secondary to penetrating injuries.

B. **Signs:**

Beck's Triad: JVD, hypotension, and muffled heart sounds.

Kussmaul's sign: Rise in venous pressure with inspiration. Pulsus paradoxus or elevated CVP may be absent when associated with hypovolemia.

C. **Work-up:** Obtain a CXR, enlarged cardiac silhouette, and a ECG, total electrical alternans, electromechanical dissociation (pulseless electrical activity), decreased voltage. Consider ultrasonic evaluation if it is available and appropriate.

7.2 RX:

A. Pericardiocentesis is indicated if the patient is unresponsive to the usual resuscitation measures for hypovolemic shock, or if there is a high likelihood of injury to the myocardium or one of the great vessels. Pericardium can be opened at thoracotomy in extremis.

B. All patients who have a positive pericardiocentesis (recovery of non-clotting blood) due to trauma require open thoracotomy with inspection of the myocardium and the great vessels. Immediately consult cardiothoracic surgery and cardiology.

C. Rule out other causes of cardiac tamponade: Pericarditis, penetration of central line through vena cava, atrium, or ventricle.

D. Consider other causes of hemodynamic instability that may mimic the signs and symptoms of cardiac tamponade (tension pneumothorax, massive pulmonary embolism, shock secondary to massive hemothorax) especially if patient is unresponsive to pericardiocentesis.

E. **Disposition:** Admit to the ICU or to the OR.

8. Esophageal Injury:

After rupture, esophageal contents leak into the mediastinum followed by an immediate or delayed rupture into the pleural space (usually on left) with resulting empyema.

8.1 Clinical Evaluation:

A. **Symptoms:** Usually associated with chest penetrating injuries or severe blunt trauma to the abdomen, or instrumentation of the esophagus with nasogastric tubes or endoscopy. Patient may complain of chest pain or shortness of breath. High index of suspicion is required.

B. **Signs:** Exam for signs of severe blows to the abdomen associated with left or sometimes right pleural effusion on CXR, subcutaneous or mediastinal emphysema and shock.

C. **Work-up:** Obtain CXR. Perform a Gastrografin swallow or endoscopic exam.

8.2 RX:

A. Surgical therapy consists of primary repair if feasible, or esophageal diversion in the neck and a gastrostomy. Start empiric broad spectrum antibiotic therapy as soon as possible.

B. **Disposition:** Admit patient to the OR or to the ICU.

9. Flail Chest:

Uncomplicated flail chest is usually well tolerated with no secondary hypoxia; however, major secondary dysfunctions may result from disrupted mechanical chest function along with possible injuries to the underlying lung parenchyma (contusion and or laceration).

9.1 Clinical Evaluation:

A. **Symptoms:** Usually secondary to severe, blunt chest injury with multiple rib fractures.
B. **Signs:** Freely moving rib segment without bony continuity with the rest of the chest wall. The segment moves in a paradoxical fashion with respect to the chest as a whole.
C. **Work-up:** Order CXR and ABGs.

9.2 RX:

A. Aggressive pulmonary toilet and close observation for any signs of respiratory insufficiency or associated major injuries. Active mechanical ventilatory support of respiration if needed.
B. **Disposition:** Admit, usually to ICU.

10. Hemothorax:

A massive hemothorax is defined as > 1500 mL blood lost into the thoracic cavity.

10.1 Clinical Evaluation:

A. **Symptoms:** Most commonly due to penetrating injuries.
B. **Signs:** Absence of breath sounds and dullness to percussion on the ipsilateral side. Signs and symptoms of hypovolemic shock.

10.2 RX:

A. **Simultaneously** decompress chest cavity with a chest tube and restore volume deficit (may use autotransfused blood). Consult cardiothoracic surgery as soon as possible.
B. **Place** two large-bore IVs or central venous line.
C. **Insert a chest tube** as described previously, but place the site of insertion at the level of the fifth or sixth intercostal space along the midaxillary line ipsilateral to the hemothorax. The chest tube should not be inserted through the injury site. Instead the tube should be positioned in a location away from the injury.
D. **Clean and close** penetrating wound to decrease the likelihood of tension pneumothorax.
E. **Consider thoracotomy** based on the rate of blood loss, i.e., > 200 mL/hour for 2-3 consecutive hours, rather than the initial blood loss volume or the color of the draining blood. If the site of wound penetration is medial to the nipple anteriorly or medial to the scapula posteriorly, there is a high probability of injury to the myocardium and the great vessels. If the great vessels or myocardium has been injured, shock may persist despite aggressive fluid resuscitation.
F. **Consider tetanus prophylaxis** and empirical antibiotic coverage in cases of penetrating injuries.
G. **Disposition:** Admit, usually to ICU.

11. Myocardial Contusion:

11.1 Clinical Evaluation:

A. **Symptoms:** Suspect with blunt trauma to chest, especially if fractures or contusion of sternum or anterior ribs.
B. **Signs:** Chest wall tenderness, bruising, and palpable rib fractures.

C. **Work-up:** Diagnosis may be made by ECG changes (myocardial injury, dysrhythmias, and bundle branch blocks), serial enzymes, and 2 D-echocardiogram (focal or regional wall motion abnormalities).

11.2 RX:

A. Place on cardiac monitor. Observe with supportive measures ensuring adequate oxygenation. Correct electrolyte abnormalities and aggressively manage emerging dysrhythmias.
B. **Disposition:** Admit to ICU or to a monitored bed.

12. Pericardiocentesis:

If an acute cardiac tamponade with hemodynamic instability is suspected, pneumothorax and hemothorax should be eliminated and emergency pericardiocentesis should be performed.

12.1 Clinical Evaluation:

A. **Symptoms:** Refer to sections that describe injuries of the chest.
B. **Signs:** Refer to sections describing injuries of the chest.
C. **DDX:** If patient does not improve, consider other problems that may resemble tamponade, such as tension pneumothorax, pulmonary embolism, or shock secondary to massive hemothorax.

12.2 RX:

A. Infusion of Ringer's lactate, crystalloid, colloid and/or blood may provide temporizing measures.
B. Protect airway, administer oxygen, and ensure that intubation and cardiopulmonary resuscitation equipment are available. If patient can be stabilized, pericardiocentesis should be performed by a specialist in the operating room or catheter lab.
C. Use the para-xiphoid approach for pericardiocentesis in most situations. Place patient in supine position with chest elevated at 30-45 degrees, then cleanse and drape peri-xiphoid area. Infiltrate lidocaine 1% with or without epinephrine (if time permits) into skin and deep tissues.
D. Attach a long, large bore (12-18 cm, 16-18 gauge), short bevel cardiac needle to a 50 cc syringe with a 3-way stop cock. Use a alligator clip to attach a V-lead of the ECG to the metal of the needle.
E. Perform a para-xiphoid approach by advancing the needle just below costal margin immediately to the left and inferior to the xiphoid process. Apply suction to the syringe while advancing the needle slowly at a 45 degrees angle to horizontal towards the mid-point of the left clavicle.
F. As the needle penetrates the pericardium, resistance will be felt, and a characteristic "popping" sensation will be noted.
G. Monitor the ECG for ST segment elevation (indicating ventricular heart muscle contact), or PR segment elevation (indicating atrial epicardial contact). After the needle comes in contact with the epicardium, withdraw the needle slightly. Ectopic ventricular beats are associated with cardiac penetration.
H. Aspirate as much blood as possible. Blood from the pericardial space usually will not clot. Blood, inadvertently, drawn from inside the ventricles or atrium usually will clot. If fluid is not obtained, redirect the needle toward the right shoulder or head.
I. Stabilize the needle by attaching a hemostat or Kelly clamp.
J. Consider emergency thoracotomy to determine the cause of a hemopericardium, especially if there is active bleeding.

13. Pneumothorax:

This condition is rarely spontaneous. It occurs primarily from blunt or penetrating trauma. (Refer also to the “Tension Pneumothorax”.)

13.1 Clinical Evaluation:

A. **Symptoms:** Dyspnea and pleuritic chest pain.
B. **Signs:** Tympanitic to percussion, decreased breath sounds, and subcutaneous emphysema.
C. **DDX:** Tension pneumothorax and hemothorax.
D. **Work-up:** Upright and expiratory CXR is more sensitive.

13.2 RX:

A. For a traumatic pneumothorax, perform a tube thoracostomy by using a #36 to #40 French CT. A smaller tube may be used with a spontaneous pneumothorax.
B. Treat small Primary Spontaneous Pneumothorax (< 10-15%) not associated with any known underlying pulmonary diseases as follows. If the patient is not dyspneic, observe for 4-8 hours and repeat CXR. If the pneumothorax does not increase in size and the patient remains asymptomatic, consider discharging him/her home with instructions, i.e., rest and curtail all strenuous activities. Instruct patient to return if there is an increase in dyspnea or recurrence of chest pain.
C. Treat secondary spontaneous pneumothorax (associated with known underlying pulmonary pathology, most commonly emphysema) or primary spontaneous pneumothorax > 15%, or if patient is symptomatic as follows.

   Administer high flow oxygen. Consider needle aspiration of the pneumothorax by using a 16 gauge needle with an internal polyethylene catheter. Insert in the anterior, second intercostal space in the midclavicular line. Otherwise, insert a chest tube.

   Anesthetize and prep the area before inserting needle. Attach a 60 mL syringe via a 3-way stopcock and aspirate until no more air is aspirated. If no additional air can be aspirated and the volume is < 4 L, occlude the catheter and observe for 4 hours.

   If symptoms abate and chest X-ray does not show recurrence of the pneumothorax, remove the catheter and discharge the patient home with instructions.

   If the aspirated air is > 4 L and additional air is aspirated without resistance, suspect an active bronchopleural fistula with continued air leak. Admission is required for insertion of a chest tube as explained below.
D. To patients with traumatic pneumothorax associated with a penetrating injury, hemothorax, mechanical ventilation, tension pneumothorax, or with pneumothorax that does not resolve after needle aspiration, administer a high flow oxygen and insert a chest tube. Also, initiate aggressive hemodynamic and respiratory resuscitation as indicated. Do not delay the management of a tension pneumothorax until radiographic confirmation. Insert a needle thoracotomy or a chest tube immediately.
E. **Chest Tube Insertion:**

   Position patient in a supine position with involved side elevated 10-20 degrees. Abduct arm at 90 degrees. The usual site of insertion is the fourth or fifth intercostal space, between the mid-axillary and anterior axillary line (drainage of air or free fluid). The point at which the anterior axillary fold meets the chest wall is a useful guide. Alternatively, the second or third intercostal space, in the mid-clavicular line, may be used for pneumothorax drainage alone.

   Clean skin with iodine solution and drape. Determine intrathoracic tube distance (lateral chest wall to the apices) and mark length of tube with a clamp.

   Infiltrate 1% lidocaine into the skin, subcutaneous tissues, intercostal muscles, periosteum, and pleura by using a 25-gauge needle. Use a scalpel to make a transverse skin incision, 2 cm wide, located over the rib just inferior to the interspace where the tube will penetrate the chest wall.

   Using a Kelly clamp, bluntly dissect a subcutaneous tunnel from the skin incision extending just over the superior margin of the lower rib. Avoid the neurovascular bundle located at the upper margin of the intercostal space.

   Bluntly dissect over the rib and penetrate the pleura with the clamp. Open the pleura 1 cm.

With gloved finger, explore the subcutaneous tunnel and palpate the lung medially. Exclude possible abdominal penetration and ensure correct location within pleural space. Use finger to disrupt any local pleural adhesions.
Using the Kelly clamp, grasp the tip of the thoracostomy tube (36 F, internal diameter 12 mm), and direct it into the pleural space in a posterior, superior direction. Guide the tube into the pleural space until the last hole is inside the pleural space.
Attach the tube to an underwater seal apparatus containing sterile normal saline and adjust to 20 cm H_2O of negative pressure or attach to suction if the leak is severe. Suture the tube to the skin of the chest wall by using O silk. Apply Vaseline gauze, 4 x 4 gauze sponges, and elastic tape.
Obtain CXR to verify correct placement and evaluate re-expansion of lung.
Consider consultation for pleurodesis sclerotherapy if clinically indicated.

F. With positive pressure ventilation, perform an immediate CT. To compensate for loss of gas through pneumothorax, an increase in total minute ventilation, tidal volume, or respiration rate may be required. For a severe leak, high frequency, low pressure ventilation or synchronized inspiratory CT occlusion may be necessary.
G. **Disposition:** Obtain a surgical consultation. Admit all patients who are traumatic. Patients with spontaneous pneumothorax may sometimes be discharged home with a unidirectional, i.e., Heimlich valve device.

14. Pulmonary Contusion:

Diagnosis is usually delayed because respiratory failure develops over time rather than occurring early. Severe forms may be indistinguishable from adult respiratory distress syndrome.

14.1 Clinical Evaluation:

A. **Symptoms:** Chest trauma.
B. **Signs:** Chest wall tenderness, bruises, and palpable fractures.
C. **Work-up:** CXR- localized alveolar and or interstitial infiltrate, usually underlying the site of blunt injury or within the trajectory of the penetrating injury. Obtain ABGs.

14.2 RX:

A. Consider conservative management with close observation in a critical care unit. Intubation is required whenever the respiratory failure is severe or if associated medical conditions predispose to early intubation, including pre-existing chronic pulmonary disease, renal failure, abdominal injury, head trauma with secondary depressed level of consciousness, prolonged immobilization, mainly secondary to skeletal injuries.
B. **Disposition:** Admit, usually to an ICU.

15. Tension Pneumothorax:

15.1 Clinical Evaluation:

A. **Symptoms:** Blunt or penetrating chest trauma.
B. **Signs:** Severe hemodynamic and/or respiratory compromise, contralateral deviated trachea, decreased or absent breath sounds and hyperresonance to percussion on the affected side, jugular venous distention, asymmetrical chest wall motion with respiration, flattening or inversion of the ipsilateral hemidiaphragm, contralateral shifting of the mediastinum, flattening of the cardio-mediastinal contour, and spreading of the ribs on the ipsilateral side.
C. **Work-up:** Obtain CXR and ABGs. Draw blood for CBC, PT, PTT, T&C, SMA-7, and toxicology screen.

15.2 RX:

A. Perform emergent chest tube placement.
B. Consider temporary ipsilateral placement of a large-bore IV catheter into the pleural space, at the level of the second intercostal space at the mid-clavicular line, until the chest tube is placed.
C. Insert 2 large-bore IVs.
D. Consider central venous pressure monitoring and arterial line.
E. Consider intubation if indicated.
F. Send pleural fluid for hematocrit, amylase and pH (in order to eliminate possible esophageal rupture).
G. **Disposition:** Arrange for cardiothoracic exploration if there is a penetrating chest injury, persistent air leak, severe or persistent hemodynamic instability despite aggressive fluid resuscitation, or persistent active blood loss from the chest tube.

16. Tracheobronchial Injury:

Suspect tracheobronchial tree injury in all upper torso, penetrating or blunt (especially decelerating) injuries.

16.1 Clinical Evaluation:

A. **Symptoms:** Hoarseness, hemoptysis.
B. **Signs:** Subcutaneous emphysema, palpable fracture, and crepitus.
C. **DDX:** Associated injuries to the esophagus, carotid arteries, or jugular veins. Tension pneumothorax (especially if large air leak through chest tube). Abnormal breathing suggestive of airway obstruction.
D. **Work-up:** Obtain CXR, CT chest, and arteriogram.

16.2 RX:

A. Maintain a high index of suspicion, secure airway and ventilation, relieve tension pneumothorax, and obtain early surgical correction of large vessel injury or esophageal disruption.
B. **Disposition:** Admit to the OR or to the ICU.

17. Eye Trauma:

17.1 Clinical Evaluation:

A. **Symptoms:** Mechanism, environment, pre-existing ocular disease, corrective lens/contact use, pain, photophobia, and vision loss.
B. **Signs:** Visual acuity, eyelids, globe (fracture or penetration), orbit (step-off deformity and crepitus), pupil (size and shape), cornea (opacity, ulceration and foreign bodies), conjunctiva (chemosis, subconjunctival emphysema, hemorrhage, and foreign bodies), anterior chamber (hyphema), iris (regular shape or reactive), lens (check displacement), vitreous (transparent unless hemorrhage), and retina (hemorrhage, tears, and detachment).
C. **Work-up:** Perform a visual field exam, slit-lamp exam, and funduscopic exam. Orbital soft tissues and CT may be helpful.

17.2 RX:

A. Consult ophthalmologist for wounds to the lid which involve the medial canthus, injury to lacrimal sac or duct, horizontal lacerations of the upper lid that may include the levator, and lid margin lacerations. Superficial lid lacerations may be closed.
B. Treat superficial abrasions to the cornea with pain medicine, antibiotic ointment (sulfacetamide, neomycin, bacitracin, polymyxin, and gentamicin), and a short-acting cycloplegic. Arrange for a close follow-up. Remove foreign bodies with irrigation or slit-lamp needle extraction in consultation with an ophthalmologist. For anterior chamber hyphema, patch, hospitalize, advise upright bed rest, prescribe analgesics, and refer to an ophthalmologist.
C. Displacement of the lens requires immediate ophthalmologist consultation.
D. For a vitreous hemorrhage, advise bed rest with patching and refer to a specialist.
E. Refer to an ophthalmologist for a retinal hemorrhage.
F. Penetration of the globe requires immediate ophthalmology referral.

G. For chemical contact/exposure, start immediate copious and continuous saline irrigation. Refer to a specialist immediately.
H. Examine carefully for evidence of entrapment in an orbital fracture. Obtain an ophthalmology consult.
I. Immediately refer to an ophthalmologist when encountered with retrobulbar hematoma.

18. Dental Trauma:

Subluxation is the abnormal loosening of a tooth. Displacement is partial to total avulsion. A fracture may involve enamel, dentin, cementum, and pulp in the crown or roof. Replace permanent teeth as quickly as possible. A percentage point for success is lost for each minute the tooth is absent from the oral cavity.

18.1 Clinical Evaluation:

A. **Symptoms:** How, when, where, and what treatment. Pain, sensitivity touch or temperature. Past dental history.
B. **Signs:** Jaw/TMJ function, occlusion, fracture, tooth coloration, and soft tissue trauma. Digital exam.
C. **Work-up:** Consider Panorex, soft tissue, or peripheral radiographs.

18.2 RX:

Transport teeth in mouth, milk, isotonic saline or specialized solution.

	Primary teeth	**Permanent teeth**
Subluxation	No stabilization. Soft diet. Dental follow up.	No stabilization. Soft diet. Dental follow up.
Displacement	Extract if: 1. Exfoliation will occur within 6 months OR intruded and close to permanent tooth 2. Extruded allow to re-erupt	Nonmobile: No treatment. Refer to dentist Mobile: Reposition. Temporary stabilization.
Avulsion	Do not reimplant.	Clean tooth and socket, NO SCRUBBING. Reimplant ASAP.
Fractures **Crown**	Hemostasis. Pain control. Remove tooth fragment to prevent aspiration. Refer to dentist.	Same.
Root	Apical/Middle 1/3: Reposition/ stabilize. Refer to dentist. Coronal 1/3: Remove crown. Protect/ stabilize. Refer to dentist.	Same. Same.
Dentoalveolar	Reposition/stabilize. Remove bone fragments. Refer to dentist.	Same.

19. Le Fort Fractures:

The Le Fort classification describes characteristic mid facial fracture lines. A free floating jaw is found in all the Le Fort type fractures.

19.1 Clinical Evaluation:

A. **Signs:**

Le Fort I: Horizontal maxillary fracture. Grasping the alveolar process between the index finger and thumb will cause anterior - posterior motion. Movement of the premaxilla signifies **at least** a Le Fort I fracture.

Le Fort II: Pyramidal fracture. Inspection may reveal significant mid face swelling, bilateral subconjunctival hemorrhages, periorbital ecchymosis, epistaxis or CSF rhinorrhea. Analyze the fluid for glucose. CSF rhinorrhea is a result of a cribriform plate fracture. The diagnosis can be confirmed by gently holding the upper dental arch while palpating the base of the nose.

Le Fort III: Craniofacial disjunction. The fracture line extends from the frontozygomatic sutures, across the orbits, and through the base of the nose and the ethmoid bones. Patient may have periorbital ecchymosis, "dishface" features. The diagnosis can be confirmed if there is movement of the zygomas and mid face.

B. **Work-up:** All fracture types require Water's projections. Computed tomography of the orbits helps confirm the diagnosis of Le Fort II and III type fractures.

19.2 RX:

A. Any patient with a suspected CSF leak requires a neurosurgical consultation prior to a maxillofacial surgery consultation.
B. Administer tetanus and antibiotic prophylaxis.
C. **Disposition:** Consult ENT, ophthalmology, or neurosurgery for admission versus outpatient treatment.

20. Mandibular Fractures:

With a "Ring" type bony structure, examine for 2 fractures. There are basically two principles of treatment for mandibular fractures: 1) restoration of form, and 2) restoration of function. The signs and symptoms of a mandibular fracture are malocclusion, bony crepitus, pain, deformity and deviation, and limited range of motion. Angle of the mandible is the most common area of fracture.

20.1 Clinical Evaluation:

A. **Signs:** Extraoral examination reveals swelling, ecchymosis, bony crepitus or step-off deformity, and point tenderness. Test for anesthesia of the lower lip. Intraoral examination may reveal blood, malalignment or deformity of the dental arches or teeth. Check for breaks in the mucosa and hematomas (especially of the sublingual area). Test for complete range of motion.
B. **Work-up:** Obtain a panoramic view of the maxilla and of the mandible; otherwise, obtain the standard 3 views: PA of the face and skull, right and left lateral oblique views. Regional classification: alveolar, condylar, angle and body.

20.2 RX:

A. NPO.
B. Initiate tetanus prophylaxis.
C. Start on antibiotics, such as penicillin, cephalosporin, or clindamycin.
D. Preserve all teeth and orthodontic devices.

E. Definitive treatment per oral surgeon- internal fixation. Alveolar fractures require stabilization via arch bars or wires.
F. **Disposition:** As per consultant.

21. Mid Facial Fractures:

Avulsed teeth should be reimplanted ASAP. Definitive treatment occurs within several days. ED treatment is supportive.

21.1 Clinical Evaluation:

A. **Signs:**

Zygomatic arch fracture: Depression of bone. Patient may not be able to open or close his/her mouth.

Zygomatic-Maxillary complex: Swelling/ecchymosis of the cheek or periorbital area, facial depression, unilateral epistaxis, anesthesia of the infraorbital nerve (cheek, upper lip, and teeth), diplopia, lateral subconjunctival hemorrhage, restriction of mandibular movements, and tissue crepitus. There may be marked tissue edema. Test for visual acuity and EOM. Perform slit-lamp and funduscopic exam prn.

Orbital floor fractures: Diplopia and inferior displacement of the globe, restriction of ocular movements secondary to tissue entrapment in the maxillary sinus. Check lids for foreign bodies, orbital rims for edema/hemorrhage, corneas for abrasions, and sclera for tears. Inspect anterior chamber for hyphema and the iris, lens, posterior chamber and retina for trauma.

B. **Work-up:**

Zygomatic arch: Basal skull view (jug handle view and submentaloccipital view).

Zygomatic-Maxillary complex: Water's projection and basal skull view. Confirmation and further evaluation of the orbital and maxillary fractures may require tomograms.

Orbital floor fractures: Water's view X-rays and tomograms.

21.2 RX:

A. Zygomatic arch fracture: Delayed surgical intervention for cosmetic defect or mandibular dysmobility.
B. Zygomatic-Maxillary complex: Open reduction and wire fixation or antral packing.
C. Orbital floor fractures: Surgical reconstruction of the orbital floor.
D. **Disposition:** Per surgical consult.

22. Head Injuries:

Raised intracranial pressure can lead to herniation of the uncus adjacent to the tentorial edge and pressure on the adjacent third nerve with ipsilateral pupil dilation. Further pressure results in a shift of the contralateral peduncle against the edge of the tentorium and pressure against the adjacent third nerve and posterior cerebral artery on the other side. Dilation of contralateral pupil occurs with cessation of spontaneous respiration because of bilateral interruption of the pathways found in the cerebral peduncles.

22.1 Clinical Evaluation:

A. **Symptoms:** Mechanism of injury, past medical history, and drug intake.

B. **Signs:**

Make initial assessment of the patient.

Assume c-spine injury in any patient with multisystem trauma especially injury involving the area above the clavicles. A normal neurologic examination does not rule out a c-spine injury.

Perform a mini neurologic examination as soon as possible and repeat frequently. Check: Level of consciousness (Glasgow Coma Scale) and eye-opening response (4-Spontaneous, 3-Voice, 2-Pain, 1-none). Best Verbal (5-Oriented, 4-Confused, 3-Inappropriate words, 2-Incomprehensible words, 1-None). Best Motor (6-Obeys commands, 5-Localizes pain, 4- Withdraws pain, 3-Flexion pain, 2-Extension pain, 1- None). [<8 Severe head injury, 9-12 Moderate head injury, 13-15 Minor head injury]. Lateralizing extremity weakness or changes in sensation. Pupillary function. Examine skull for clinically detectable depressed skull fracture, Battle's sign (ecchymosis over mastoid process), Raccoons eye (periorbital ecchymosis), and CSF rhinorrhea or otorrhea.

C. **Work-up:** Indications for CT include: 1) Patient with transient or persistent unconsciousness with evidence of head injury or coma from toxins or metabolic causes, and 2) patients with skull fractures include depressed and basal. Draw blood for CBC, PT, PTT, Chem 18; T&C; toxicology screen.

22.2 RX:

A. **General Management Considerations:**

Support airway, IV, O_2, and monitor.

Consider central venous pressure monitoring (CVP line or pulmonary artery catheter); consider insertion of arterial line.

Aggressively resuscitate shock, and search for underlying causes (head injuries do not usually cause shock except in terminal stages).

B. Consider a minor concussion if Glasgow Coma Scale (GCS) is > 13, pupils are equal, there are no lateralizing deficits, there are no open head injuries, and the patient is neurologically intact with no loss of consciousness, or loss of consciousness less than 5 minutes, and has no major underlying medical problems. The patient may be eligible for discharge to home with instructions, provided there is adequate support available and access for return is possible.

C. If GCS is > 9, the pupils are equal, no lateralizing deficits are evident, and no open head injuries were sustained, but neurologically is not intact, the condition is probably a contusion or a small mass lesion, such as subdural or epidural hematomas.

D. If GCS is > 9 but the patient has either unequal pupils or any lateralizing deficit, a possible mass effect is evident, such as a large subdural or epidural hematomas or an intracerebral bleed. Each of these conditions requires admission after a neurosurgical consultation and head CT is obtained.

E. If GCS is < 8, with or without unequal pupils, with lateralizing deficits, or with open head injuries, the most likely cause is a large intracerebral mass or a diffuse axonal injury. Obtain a STAT CT of head and a STAT neurosurgical consultation. Emergency intubation may be indicated, usually with rapid sequence induction (secondary concern for elevated ICP) for airway control with or without hyperventilation. The intubation should be done with in-line-immobilization, cricothyroidotomy prn.

F. Intravenous resuscitation solutions should be isotonic (LR or NS).

G. Except for shock management, consider restricting fluid intake to maintenance levels, or as indicated by hemodynamic monitoring.

H. Supply high flow oxygen.

I. Maintain NPO.

J. Give stress ulcer prophylaxis in the form of H_2-blockers (ranitidine and cimetidine), or sucralfate.

K. Consider hyperosmolar therapy, such as mannitol 1 mg/kg IVP, or hyperventilation by maintaining a pCO_2 of 30 mm Hg.

L. If seizures occur, treat with lorazepam, 4-8 mg IVP, repeated until seizures are controlled, followed by phenytoin, 17 mg/kg IV loading at a rate of 50 mg/minute.

M. Avoid excitement, agitation, administration of sedative- hypnotics, narcotics, or neuromuscular blockers, unless necessary.

N. Control temperature.

O. Clean and repair open head wounds.

P. Initiate tetanus prophylaxis.
Q. Administer Lidocaine 1 mg/kg IV during rapid sequence intubation to prevent a rise in the intracranial pressure.

23. Acute Subdural or Epidural Hematoma:

23.1 Clinical Evaluation:

A. **History/Signs:**

Subdural: Acute is usually caused by torn cortical vessels from contusions or cortical lacerations. Chronic is usually produced by tearing of bridging veins. More common in elderly. Clinical course is usually slow in onset.

Epidural: Clinical course is typically biphasic, injury, loss of consciousness, lucid interval, and secondary depression in consciousness. Rapid accumulation of a hematoma due to a tear of the middle meningeal artery with a rapid rise of the ICP, ipsilateral uncal herniation, and peduncle and third nerve compression. Survival depends on immediate decompression prior to final stages, not when both pupils are dilated. Rapid surgical intervention is mandatory. No time should be spent on diagnostic tests if the patient has clinically evident symptoms. Consider emergency trephination for decompression.

B. **Work-up:** If time permits, obtain an emergency CT scan.

23.2 RX:

A. Support airway, IV, O_2, and monitor. Include rapid sequence induction and hyperventilation for signs of increased ICP or imminent herniation. Implement a "change in mental status" management.
B. Obtain a neurosurgical consultation STAT.
C. If patient is in a frank coma or shows signs of increased intracranial pressure, neurosurgeon may consider emergency burr hole placement and evacuation of clot. Consider intracranial pressure monitoring if indicated.
D. **Disposition:** Admit to the OR or to the ICU.

24. Cerebral Contusion:

24.1 Clinical Evaluation:

A. **History/Signs:** Persistent neurologic deficit following head trauma with altered level of consciousness.
B. **Work-up:** Obtain a CT head.

24.2 RX:

A. Support airway, IV, O_2, and monitor. Include rapid sequence induction and hyperventilation to maintain pCO_2 between 25-30 mm Hg. Watch for signs of increased ICP or imminent herniation. Change in mental status management.
B. Obtain a neurosurgery consultation STAT.
C. Administer isotonic fluids at kvo rate.
D. If patient is not significantly volume depleted and is not in shock, administer mannitol 1 g/kg IV. Prescribe dexamethasone, 10-20 mg IV x 1 dose. Monitor urine output.
E. Initiate prophylaxis and treatment of seizures with diazepam (Valium), 5-10 mg given slow IV (not faster than 1 mg/minute). Repeat dose q 10-15 minutes if needed.
F. Administer phenytoin, 1 g (15-20 mg/kg) loading does at 50 mg/minute IV.
G. **Disposition:** Admit to ICU. Obtain an immediate neurosurgical consultation.

25. Concussion:

25.1 Clinical Evaluation:

A. **History/Signs:** Transient neurological dysfunction following blunt trauma to the head.

B. **Work-up:** Acquire a CT of the head.

25.2 RX:

A. Support airway, IV, O_2, and monitor prn.

B. Obtain a trauma/neurosurgical consultation.

C. Hold narcotics, sedatives, or aspirin when possible. NPO initially. Start maintenance IV and insert a NG prn.

D. **Disposition:** Patients with loss of conscious, amnesia, or other severe CNS symptoms should be hospitalized for at least 24-48 hours and observed for serial reassessments of neurological function and mental status.

UROGENITAL

1. Acute Urinary Retention:

Acute urinary retention is the inability to urinate. It is a problem that occurs primarily in adult males. The most prevalent cause of this condition is benign prostatic hypertrophy (BPH). Other common causes include prostatic carcinoma, bladder carcinoma, UTI, urethral stricture, spinal cord disease/trauma, and clots of blood. Atypical sources of acute urinary retention are phimosis, paraphimosis, urethritis, urethral calculus, foreign body, or medications (primarily anticholinergics but also narcotics, phenothiazines, anticholinergics, cyclic antidepressants, antihistamines, antihypertensives and muscle relaxants).

1.1 Clinical Evaluation:

A. **Symptoms:** Low abdominal pain and inability to void. Obtain history of medication, neurologic disease/trauma, and prior episodes.

B. **Signs:**

Abdomen: Palpate for tenderness and distention of suprapubic region.
Rectal: Prostate size and consistency.
Pelvic: masses and tenderness.
Neurologic abnormalities.

C. **Work-up:** Order U/A and C&S, CBC, and chemistries.

1.2 RX:

A. Pass a 16-French Foley catheter if there are numerous blood clots. If unable to pass Foley, then use a 16-French coude. If still unable to pass, try another size. Refer to a urologist or perform a suprapubic catheterization. If UTI, treat as indicated for UTI.

B. **Disposition:** Consider admission for patients with acute retention. Otherwise, discharge home with a catheter and leg drainage bag for chronic conditions.

2. Dialysis-Related Emergencies:

Patients in chronic renal failure may have a surgically created arteriovenous fistula or artificial vascular graft placed in the arm. Dialysis is performed several times per week for several hours. These patients are at increased risk for cardiac disease, including non-infectious pericarditis. NOTE: Do not use involved arm for BP, IV access, or for taking blood.

2.1 Clinical Evaluation:

A. **Symptoms:** Common complaints are faintness and dizziness, particularly after dialysis, shortness of breath, chest pain, bleeding, pain and swelling at access site, and constipation.

B. **Signs:** Hypotension usually occurs during and immediately after dialysis. Hypertension is typically the result of volume overload, indicating the need for dialysis. Examine for cardiac rhythm, heart sounds, and for friction rub. Dyspnea and rales may indicate pneumonia or congestive heart failure. Bruising and bleeding from access site may be the result of thrombocytopenia. Common problem at access site is infection. Signs are a warm red arm and fever. Loss of a thrill indicates possible thrombosis.

C. **Work-up:** Obtain ECG (peaked T-waves and/or widened QRS suggest hyperkalemia; diffuse upward concave ST elevations suggest pericarditis), CXR, ABG, SMA-7, and blood culture (if fever and infection suspected).

2.2 RX:

A. Support airway, IV, O_2, and monitor.
B. Hypotension commonly responds to rapid infusion of NS. Vasopressors are seldom necessary.
C. Hypertension and dyspnea are usually the result of volume overload and indicate the need for dialysis. Treat with oxygen, 4 L/minute by NC, or 6 L by mask. NTG, 0.4 mg sublingually q 30 minutes prn, reduces preload and afterload. Severe hypertension is controlled by sodium nitroprusside, 0.5 μg/kg/minute, and titrated to diastolic of > 80-100 mm Hg.
D. Treat cardiac arrhythmias, pulmonary edema and bleeding abnormalities in the standard fashion.
E. Pericarditis usually does not result in cardiac tamponade, and pericardiocentesis is rarely necessary.
F. Treat infection of access site with vancomycin, 1 g IV as loading dose. Thrombosis of access site requires immediate surgical consultation.
G. Treat severe hyperkalemia, such as ECG manifestations, chest pain, and/or K^+ > 7.5 mEq/L, with calcium gluconate, 10 mL of 10% solution over 5 minutes, followed by 50 mL of 50% glucose +20 units of regular insulin, then 50 mEq of sodium bicarbonate IV. A definitive treatment is dialysis.
H. Constipation usually responds to docusate sodium (Colace), 200 mg po daily.
I. **Disposition:** Admit and perform emergency dialysis for patients with volume overload and/or pulmonary edema.

3. Epididymitis:

Epididymitis is an infection/inflammation of epididymis from retrograde spread of organisms up the vas deferens. It is the most common cause of an acute scrotal mass in adults. This condition is usually contracted by sexually transmitted diseases, chronic prostatitis, and urethral instrumentation. Males under age 35 are typically infected by *Chlamydia trachomatis* and *Neisseria gonorrhoeae* whereas the condition in males over 35 is usually caused by *E. coli, Enterococci, Pseudomonas* and *Proteus*.

3.1 Clinical Evaluation:

A. **Symptoms:** Acute onset of scrotal pain and swelling on one side over several hours. Severe pain in back part of testicle, relieved by elevation (Prenh sign). Sometimes earlier history of sexually transmitted disease and/or penile discharge. Intercourse with new sexual partners.
B. **Signs:** Fever. Palpate for abdominal tenderness and auscultate for bowel sounds. Observe for penile discharge, genital lesions, hernia, and lymphadenopathy. Gently palpate both testes lying and standing. Affected testis low-riding, with posterior induration and exquisite point tenderness.
C. **DDX:** Testicular torsion, orchitis, torsion of appendix testis, tumor, and hernia.
D. **Work-up:** Obtain U/A (usually shows pyuria or bacteriuria), urine C&S, CBC, and blood culture (if sepsis suspected).

3.2 RX:

A. Treat with ceftriaxone (Rocephin), 250 mg IM, plus doxycycline, 100 mg q 12 hours for 10 days.
B. **Disposition:** Admit the febrile toxic patient. Scrotal elevation with a towel.

4. Hematuria:

Hematuria occurs when the RBCs are > 5 per high power field of a urine sediment of 10 mL. Urine dipstick detects less than 5 RBCs. Most cases are caused from UTI. Sudden severe back pain suggests a ureteral stone. Most common causes in the < 20 year old age group is urinary tract infection and glomerulonephritis. The > 20 year old group suffers from UTI and stone. Lastly, the > 50 year old group are affected by UTI, stone, BPH, bladder and kidney cancer.

Renal causes: IgA nephropathy (Berger's disease) is common, glomerulonephritis (GN) (from streptococcal infection, SLE, Goodpasture's, and vasculitis), pyelonephritis, trauma, renal epithelial or vascular tumors, and SBE.
Lower urinary tract causes: Calculus, tumor, infection, and prostatitis.
Hematologic causes: Coagulopathy, sickle cell disease.
Other causes: AAA, renal artery aneurysm rupture, cyclophosphamide, FB, and HSP. Clots of blood can cause secondary obstruction.

4.1 Clinical Evaluation:

A. **Symptoms:** Hemorrhagic cystitis and pyelonephritis are indicated by the presence of a fever, dysuria, frequency, urgency, and retention. Renal colic pain suggests calculus or mimicking AAA. History of sickle cell, coagulopathy or anticoagulant use suggests a hematologic etiology. Sparse history may indicate a neoplasm. Streptococcal pharyngitis within past few weeks implies glomerulonephritis.
B. **Signs:** Mass or bruit on abdominal exam suggests renal artery or AAA. Fever, tachycardia, ill appearance suggest infectious cause. For the age group > 40, consider a malignancy.
C. **DDX:** Pigmenturia caused by porphyria, myoglobin, free hemoglobin, beets, rhubarb, and some medications.
D. **Work-up:** Verify true hematuria with microscopic analysis of spun urine. RBC casts suggest GN, SLE, and SBE. WBCs indicate infection. WBC casts suggest pyelonephritis. Examine for prostatitis. Proteinuria suggests pyelonephritis, GN, and nephrotic syndrome. If GN is suspected, especially in children, examine for the other components of nephritis syndrome- edema, HTN, and renal insufficiency. Order CBC and SMA-7. IVP is appropriate in the ED to evaluate hematuria after trauma or for suspected renal stone. CT for suspected aneurysm. Further evaluation of hematuria may be appropriately managed on an outpatient basis; possible cancer, ongoing bleeding may require inpatient evaluation and intervention.

4.2 RX:

A. Customize treatment according to etiology.
B. **Disposition:** Admit for patients complicated by severe illness, dehydration, renal insufficiency or failure, diabetes, obstruction, and new GN.

5. Prostatitis:

Prostatitis is an acute or chronic inflammation of the prostate gland. Most cases are caused by bacterial infection with the same organisms that cause urinary tract infections, i.e., *E. coli* (most common), *Pseudomonas*, and *Enterococci*. Chronic prostatitis is the most common cause of recurrent urinary tract infection in males. In some chronic cases, cultures are negative. Younger males are more prone to acute prostatitis whereas older males exhibit chronic prostatitis with exacerbations.

5.1 Clinical Evaluation:

A. **Symptoms:**

Acute prostatitis: Fever, chills, dysuria, frequency, urgency and recent onset of low back or groin pain.
Exacerbations of chronic prostatitis: Low-grade fever, chronic low back pain, frequency and dysuria.

B. **Signs:**

Fever. Palpate abdomen, flanks, lumbar region for tenderness (suprapubic or costovertebral angle tenderness).
Genitalia: Urethral discharge, lesions, and inguinal adenopathy. Palpate testes for swelling, tenderness or masses.

Rectal: Tender soft prostate in acute prostatitis; slightly tender prostate with normal consistency in chronic prostatitis. NOTE: do not massage gland since bacteremia may result.

C. **Work-up:** Order CBC, U/A and C&S, and blood culture (if applicable).

5.2 RX:

A. For acute prostatitis, treat with ciprofloxacin (Cipro), 200 mg IV q 12 hours, or ofloxacin (Floxin), 200 mg IV q 12 hours. Treat outpatients with the same therapy recommended for chronic prostatitis for at least 1 month.

B. Treat chronic prostatitis with ciprofloxacin, 250 mg po tid for 4 weeks, or ofloxacin, 200 mg bid for 4 weeks.

C. **Disposition:** Consider admission for acute prostatitis. Arrange outpatient therapy and obtain a urology consultation for chronic prostatitis.

6. Renal Colic:

Renal colic induces severe pain from an obstruction of urinary outflow tract by one or more calculi. Eighty percent of the stones are calcium salts.

6.1 Clinical Evaluation:

A. **Symptoms:** Abrupt onset of severe abdominal or flank pain, usually at night or early morning. Pain is usually intermittent and sometimes accompanied by nausea and vomiting. Inquire about family history of stones.

B. **Signs:**

Vitals: Tachypnea, tachycardia and HTN related to discomfort.

Patient writhing in pain, unable to find comfortable position (a patient with peritonitis lies curled up, as any movement aggravates pain).

Abdomen: Moderate abdominal or flank tenderness over site of obstruction. No point tenderness or rebound. Sometimes decreased bowel sounds. Examine carefully for bruits and pulsatile mass (renal colic in elderly must be differentiated from leaking or ruptured abdominal aortic aneurysm, a lethal condition).

C. **DDX:** Most common cases are associated with pancreatitis, biliary colic, pyelonephritis, bowel obstruction, and appendicitis. Less common are perforated peptic ulcer or diverticulum, rupture of abdominal aorta, mesenteric artery occlusion, cervical cancer, and endometriosis.

D. **Work-up:** Order U/A (almost always shows large amount of blood), CBC, chemistries, KUB (many calcium stones evident on plain film), intravenous pyelogram (IVP shows delayed filling and dilatation on involved side), and renal ultrasound prn.

6.2 RX:

A. Start IV, O_2, and monitor prn.

B. Control pain with meperidine (Demerol), 25-50 mg IV q 10 minutes, **or** meperidine, 50-100 mg IM q 3-6 hours, **or** consider ketorolac, 30-60 mg IM or IV.

C. Hydrate patient with IV NS.

D. **Disposition:**

Admit patients with severe infection/fever, high-grade obstruction, and intractable pain.

Obtain urologic consultation for stones > 6 mm.

Discharge a patient home with a prescription of acetaminophen/codeine or NSAIDS. Advise outpatient to increase fluids, strain urine, and arrange for a follow-up in 2 days.

7. Renal Failure:

In renal failure, the kidneys no longer adequately filter nitrogenous wastes, and BUN and creatinine accumulate in bloodstream (azotemia). "Uremia" is the effect of renal failure on organ systems.

7.1 Clinical Evaluation:

A. **Symptoms:** There are a few specific symptoms. Acute abdominal pain with nausea and vomiting may suggest prerenal causation. Acute onset of decreased urine output (oliguria < 500 mL), high blood pressure and shortness of breath may represent nephritis. Oliguria plus suprapubic pain may indicate postrenal cause.

B. **Signs:** Vitals are important. Check for hypotension/hypertension and orthostatics. Note skin turgor, color, and edema. Examine cardiac and respiratory signs. Abdominal and flank tenderness may suggest postrenal cause. Perform prostate and pelvic exams.

C. **DDX:**

Prerenal: Reduction in cardiac output (congestive heart failure and cirrhosis), hypovolemia (fluid loss).

Renal: Acute tubular necrosis (ATN) secondary to shock, hemorrhage, some antibiotics; acute interstitial nephritis (AIN) from drugs, including some antibiotics, and NSAIDS.

Postrenal: Obstruction of collecting system, urethra, bladder, and ureters.

D. **Work-up:** Order CBC, electrolytes, glucose, calcium, phosphorous, BUN, creatinine, U/A and urine sediment, ECG, and CXR. Measurement of urinary and serum Na and Cr (mostly helpful beyond ED).

7.2 RX:

A. Support airway, IV, O_2, and monitor prn.

B. For prerenal, hypovolemia is managed with NS or RL infused rapidly.

C. For renal, implement dialysis and administer a low dose of dopamine, 2 μg/kg/minute. This treatment may increase renal blood flow in ATN.

D. A Foley catheter may relieve bladder outlet obstruction for postrenal conditions.

E. **Disposition:** Admit.

8. Testicular Torsion:

Torsion is twisting of the spermatic cord and testis, occluding the venous system and decreasing arterial flow. It commonly occurs during puberty at an average of 17 years of age. The cause of testicular torsion is related to an abnormally developed tunica vaginalis. To salvage testis, detorsion needs to take place in less than 6 hours.

8.1 Clinical Evaluation:

A. **Symptoms:** Sudden onset of pain in scrotum, which may radiate to abdomen. Sometimes previous milder attacks. Frequently occurs during sleep or after physical activity. Nausea and vomiting sometimes present.

B. **Signs:** Palpate abdomen for tenderness/auscultate for bowel sounds. Observe for penile discharge, genital lesions, hernia and lymphadenopathy. Gently palpate both testes with patient lying and standing. Affected testis is tender, high-riding, slightly swollen, sometimes lying horizontally or malrotated anteriorly. Feel posteriorly for enlarged tender spermatic cord (epididymitis) or other masses. Transilluminate for hydrocele.

C. **DDX:** Epididymitis, orchitis, torsion of appendix testis, tumor, hernia, hydrocele, and hematocele.

D. **Work-up:** Obtain U/A (neg), CBC (1/3 of patients have leukocytosis). Although radionuclide scanning is test of choice for diagnosis, no delay should be made for this test. Laboratory preparation for surgery.

8.2 RX:

A. Brief attempt at manual detorsion may be attempted in the ED.
B. **Disposition:** Obtain a urology consultation and prepare for immediate surgical detorsion.

WOUNDS

1. Wounds:

1.1 Clinical Evaluation:

A. **Symptoms:** Mechanism of injury (simple laceration, crushing injury, closed fist injuries (CFI), bite wounds, or Puncture), age of the wound (Golden Period for closing < 6 to 12 hours depending on location), environmental factors (clean or contaminated environment), age of the patient (increased infection if < 2 years or > 50 years), pre-existing health problems (diabetes, alcoholism, or immunosuppression), nutritional status, smoking (delays distal extremity healing), medications (steroids), allergies, and tetanus immunization.

B. **Signs:** Location of the wound (vascular vs low vascularity, stress on the wound, or high bacteria count skin area), underlying structures (nerves, tendons, vascular structures, and bone/joints), sensory-motor function of affected area (2 point discrimination, range of motion, and strength), circulation (distal pulses, capillary refill time, and color/temperature).

C. **DDX:** Simple laceration, stellate laceration, avulsion, punctures, bites, and closed fist injuries (CFI).

D. **Work-up:** Obtain a X-ray if possible to check for foreign body or underlying fracture.

Skin Preparation: It is necessary to disinfect the skin before performing any procedure. There are various soaps and disinfectants on the market. Povidone-iodine (Betadine) and chlorhexidine (Hibiclens) are two common and excellent skin disinfectants. The disinfecting agent should be used on the skin only and not in the wound. Disinfectants are known to be toxic to wound tissue and may hinder the healing process while increasing the infection rate. Hair may be cut but should not be shaved. Never shave eyebrows.

Anesthetizing the wound: Direct infiltration (through the wound edge), parallel margin infiltration (field block), or regional blocks (digital blocks being the most common) should be considered. If the patient is allergic to one group of local anesthesia, use one from the other category. Amides include lidocaine (Xylocaine), mepivacaine (Carbocaine), bupivacaine (Marcaine). Esters are procaine (Novocaine), tetracaine (Pontocaine), chloroprocaine (Nesacaine), benzocaine, and cocaine (not for injection). Benadryl (an amide antihistamine) can be used as a local anesthesia in patients who are allergic to esters. Epinephrine in the anesthetic solution will increase the time of anesthesia and decrease bleeding. There is some increase in infection rate, so avoid epinephrine in infection-prone wounds. **Epinephrine should also be avoided in areas of distal vascularity (fingers, toes, penis, nose, and ears)**. Topical anesthetics consist of TAC (TEC), tetracaine and adrenaline (epinephrine). Cocaine is also a good local anesthetic. There has been concern about increased infection rates and severe reactions if the anesthetic is exposed to mucus membranes. DO NOT ALLOW TAC TO COME IN CONTACT WITH MUCUS MEMBRANES! Buffering anesthetics with sodium bicarbonate (1 mEq/mL) at a ratio of 1 mL of sodium bicarbonate per 10 mL of 1% anesthetic will raise the pH of the solution to near neutral and decrease the pain of injection. Warmed anesthetics also decrease pain.

1.2 RX:

A. **INSPECT THE WOUND IN A BLOODLESS FIELD:** (Foreign bodies, deep structures involved: Tendons, joints, nerves, vascular structures, bone, and organs). Culture all infected wounds. Uninfected (fresh) wounds do not need to be cultured. Debride all devitalized tissue and remove all foreign bodies.

B. **IRRIGATE THE WOUND:** Nearly all wounds need to be irrigated with high pressures and large volumes (250 mL to 2000 mL) of irrigating solution (usually sterile normal saline). Betadine, other soaps, and peroxide should not be used inside the wound. However, they can be used on surrounding skin. THE TWO MOST IMPORTANT ITEMS IN WOUND CARE ARE INSPECTING THE WOUND AND IRRIGATING THE WOUND!

C. **CLOSURE:** Most wounds can be closed with nylon sutures through the skin. If a wound involves deep tissue, subcutaneous sutures may be needed to bring the deep tissue together. However, subcutaneous sutures may increase the infection rate for wounds. It is impossible to describe how to suture in a brief presentation, as is the intent of this book. Please refer to larger texts or ask for demonstrations. Dressings should absorb fluids from the wound and protect the wound from contamination. An antibiotic ointment is helpful in maintaining skin softness and promoting healing. Immobilization of a joint with a splint may be necessary to prevent the wound from opening.

D. **Disposition:** Large or deep wounds that involve underlying structures should be referred to an appropriate surgical specialty. Otherwise, instruct patient to watch for infection (redness, swelling, pain, and drainage). Wounds should be kept clean and dry for 1 day and be regularly cleaned thereafter. About 2% to 5% of all wounds become infected. The bandage should be changed every day. The wound may be gently cleaned at dressing change and a fresh antibiotic ointment should be applied. **Sutures should be removed from a face wound after 3-5 days, 7-10 days for scalp wound, 7-10 days for a trunk wound, 10-14 days for arm and leg wounds, and 14 days for joint wounds.** Pain medications, such as acetaminophen with codeine or hydrocodone, NSAIDS, should be prescribed for pain expected when local anesthesia wears off.

2. Special Wounds:

A. **Puncture Wounds:** Most puncture wounds occur to the feet. If the puncture impinges through a tennis shoe, *Pseudomonas aeruginosa* infections are possible. Soaking a puncture wound is not an adequate treatment. The puncture should be opened, inspected, debrided, irrigated, and allowed to remain open. Prophylactic antibiotics are usually not required. Frequent follow-up visits on days 1, 3, 5, and 7 to inspect for infection are a must.

B. **Bite Wounds:** Eighty to ninety percent of these types of wounds are dog bites, 5% to 10% are cat bites, 2% to 3% are human bites, 2% to 3% other (rats, hamsters, etc.). Cat bites have the highest infection rate, human bites are second, and dog bites are third. All bite wounds should receive proper wound inspection, debridement, and irrigation. Bite wounds, for the most part, should not be sutured closed. If these wounds need to be closed, the procedure can be accomplished in a delayed manner within 2 to 4 days. Consider X-rays for evaluation of deep structures and retained foreign bodies. Antibiotics should be prescribed for most bite wounds, such as penicillin and a cephalosporin. If a patient is allergic to penicillin, consider erythromycin and tetracycline. Advise frequent follow-up visits to inspect the wound for infection.

C. **Closed Fist Injuries:** There is a high rate of infection for closed fist injuries. Inspection, debridement and irrigation may need to be performed in the OR. All closed fist wounds should be X-rayed. IV antibiotics must be started on all patients with this type of injury. Most of these individuals will need to be admitted for close follow-up and continued antibiotic treatments. In addition, splinting is important to prevent infection.

3. Tetanus Immunization:

3.1 Clinical Evaluation:

All patients with a wound should be evaluated for tetanus immunization. The most significant step in preventing tetanus is proper wound management (debridement and irrigation).

3.2 RX:

HISTORY	NON-TETANUS PRONE WOUNDS	*TETANUS PRONE WOUNDS
Unknown or less than 3 shots	Td	Td + TIG
3 or more shots: last shot: 0-5 years.	None	None
3 or more shots: last shot: 5-10 years.	None	Td
3 or more shots; last shot: 10+ years.	Td	Td

*Tetanus prone wounds: > 6 hours old, contaminated, infected, nonviable tissue, punctures, crushes, missiles, burns, and frostbite.

Tetanus immunizations are safe in pregnancy.

PROCEDURE PEARLS

"The environment is everything that isn't me."

Albert Einstein

PROCEDURE PEARLS

❑❑ What are the indications for intubation?

A respiratory rate > 40, excessive use of accessory muscles of breathing, pO_2 of < 100 on 40% O_2, pCO_2 > 50, decreased mental status, GCS < 8, and trauma patients with potential upper airway obstruction and/or facial burns.

❑❑ What are the indications for performing a cricothyrotomy?

Immediate airway management in a patient in whom oral or nasal intubation is contraindicated or cannot be established. It may be required for maxillofacial or laryngeal trauma, upper airway obstruction, or cervical spine precautions.

❑❑ What are the absolute contraindications to performing a cricothyrotomy?

Children < 12 years of age, coagulopathy, transection of trachea with retraction of distal end into the mediastinum, a fractured larynx, and an easy endotracheal intubation in the absence of contraindications.

❑❑ How is a cricothyrotomy performed?

Position the patient in a neutral position with c-spine immobilization or extend the neck if there is no risk of a spine injury. Identify the cricothyroid membrane, make a 2 cm transverse skin incision through the membrane into the trachea, dilate the opening, and insert a tracheostomy tube or endotracheal tube.

❑❑ What are the potential complications of a cricothyrotomy?

Hemorrhage, infection, subcutaneous or mediastinal emphysema, pneumothorax, laceration of the trachea or esophagus, subglottic or laryngeal stenosis, prolonged hypoxia due to prolonged unsuccessful attempts, creation of a paratracheal tract, and right mainstem bronchus intubation.

❑❑ What are the advantages of a cricothyrotomy compared to a tracheostomy?

A cricothyrotomy is easier and faster to perform, does not require the OR, and manipulations of the neck are not required as much. This procedure also decreases the incidence of early and late complications.

❑❑ What is the complication rate of an emergency cricothyrotomy?

10-40%.

❑❑ What are the <u>most</u> <u>common</u> complications of an emergency cricothyrotomy?

Bleeding, unsuccessful tube placement, and prolonged procedure time.

❑❑ What is the <u>most</u> <u>common</u> cause of subglottic stenosis?

Endotracheal intubation, not cricothyrotomy or tracheostomy.

❑❑ How is a needle cricothyrotomy performed?

Insert a large (14 g) intravenous cannula through the inferior part of the cricothyroid membrane, with the needle at a 45 degree angle to the skin, and oriented caudad. Once in the trachea, insert the catheter and confirm by aspirating air with a syringe. Ventilate for one second and allow exhalation for 4 seconds.

❑❑ What are the indications for a needle cric?

1) When an orotracheal or nasotracheal intubation cannot be performed.
2) When intubation cannot be performed in a timely manner.
3) When intubation is contraindicated.
4) When temporary relief of hypoxemia is required due to an airway obstruction.

❑❑ What are the absolute contraindications to a needle cric?

1) When endotracheal intubation is not contraindicated and can be accomplished easily and rapidly.
2) When the trachea has been transected and retracted.
3) When there is direct damage to the cricoid cartilage or larynx.

❑❑ What is the <u>most</u> <u>common</u> complication of percutaneous translaryngeal ventilation?

Subcutaneous emphysema.

❑❑ What are the indications for an endotracheal intubation?

Protection of the airway (loss of gag reflex, obstruction, pharyngeal hemorrhage), delivery of CPAP (ARDS, hyaline membrane disease), respiratory failure (asthma, pulmonary edema, neuromuscular disease), flail chest, and cardiopulmonary arrest.

❑❑ How is the appropriate endotracheal tube size in children determined?

Tube diameter = (patient age + 16/4)
= diameter of patient's fifth finger
= thumbnail width

❑❑ What are the complications of endotracheal intubation?

Esophageal intubation, right mainstem bronchus intubation, pharyngeal laceration, vocal cord damage, tracheal laceration, vomiting with aspiration, hypoxia from prolonged attempt times, dental fractures, transient increase in intracranial pressure, tachycardia, and bradycardia.

❑❑ How is a patient with a possible c-spine injury intubated?

Place the head and neck in a neutral position with a collar in place. An assistant should provide in-line stabilization.

❑❑ What are the contraindications to nasotracheal intubation?

Apnea, severe facial fractures, blunt laryngeal trauma with suspected tracheal disruption, and coagulopathy.

❑❑ **What are the advantages of a nasotracheal intubation over an orotracheal intubation?**

The tube can be passed with the patient sitting upright and with minimal neck manipulation. Tube fixation is more secure and the patient cannot bite down on the tube.

❑❑ **What is the <u>most</u> <u>common</u> complication from nasotracheal intubation?**

Epistaxis.

❑❑ **What are the complications of nasotracheal intubation?**

Epistaxis, turbinate fractures, nasal necrosis, intracranial placement through a basilar skull fracture, retropharyngeal laceration or dissection, and unsuccessful placement.

❑❑ **For which type of patient would a Venturi mask be used?**

A patient with respiratory failure secondary to COPD or any patient in whom it would be dangerous to administer an unpredictable volume of oxygen that may induce respiratory arrest by suppressing the respiratory center.

❑❑ **What is the contraindication to an oropharyngeal airway?**

A patient with an intact gag reflex.

❑❑ **What is the <u>most</u> <u>common</u> complication from inserting a nasopharyngeal airway?**

Nasal bleeding.

❑❑ **What are the contraindications associated with using a bag-valve-mask device for artificial ventilation?**

Oropharyngeal bleeding, severe maxillofacial fractures, and upper airway obstruction or injury.

❑❑ **What percent of FiO_2 can be delivered by the bag-valve-mask system?**

If a tight seal is obtained, the bag-valve-mask system can deliver a 40% FiO_2 at 12 L/min. If an oxygen reservoir is attached, oxygen concentration approaches 90%.

❑❑ **What should be done if laryngospasm occurs while intubating?**

Hold constant pressure on the cords with the tip of the endotracheal tube, laryngospasm usually resolves quickly. If it persists, insert lidocaine through the tube.

❑❑ **How is the correct positioning of an endotracheal tube determined?**

Auscultate in the anterior or midaxillary line bilaterally then over the stomach, check chest X-ray placement, (tube 2 cm above the carina), and use a CO_2 detector.

❑❑ **What are the anatomic differences in children that make intubation more challenging?**

Small mandible, big tongue, large head, the larynx is more anterior and cephalad, and the angle between the laryngeal opening and the pharynx is more acute.

❑❑ **How should the head of a pediatric patient be positioned for intubation?**

Due to the large size of the head in relationship to the body, intubation should be performed with the head in the neutral position.

❑❑ **What are the indications for a pericardiocentesis?**

The diagnosis and relief of cardiac tamponade, including patients with suspected cardiac injury who do not respond to volume replacement.

❑❑ **How reliable is a pericardiocentesis?**

The false-negative rate is 20-40%.

❑❑ **How is a pericardiocentesis performed?**

Attach a limb lead to an 18-gauge spinal needle connected to a 20 cc syringe. Place the patient at a 30 degree angle with his/her head up. Insert the needle at a 30 degree angle at the left xiphosternal angle aiming for the ipsilateral shoulder or nipple. Once you enter the pericardium, begin aspirating. Admit the patient to a monitored floor for 24 hours.

❑❑ **What are the complications of a pericardiocentesis?**

Laceration of the myocardium or a coronary artery, pneumothorax, arrhythmias, and pneumopericardium.

❑❑ **What arrhythmias can occur after a pericardiocentesis?**

PVCs are the most common followed by asystole, V-F if, and trachycardia.

❑❑ **What are the indications for chest tube insertion?**

Tension pneumothorax, simple pneumothorax of > 20%, hemothorax, and hemopneumothorax.

❑❑ **What are the potential complications of inserting a chest tube too low, i.e., below the 5th intercostal space?**

Perforation of the liver or spleen and insertion into the abdominal cavity, and diaphragmatic trauma.

❑❑ **How is a chest tube inserted?**

Select the appropriate site, (best site being the 4th intercostal space, midaxillary line), prep and drape, infiltrate with local anesthetic if time permits, and make a linear incision along the rib one interspace below the site of tube insertion. Insert a curved clamp and tunnel superiorly to an interspace and push the clamps through the intercostal muscles into the thoracic cavity just over a rib. Insert a finger to check for adhesions. Direct the tube posteriorly, superiorly, and laterally. Suture in place and attach to underwater seal with suction.

❑❑ **What are the complications from a chest tube insertion?**

Bleeding from the chest wall, occlusion of the chest tube, continuing air leak, subcutaneous emphysema, persistent pneumothorax, laceration to the lung, liver or spleen, subcutaneous insertion, and intraabdominal insertion.

❑❑ **What are the potential complications from a thoracentesis?**

Laceration of an intercostal artery or vein, pneumothorax, pulmonary edema, hypoxia, infection and puncture of the liver or spleen.

❑❑ **What are the advantages of transcutaneous pacing?**

Can be instituted quickly, easy to use, and is noninvasive.

❑❑ **What conditions can render transcutaneous pacing ineffective?**

Dilated cardiomyopathy, obesity, emphysema, kyphoscoliosis, and a pericardial effusion.

❑❑ **What are the indications of transthoracic pacing?**

Unable to insert a transvenous pacemaker, early in asystole, bradycardia with altered hemodynamic state, Mobitz type II with symptoms, myocardial infarction with a type II second degree heart block and third degree heart block, symptomatic bundle branch blocks, and a malfunction of an implanted pacemaker.

❑❑ **What are the potential complications from a transthoracic pacemaker insertion?**

Coronary artery laceration, pericardial tamponade, laceration of the myocardium, and fracture of the pacing wire. Transthoracic pacemakers are no longer commonly used for these reasons.

❑❑ **How is a transvenous pacemaker blindly inserted?**

Cannulate a central vein (internal jugular, subclavian,) in the standard fashion. Insert the electrode catheter into the superior vena cava. Attach the pacemaker catheter to the generator and set the output to its maximum (mA) and a rate of 70/minute. Turn the generator on and advance until ventricular pacing occurs. Confirm placement by chest X-ray.

❑❑ **What complications may occur from a transvenous pacemaker insertion?**

Myocardial perforation, perforation of the ventricular septum, malposition into the hepatic vein or inferior vena cava, failure to capture, arrhythmias, diaphragmatic pacing, and muscle spasm.

❑❑ **What findings indicate a possible interventricular septum perforation?**

Catheter tip in the left ventricle on a chest X-ray, increased pacing threshold, and the conversion of a left bundle branch block to a right bundle branch block.

❑❑ **What arrhythmias may occur with transvenous pacing?**

Ventricular fibrillation or ventricular tachycardia.

❑❑ **What are the indications for a burr hole?**

Unilateral neurologic findings with deterioration despite standard treatment, (hyperventilation and mannitol), unavailable neurosurgeon, and an impending herniation.

❑❑ **What are the indications for a lumbar puncture?**

Diagnosis of infections (meningitis, encephalitis, abscesses), cancer (metastatic carcinoma, leukemia), subarachnoid hemorrhage, and relief of intracranial pressure (pseudotumor cerebri).

❑❑ **What are the contraindications to performing a lumbar puncture?**

Coagulation defect, anticoagulation therapy, history of progressively increasing headache (perform a CT first), presence of localizing neurologic signs or symptoms (CT first), presence of papilledema (CT first), and infection at the site of the puncture.

❑❑ **What are the complications associated with a lumbar puncture?**

Headache, epidermoid tumor, spinal subdural and epidural hematoma, infection, and herniation.

❑❑ **How are Gardner tongs applied?**

Shave the hair where the tong is to be applied, prep the skin, and insert the tong above the ears and below the "equator" at ~5 cm superior to the mastoid bone. When bone is encountered, continue inserting the screws until 5 mm of excursion is noted. The points should be just below the temporal ridges.

❑❑ **What are the indications for the insertion of a cervical traction device?**

Unstable cervical spine injuries, fracture dislocations requiring reduction, unilateral and bilateral locked facets (C3-C7), Hangman's fracture, Jefferson's fracture, and a severe ligamentous injury associated with a teardrop fracture.

❑❑ **What are the indications for a culdocentesis?**

Identify the presence of peritoneal fluid, blood, or pus in the cul-de-sac.

❑❑ **How is a culdocentesis performed?**

Grasp the posterior lip of the cervix with a tenaculum, cleanse the posterior vaginal fornix, insert an 18-gauge spinal attached to a 20 cc syringe in the midline of the posterior fornix, aspirate as the needle is being inserted, and advance no further than 2 cm.

❑❑ **What constitutes a positive tap?**

The aspiration of nonclotted 2 mL of blood.

❑❑ **How is a dislocated knee reduced?**

One person applies traction longitudinally in the line of the deformity to the involved extended knee while an assistant applies countertraction above the knee.

❑❑ **After the knee is reduced, what must be done?**

An arteriogram should be performed to evaluate the popliteal artery.

❑❑ **What are the indications for bladder catheterization?**

Relief of acute urinary retention, the evaluation of urine output for the critically ill or for injured patients, neurogenic bladder, urethral or prostatic obstruction leading to hydronephrosis and decreased renal function, and an urologic study of the anatomy of the urinary tract.

❑❑ **What are the contraindications to bladder catheterization?**

Prostatic displacement on rectal exam, perineal hematoma, and blood at the urethral meatus.

❑❑ **What complication can occur from catheterizing a patient with pelvic trauma?**

A partial urethral disruption may be converted to a complete injury.

❑❑ **What are the complications of bladder catheterization?**

Creation of a false passage, cystitis, urethritis, pyelonephritis, hemorrhage, urethral trauma, and epididymitis.

❑❑ **What is the indication for suprapubic catheterization?**

Urinary obstruction in a patient where catheterization cannot be done.

❑❑ **What is the indication for suprapubic aspiration?**

For diagnostic purposes in pediatric patients.

❑❑ **What are the contraindications to the placement of a suprapubic catheter?**

Unable to define the bladder, lower abdominal scarring, history of intraperitoneal surgery or irradiation, and bleeding disorders.

❑❑ **What complications are associated with suprapubic catheterization?**

Puncture of a large vessel, puncture of the large or small bowel, leakage around the catheter, hematuria, abdominal wall abscess, extraperitoneal extravasation, intraperitoneal extravasation, and ureteral catheterization.

❑❑ **How is a suprapubic aspiration performed?**

Percuss or use ultrasound to determine the level of the bladder. Insert a 22-gauge 1 inch needle, 2 cm above the symphysis pubis at a 45-60 degree angle. Aspirate urine for analysis.

❑❑ **Describe the technique for a suprapubic catheter insertion.**

Percuss to determine the location of the bladder, prep and anesthetize the area, and insert the trocar-catheter system at a 30 degree angle 3-4 cm cephalad to the symphysis pubis. Insert the catheter 3 cm over the trocar and suture in place.

❑❑ **Describe how to detorse a testicle.**

Perform a spermatic cord block and grasp the testicle and attempt to rotate laterally and superiorly. If successful, the testicle will drop into a normal position.

❑❑ **What are the indications for insertion of a central venous catheter?**

Emergency IV route in a seriously ill or injured patient, transvenous pacemaker insertion, rapid administration of large volumes of fluid, Swan-Ganz insertion, and the infusion of concentrated solutions, such as hyperosmolar or irritating solutions that have a potential for thrombophlebitis. Additional indications include the inability to obtain a peripheral IV, and central venous pressure monitoring.

❑❑ **What are the contraindications to subclavian venipuncture?**

Chest wall deformity, distorted local anatomy, extreme weight, radiation therapy to region, vasculitis, coagulopathy, agitated uncooperative patient, prior long-term subclavian cannulation, possible superior vena cava injury, and suspected subclavian vessel injury.

❑❑ **What is the technique for inserting a subclavian line?**

Place the patient in 10-20 degrees of Trendelenburg with a folded sheet between the shoulder blades, locate the site and turn the patient's head to the opposite direction, prep, drape, and anesthetize, enter at the junction between the middle and lateral one-third of the clavicle 1 cm below the clavicle, insert the needle walking down the clavicle until the subclavius muscle is entered, aim the needle for the sternal notch until blood is aspirated, remove the syringe and place a finger over the hub, perform the Seldinger technique to cannulate and dilate for catheter insertion, and suture in place. Aspirate from each port, obtain a chest X-ray for placement, and auscultate for bilateral breath sounds.

❑❑ **Why should a finger be placed over the needle hub once the syringe is removed?**

If the hub is left open, air may enter with each inspiration causing a potential air embolism.

❑❑ **When do most complications from a subclavian line occur?**

Forty percent of complications occur when the procedure is performed as an emergency.

❑❑ **What complications are associated with insertion of a subclavian line?**

Pneumothorax, hemothorax, tracheal perforation, catheter fragmentation, air embolus, thoracic duct laceration, pericardial tamponade, subclavian artery puncture, local hematoma, local cellulitis, generalized sepsis, phrenic nerve injury, dysrhythmias, catheter malposition, chest pain, and hydrothorax.

❑❑ **Which type of patient has a particular risk for a pneumothorax during a subclavian line insertion?**

A patient receiving mechanical ventilation or undergoing multiple attempts at cannulation. Children (pleural reflection is higher), and emphysematous patients also are at risk.

❑❑ **If a patient becomes cyanotic, tachypneic, hypotensive, with a new holosystolic murmur heard over the precordium during a subclavian line insertion, what complication must be considered?**

An air embolism.

❑❑ **Why should the right side be attempted first when inserting a subclavian line?**

There is a danger of injury to the thoracic duct on the left. In addition, the right subclavian has a straighter course in relation to the innominate and superior vena cava, resulting in a more successful cannulation when compared to the left side.

❑❑ **Why try a supraclavicular approach when cannulating the subclavian vein?**

The complication rate is lower because the needle is directed away from the pleural dome and subclavian artery.

❑❑ **What are other advantages of the supraclavicular approach over the infraclavicular approach?**

The subclavian and internal jugular is the target used, it is less painful, the distance between the skin and vein is shorter, and the variability of the space between the first rib and the clavicle is avoided.

❑❑ **Describe the supraclavicular approach to subclavian vein cannulation?**

Place the patient in a Trendelenburg position, prep, drape, and anesthetize. Insert a 14-gauge needle, at a 45 degree angle to the sagittal plane, at the junction of the lateral aspect of the clavicular head of the sternocleidomastoid muscle with the superior border of the clavicle. Use the Seldinger technique to cannulate and secure the catheter in place.

❑❑ **What are the advantages of an internal jugular vein cannulation?**

There is a low risk of pleural puncture, hematomas are easier to compress, malpositioning is rare, may be used in a patient with a coagulopathy (only if absolutely necessary), and is useful in patients with a short, thick neck.

❑❑ **What are the disadvantages of an internal jugular line?**

Insertion failures are higher compared to infraclavicular attempts. In addition, an internal juglar line is more uncomfortable for the patient, is easier to become dislodged and kinked, and is contraindicated in a patient with a c-spine injury.

❑❑ **Describe the insertion procedure of an internal jugular line.**

Place the patient in 20 degrees of Trendelenburg with his/her head pointed away from the insertion side, prep, drape, and anesthetize. Insert the needle at a 30 degree angle at the apex of the triangle formed by the junction of the sternal and clavicular heads of the sternocleidomastoid muscle, aim for the ipsilateral nipple, cannulate by the Seldinger technique, and suture in place.

❑❑ **What complications are associated with the insertion of an internal jugular line?**

Hematoma, thoracic duct injury, hemo/pneumothorax, air embolism, phlebitis, infection, nerve damage, and myocardial puncture.

❑❑ **Describe the technique for inserting a femoral venous catheter.**

Prep, drape, and anesthetize the skin. Insert the needle at a 45-degree angle 1 cm medial to the femoral artery and two fingerbreadths (2-3 cm) below the inguinal ligament. Direct the needle toward the umbilicus, insert, and secure via the Seldinger technique.

❑❑ **What are the indications for femoral venous cannulation?**

Rapid volume replacement, unable to obtain peripheral access, and radiographic procedures.

❑❑ **What are the contraindications to femoral venous cannulation?**

Trauma to the inguinal region, possible injury to the inferior vena cava or iliacs, and skin abnormalities, such as burns, deep abrasions, or severe dermatitis.

❑❑ **What complications are associated with femoral venous cannulation?**

Femoral nerve injury, septic arthritis, hematoma, catheter insertion into the abdominal cavity, psoas abscess, thrombosis, and phlebitis.

❑❑ **Which is the most common organism that causes septic arthritis due to femoral line insertion?**

Staphylococcus aureus.

❑❑ **Describe the procedure for performing a saphenous vein cutdown at the ankle.**

Prep, drape, and anesthetize an area two fingerbreadths above the medial malleolus. Make a transverse incision over the vein, dissect down to the vein with curved hemostats, isolate the vein between two ligatures tying off the distal portion, make a longitudinal incision between the two sutures and insert a catheter into the vein. Secure the proximal ligature around the cannula, close the wound, and suture the cannula to the skin.

❑❑ **What are some advantages of a saphenous vein cutdown?**

Only vessel of significance in that area, always found just anterior to the medial malleolus, and easy to access.

❑❑ **What are the indications for a saphenous vein cutdown?**

Unable to insert a peripheral line, the need for rapid volume replacement, and cardiac arrest in infants and small children in whom access to a central line is unsuccessful.

❑❑ **What are the contraindications to a saphenous vein cutdown?**

When less invasive alternatives exist, when more rapid access is required, coagulation disorders, compromised host-defense mechanisms, or impaired healing.

❑❑ **What are the complications associated with a saphenous vein cutdown?**

Local hematoma, infection, sepsis, phlebitis, embolization, wound dehiscence, and injuries to associated arteries/nerves.

❑❑ **Describe the technique for inserting an interosseous line.**

Prep, anesthetize and drape the lower leg. Choose a site 1-3 cm below the tibial tuberosity on the anterior flat surface of the tibia, direct the needle 90 degrees, and advance until marrow contents are aspirated.

❑❑ **What are the indications for an interosseous line?**

When fluids or drugs must be introduced into the circulation rapidly and when the venous access is not available. Other indications include cardiac arrest in an infant or child, shock, severe burns, dehydration, status epilepticus, or any condition requiring emergency administration of fluids and drugs.

❑❑ **What are the contraindications to the placement of an interosseous line?**

Infection at the intended site and a fracture to the tibia.

❑❑ **What is the <u>most</u> <u>common</u> complication of interosseous infusion?**

Subcutaneous and subperiosteal infiltration of fluid or leakage from the puncture site.

❑❑ **What are the indications for a nasogastric tube?**

To aspirate gastric contents for diagnostic or therapeutic reasons, the presence of an ileus or mechanical obstruction, to prevent gastric aspiration in a trauma patient before doing a peritoneal lavage, for feeding purposes, and for the administration of therapeutic substances such as charcoal.

❑❑ **What are the contraindications to nasogastric tube insertion?**

Facial fractures with possible cribriform plate fracture, esophageal perforation, strictures or history of alkali ingestion, comatose state with an unprotected airway, and penetrating neck wounds in an awake trauma patient.

❑❑ **Describe the technique for inserting a nasogastric tube.**

Insert the tube along the floor of the nose directed posteriorly. After the tube passes the posterior pharynx continue inserting to the stomach.

❑❑ **What procedure(s) should be performed to ensure that a nasogastric tube is in place?**

Aspirate gastric contents, inject 20-30 cc of air while listening over the stomach, or obtain a chest X-ray for placement.

❑❑ **What are the indications that a nasogastric tube was inserted into the trachea?**

The patient will cough or is unable to speak.

❑❑ **What complications are the associated with nasogastric tube insertion?**

Epistaxis, rupture of the esophagus or stomach, perforation of the esophagus, intracranial insertion, insertion in the submucosa of the posterior pharynx, ulceration of the nasal mucosa, sinusitis, otitis media, and tracheal insertion.

❑❑ **Describe the procedure for performing a diagnostic peritoneal lavage.**

Insert a bladder catheter and nasogastric tube, prepare, drape, and anesthetize the area. Make a vertical incision one third the distance from the umbilicus to the symphysis pubis, insert a peritoneal dialysis catheter, aspirate for blood and infuse 1 L of LR or NS, allow the fluid to drain out.

❑❑ **What are the indications for a diagnostic peritoneal lavage (DPL)?**

To detect intra-abdominal injury in a patient with potential abdominal trauma requiring surgery, when a patient is unconscious due to a head injury or substance abuse, when there is a recent or preexisting paraplegia, and when there is a penetrating trauma to the thoracoabdominal, pelvic, back and flank region.

❑❑ **What are the indications for a DPL in children?**

Unexplained shock following trauma, altered level of consciousness, major thoracic injury, multiple trauma, and major orthopedic injuries, such as a fractured pelvis, femur, or hip.

❑❑ **What are the absolute contraindications to a DPL?**

An unstable patient requiring immediate surgery is the only absolute contraindication. Previous surgeries to the abdomen, pregnant patient, and inability to catheterize the bladder are relative contraindications.

❑❑ **What approach should be used when performing a DPL on a pregnant patient?**

Supraumbilical approach.

❑❑ **What constitutes a positive DPL?**

Aspiration of > 10 cc of blood, WBC > 500, RBCs > 100,000 (blunt), > 10,000 (penetrating), elevated amylase, bile, or intestinal contents.

❑❑ **What are the indications for a thoracentesis?**

Emergency diagnosis and treatment of a tension pneumothorax
Evacuation of a simple pneumothorax.
Evacuation of a large symptomatic pleural effusion.
Diagnostic analysis of a pleural effusion.

❑❑ **What are the contraindications to performing a thoracentesis?**

Bleeding diathesis.
Anticoagulant use.
Rupture diaphragm.
Infection of the chest wall.

❑❑ **What are the complications associated with a thoracentesis?**

Pulmonaty edema, puncture of the liver or spleen, hypoxia laceration of an intercoatal artery and pneumothorax.

RANDOM PEARLS

❑❑ What are characteristics of an abusive relationship?

The abusive relationship evolves over time usually escalating from jealousy and a desire to control a partner's behavior into humiliation, degradation, and use of the fear of physical violence. He may or may not have to actually hit her if she knows that he is capable of hurting her or her children. The end result is low self-esteem, control, isolation and entrapment.

❑❑ How is a dystonic reaction treated?

Diphenhydramine (Benadryl, 25-50 mg IM or IV, or benztropine (Cogentin), 1-2 mg IV or PO. Remember that dystonias can recur acutely.

❑❑ Describe symptoms of alcohol withdrawal.

1) Autonomic hyperactivity: tachycardia, hypertension, tremors, anxiety, agitation; 6-8 hours after drinking.
2) Hallucinations: auditory, visual, tactile; 24 hour after drinking.
3) Global confusion: 1-3 days after drinking.

❑❑ List some life-threatening causes of acute psychosis.

WHHHIMP: Wernicke's Encephalopathy, Hypoxia, Hypoglycemia, Hypertensive encephalopathy, Intracerebral hemorrhage, Meningitis/Encephalitis, and Poisoning.

❑❑ What are the clinical findings that suggest acute glomerulonephritis (GN)?

Oliguria, hypertension, pulmonary edema, and urine sediment containing red blood cells, white blood cells, protein, and red blood cell casts.

❑❑ What is the <u>most</u> <u>common</u> cause of intrinsic renal failure?

Acute tubular necrosis (80%-90% of cases), resulting from an ischemic injury (the most common cause of ATN), or a nephrotoxic agent. Less frequent causes of intrinsic renal failure (10%-20% of cases), are vasculitis, malignant hypertension, acute GN, or allergic interstitial nephritis.

❑❑ Name some common nephrotoxic agents/substances.

Aminoglycosides, NSAIDs, contrast dye, and myoglobin.

❑❑ What is the eponym for idiopathic scrotal edema, and how is this disease treated?

Fournier's gangrene is a polymicrobial infection of the subcutaneous tissue that is characterized by widespread tissue necrosis. Treatment consists of broad-spectrum parenteral antibiotics and immediate surgical debridement.

❑❑ **How does the pain associated with epididymitis differ from that of prostatitis?**

Epididymitis: The pain begins in the scrotum or groin and radiates along the spermatic cord. It intensifies rapidly, is associated with dysuria, and is relieved with scrotal elevation (Prehn's sign).

Prostatitis: Patients will have frequency, dysuria, urgency, bladder outlet obstruction, and retention. They may have low back pain, perineal pain associated with fever, chills, arthralgias, and myalgias.

❑❑ **How does the treatment of epididymitis differ according to age?**

In patients less than 40 years old, the most common pathogens are Chlamydia and gonorrhea that are treated with ceftriaxone IM and doxycycline po. In patients over 40 years of age, the common causes are urinary pathogens such as *Escherichia coli (E. coli)* and *Klebsiella* that are treated with TMP-SMX.

❑❑ **Which are the causative organisms of prostatitis?**

E. coli in 80% and *Klebsiella, Enterobacter, Proteus*, or *Pseudomonas* in 20%.

❑❑ **When are the two peaks in the incidence of testicular torsion?**

The first year of life and at puberty.

❑❑ **What is the definitive diagnostic test for testicular torsion?**

Emergent surgical exploration. Although radionuclide imaging and Doppler ultrasonography may be helpful, they are time-consuming and their accuracy is operator dependent. The warm ischemia time for testicular salvage may be as short as 4 hours. Therefore, once the diagnosis is entertained, immediate urologic consultation and surgical exploration are necessary.

❑❑ **When is a retrograde urethrogram necessary in the evaluation of a patient with a penile fracture?**

A penile fracture is rupture of the corpus cavernosum with tearing of the tunica albuginea that results from blunt trauma to the erect penis. Urethral injury occurs in approximately 10% of patients with a penile fracture. Patients with hematuria, blood at the urethral meatus, or inability to void should undergo retrograde urethrography to rule out a urethral injury.

❑❑ **What is the initial treatment for priapism?**

Terbutaline, 0.25-0.5 mg, subcutaneously.

❑❑ **Describe acute glomerulonephritis (GN).**

Hematuria, proteinuria, oliguria or anuria, edema, and hypertension.

❑❑ **What is the proper position to transport a pregnant trauma patient?**

With spinal backboard tilted 30 degrees to the left in order to prevent the supine hypotension syndrome.

❑❑ **What is the clinical significance of fixed and dilated pupils in a drowning victim?**

Don't give up the ship! Ten to twenty percent of patients presenting with coma and fixed and dilated pupils recover completely. Asymptomatic patients should be observed for a minimum of 4 to 6 hours.

❑❑ **What percentage of dog and cat bites become infected?**

About 10% of dog and 50% of cat bites become infected. *Pasteurella multocida* infects 30% of dog bites and 50% of cat bites.

❑❑ **A six year old child presents with headache, fever, malaise, and tender regional lymphadenopathy about a week after a cat bite. A tender papule develops at the site. What is the diagnosis?**

Cat-scratch disease. Usually develops 3 days to 6 weeks following a cat bite or scratch. The papule typically blisters and heals with eschar formation or a transient macular or vesicular rash may develop.

❑❑ **Describe the presentation of a black widow spider versus a scorpion envenomation.**

Black widow victims typically stay in one position for a few seconds to minutes before moving, they also have a halo lesion. Scorpion victims present with a constant writhing and abnormal eye movements.

❑❑ **What are the indications for giving antivenin in a black widow spider envenomation?**

Severe pain, dangerous hypertension, pregnant women with moderate to severe envenomations, and pregnant women threatening abortion who are mildly symptomatic after an envenomation. Antivenin should be avoided in patients taking b-adrenergic blocking agents as if anaphylaxis occurs, it will be difficult to treat.

❑❑ **A patient is brought to the ED with a history of a bite wound inflicted at a mental ward. What bacterium is likely?**

Eikenella corrodens is more common in hospitalized and institutionalized patients. Most human bite infections are due to *Staphylococcus aureus* or *Streptococcus.*

❑❑ **What is the frequency of eye injuries in lightning strike victims?**

Half develop structural eye lesions. Cataracts are the most common and develops within days to years. Unreactive dilated pupils may not equal death because transient autonomic instability may occur.

❑❑ **What is the most common otologic injury in a lightning strike victim?**

Fifty percent have tympanic membrane rupture. Hemotympanum, basilar skull fracture, and acoustic and vestibular deficits may also occur.

❑❑ **What is the first-line treatment of ventricular fibrillation in a hypothermic patient?**

Bretylium NOT lidocaine.

❑❑ What is the most common arrhythmia found in a patient with hypothermia?

Atrial fibrillation. Other ECG findings include PAT, prolongation of the P-R, QRS, or Q-T, decreased P-wave amplitude, T-wave changes, PVCs, or humped ST segment adjacent to the QRS complex (Osborn wave).

❑❑ A 14 year old football player presents to the ED with a history of light-headedness, headache, nausea, and vomiting. On exam, the patient has a HR of 110, RR 22, BP of 90/60, and is afebrile. Profuse sweating is noted. What is the diagnosis?

Heat exhaustion. Treat with 0.9 NS IV fluid.

❑❑ What is the treatment for heatstroke?

Cool sponging, ice packs to groin and axilla, fanning, and iced gastric lavage. Antipyretics are not useful.

❑❑ An Osborn (J) wave displayed by an ECG is associated with what disorder?

Hypothermia.

❑❑ Compare the entrance and exit wounds of AC and DC.

AC: Entrance and exit wounds are the same size.
DC: Small entrance and large exit.
NB: Not all texts agree!

❑❑ What treatment options are available for patients who are bleeding and have liver disease?

1) Transfusion with PRBCs, (maintains hemodynamic stability).
2) Vitamin K.
3) Fresh frozen plasma.
4) Platelet transfusion.
5) DDAVP (Desmopressin).

❑❑ What options are available for the treatment of patients with renal failure and coagulopathy?

Dialysis.
Optimize hematocrit
-recombinant human erythropoietin
-transfusion with PRBCs.
Desmopressin.
Conjugated estrogens.
Cryoprecipitate and platelet transfusions if hemorrhage is life-threatening.

❑❑ What two conditions are associated with the most devastating form of DIC?

Neisseria meningitidis sepsis and acute myelogenous leukemia (promyelocytic (M3) type).

❑❑ **What are the clinical complications of DIC?**

Bleeding, thrombosis, and purpura fulminans.

❑❑ **What three laboratory studies would be most helpful in establishing the diagnosis of DIC?**

Prothrombin time - Prolonged.
Platelet count - Usually low.
Fibrinogen level - Low.
Fibrin split products - Elavated.
D - diner - Elavated.

❑❑ **What are the most common hemostatic abnormalities in patients infected with HIV?**

Thrombocytopenia and acquired circulating anticoagulants, which causes prolongation of aPTT.

❑❑ **What is the pentad of Thrombotic Thrombocytopenic Purpura (TTP)?**

Fever, thrombocytopenia, neurologic symptoms, renal insufficiency and microangiopathic hemolytic anemia (MAHA).

❑❑ **What is the leading cause of death in hemophiliacs?**

AIDS.

❑❑ **Which types of clinical crises are seen in patients with sickle cell disease?**

Vasoocclusive (Thrombotic).
Hematologic
-Sequestration
-Aplastic.
Infectious.

❑❑ **Which is the most common type of sickle cell crisis?**

Vasoocclusive, with an average of 4 attacks/year.

❑❑ **What percentage of patients with sickle cell disease have gallstones?**

75%. However, only 10% are symptomatic.

❑❑ **Which is the only type of vasoocclusive crisis that is painless?**

CNS crisis. Most commonly children are afflicted with cerebral infarction and cerebral hemorrhage develops in adults.

❑❑ **What are the major causes of GI bleeding in cancer patients?**

Hemorrhagic gastritis and peptic ulcer disease.

❑❑ **What are the mainstays of therapy for a patient with sickle cell crisis?**

Hydration, analgesia, oxygen, (only beneficial if patient is hypoxic), and cardiac monitoring, (if patient has history of cardiac disease or is having chest pain).

❑❑ **What is the single most useful test in ascertaining the presence of hemolysis and a normal marrow response?**

The reticulocyte count.

❑❑ **What is the most common clinical presentation of TTP (Thrombotic thrombocytopenic purpura)?**

Neurologic symptoms: headache, confusion, cranial nerve palsies, coma, seizures.

❑❑ **What is the currently approved emergency replacement therapy in the ED for massive hemorrhage?**

Type-specific, uncrossmatched blood, available in 10-15 minutes. Type O negative, although immediately life saving in certain situations, carries the risk of life-threatening transfusion reactions.

❑❑ **In current practice, which blood components are routinely infused along with PRBCs in a patient receiving a massive transfusion?**

None. The practice of routinely using platelet transfusion and FFP is costly, dangerous, and unwarranted.

❑❑ **What condition should be suspected in a patient with multiple myeloma who presents to the ED with paraparesis, paraplegia, and urinary incontinence?**

Acute spinal cord compression. This condition occurs primarily with multiple myeloma and lymphoma, but it is also encountered with carcinomas of the lung, breast and prostate.

❑❑ **What are the lab abnormalities in DIC?**

Increased PT, elevated fibrin split products, decreased fibrinogen, and thrombocytopenia.

❑❑ **What is appropriate treatment for a life threatening level of hypercalcemia of 16 mg per deciliter?**

Start giving the patient 0.9 NS at 5 to 10 L per day. In addition, administer furosemide. A typical dose of Lasix is 80 mg IV every 1 to 2 h. Watch out for hypokalemia. Consider glucocorticoids if the patient is obtunded or comatose. The admitting internist may also administer agents to counteract parathyroid hormone, including calcitonin and mithramycin.

❑❑ **How may hemophilia A be clinically distinguished from hemophilia B?**

Hemophilia A is not clinically distinguishable from Christmas disease (Hemophilia B).

❑❑ Which blood product is given when the coagulation abnormality is unknown?

FFP.

❑❑ Which agent can be used for treating mild hemophilia A and von Willebrand's disease type 1?

D-Amino-8. D-arginine vasopressin (DDAVP) induces a rapid rise in factor VIII levels.

❑❑ What is the minimal ß-hCG titer for which an experienced ultrasonographer should be able to visualize a viable intrauterine pregnancy?

Transvaginal, > 2000 hCG mIU/mL. Transabdominal, 6500.

❑❑ Which type of patient is eligible for methotrexate treatment for an ectopic pregnancy?

The hemodynamically stable and patients with unruptured gestations of less than 4 cm in diameter by ultrasound.

❑❑ Transient pelvic pain frequently occurs 3-7 days after methotrexate therapy for ectopic pregnancy. What is your concern?

Rupture may be difficult to differentiate from this pain presumed due to tubal abortion, typically lasting 4-12 hours.

❑❑ What is the number one cause of maternal mortality?

Thromboembolism. The risk progressively increases throughout pregnancy, peaking at > 5 times non-pregnant controls during the post-partum period.

❑❑ What is the indication for RhoGAM in the first trimester?

An unsensitized Rh-negative woman with any vaginal bleeding.

❑❑ Against how much fetomaternal hemorrhage (FMH) does the standard 300 microgram dose of RhoGAM protect?

Approximately 30 mLs of whole blood. Following trauma, FMH should always be considered. In the setting of trauma, order a quantitative Kleihauer-Betke assay to determine the amount of FMH. and then calculate the appropriate RhoGAM dose.

❑❑ What is the most common presentation of ectopic pregnancy?

Amenorrhea followed by pain.

❑❑ How does a spontaneous abortion most commonly present?

Pain followed by bleeding.

❑❑ **What is the most common finding on pelvic exam in a patient with an ectopic pregnancy?**

Unilateral adnexal tenderness.

❑❑ **When can abdominal ultrasound find an intrauterine gestational sac?**

5th week. Fetal pole, 6th week. Embryonic mass with cardiac motion, 7th week.

❑❑ **What is the most common cause of toxic shock syndrome?**

The most common cause is *S. aureus*. Other causes which are clinically similar include group A *Streptococci, Pseudomonas aeruginosa*, and *Streptococcus pneumoniae*.

❑❑ **What criteria are necessary for the diagnosis of toxic shock syndrome?**

All of the following must be present: T > 38.9°C (102° F), rash, systolic BP < 90 and orthostasis, involvement of three organ systems (GI, renal, musculoskeletal, mucosal, hepatic, hematologic, or CNS), and negative serologic tests for such diseases as RMSF, hepatitis B, measles, leptospirosis, VDRL, etc.

❑❑ **Which type of rash develops with TSS?**

Blanching erythroderma which resolves in 3 days and is then followed by a desquamation (full thickness). This typically occurs between the 6th and 14th day with peeling prominent on the hands and feet.

❑❑ **How should a patient with toxic shock syndrome be treated?**

FLUIDS, pressure support, FFP or transfusions, vaginal irrigation with iodine or saline, and antistaphylococcal penicillin, or cephalosporin with anti-ß-lactamase activity, such as nafcillin or oxacillin. Rifampin should be considered to eliminate the carrier state.

❑❑ **Define preeclampsia.**

HTN after 20 weeks EGA with generalized edema or proteinuria.

❑❑ **Define eclampsia.**

Preeclampsia plus grand mal seizures or coma.

❑❑ **Should BP be lowered acutely in a preeclampsia patient?**

Dangerous HTN (> 170/110), should be gradually lowered with hydralazine, 10 mg IV, followed by a drip. Definitive treatment for preeclampsia and eclampsia is delivery.

❑❑ **Why is Rh status important in a pregnant patient?**

Rh negative with Rh positive fetus can result in fetal anemia, hydrops, and fetal loss. Rh immunoglobulin should be given to all Rh negative patients. The usual amount of RhoGAM may be inadequate in the setting of trauma; a Kleihauer-Betke assay can quantitate fetomaternal hemorrhage.

❑❑ **When can a transvaginal and an abdominal ultrasound identify an intrauterine sac?**

Transvaginal, 31-32 days. Abdominal, 5 weeks.

❑❑ **A 24 year old, 10 week pregnant patient presents with bleeding per vagina. She also complains of nausea, vomiting, and abdominal pain. The physical findings reveal a blood pressure of 150/100 and a uterus which is larger than dates. The lab studies indicated proteinuria. What is the diagnosis?**

Molar pregnancy. Uterus may be larger or smaller than expected dates.

❑❑ **What are the risk factors for placenta previa?**

Previous cesarean section, previous placenta previa, multiparity, multiple induced abortions, and multiple gestations.

❑❑ **What are the risk factors for abruptio placenta?**

Smoking, hypertension, multiparity, trauma, and previous abruptio placenta.

❑❑ **What are the presenting signs and symptoms of abruptio placentae?**

Placental separation before delivery is associated with vaginal bleeding, (78%), abdominal pain, (66%), as well as tetanic uterine contractions, uterine irritability, and fetal death.

❑❑ **Is life threatening hemorrhage due to trauma during pregnancy most often intra- or retroperitoneal?**

Retroperitoneal.

❑❑ **What are the two distinct causes of toxic epidermal necrolysis (Scalded Skin Syndrome)?**

Staphylococcal and drugs or chemicals. Both begin with appearance of patches of tender erythema followed by loosening of the skin and denuding to glistening bases.
Staphylococcal scalded skin syndrome is commonly found in children less than 5 years and is due to toxin that cleaves within the epidermis under the stratum granulosum.

❑❑ **How is SSSS distinguished from scalded skin syndrome that is caused by drugs or chemicals?**

Pull out your microscopes and call in the pathologists trivia fans. In drug or chemical etiologies, the skin separates at the dermoepidermal junction. This drug-induced TEN carries up to 50% mortality as a result of fluid loss and secondary infection. On a microscopic exam of SSSS, intraepidermal cleavage occurs along with a few acantholytic keratinocytes. In non-staphylococcal type, cellular debris, inflammatory cells, and basal cell keratinocytes are present.

❑❑ **What is the treatment for SSSS?**

Oral or IV penicillinase-resistant penicillin, baths of potassium permanganate or dressings soaked in 0.5% silver nitrate, and fluids. Corticosteroids and silver sulfadine are contraindicated.

❑❑ What is the mechanism of action of tetanospasmin?

Enters peripheral nerve endings and ascends the axons to reach the brain and spinal cord. At this point it binds four areas of the nervous system:

1) Anterior horn cells of the spinal cord: Impairs inhibitory interneurons resulting in neuromuscular irritability and generalized spasms.
2) Sympathetic nervous system: Resulting in sweating, labile blood pressure, tachycardia, and peripheral vasoconstriction.
3) Myoneural junction: Inhibits release of acetylcholine.
4) Binds to cerebral gangliosides: Thought to cause seizures.

❑❑ What is the treatment for a tetanus prone wound?

Surgical debridement, 3,000 to 10,000 units of human tetanus immune globulin [TIG (h), (Hyper-tet)] IM (Do Not Inject Into Wound), penicillin G, or metronidazole.

❑❑ What is the most common cause of gas gangrene?

C. perfringens. The first symptom is a sensation of weight or heaviness in the muscle followed by severe pain. The DOC is penicillin G, an alternative is chloramphenicol.

❑❑ What is an ABI and what is its significance?

1) ABI = ankle/brachial index. The ankle systolic pressure (numerator) is compared to the higher of the two brachial arterial pressures (denominator). It is used to determine if arterial obstruction is present.
2) Normal ABI = greater than or equal to 1.
3) ABI 0.5-0.9 = obstructive disease of a single peripheral arterial segment, i.e., claudication.
4) ABI < 0.5 indicates multiple arterial segments are obstructed.

❑❑ Which technical factors can effect the accuracy of the ABI?

Probe pressure, probe placement which should be longitudinal to the vessel and 30-60 degree angle to the skin surface, too rapid deflation of the BP cuff, and arterial wall calcifications

❑❑ Which is the diagnostic test of choice for documenting DVT?

Duplex ultrasound. Although it is highly operator dependent and not utilized in all centers, its sensitivity and specificity are virtually identical to venography. In addition, its benefits include being noninvasive and not utilizing contrast dye. The accuracy of physical examination for DVT is generally quoted to be approximately 50%.

❑❑ Name some ultrasonographic abnormalities seen in patients with acute cholecystitis.

Wall thickening, gallstones, surrounding fluid, US Murphy's sign, air in the biliary tree.

❑❑ Where is the most common site for an ectopic implantation?

The ampullae of the fallopian tube.

❑❑ List some of the advantages/disadvantages of CT, ultrasound, and DPL for assessing trauma patients?

	Advantages	Disadvantages:
DPL	Low complication rate, done at bedside.	Invasive, time consuming, can't ID retroperitoneal injury, significant false positive rate.
CT	IDs location/extent injury, including the retroperitoneum.	Cost, time consuming, interpretation expertise, patient monitoring not optimal, requires travel.
US	Cheap, noninvasive, done at bedside, good for hemoperitoneum, fast.	Operator dependent, not good for IDing specific organ injury,

❑❑ Name 6 risk factors for an ectopic pregnancy.

Advanced maternal age, PID, prior ectopic, history of pelvic surgery or tubal ligation, IUDs, in vitro fertilization.

❑❑ What is the primary use of ultrasonography in females with a positive hCG who present with abdominal pain and/or vaginal bleeding?

To verify the presence of an intrauterine pregnancy. The incidence of simultaneous intrauterine and extrauterine pregnancies is approx. 1 in 30,000. Ultrasound may not be able to definitively verify that an ectopic pregnancy exists.

❑❑ What is the only true diagnostic sign of an ectopic pregnancy with ultrasound?

A fetus with cardiac activity outside the uterus. Complex masses and fluid in the cul-de-sac can be seen in other conditions, i.e., pelvic abscess, ruptured ovarian cyst.

❑❑ What is the role of ultrasound in detecting placenta previa and abruption?

Ultrasound is not sensitive for detecting placental abruption. However, in the patient with third trimester vaginal bleeding, ultrasound is used primarily to rule out placenta previa. An experienced ultrasonographer can detect a placenta previa. Uterine contraction, incorrect scanning techniques and an overfilled bladder can result in false positives.

❑❑ Describe the typical shape and vessel origin of subdural hematomas (SDH) and epidural hematomas (EDH)?

SDH are typically crescent-shaped and although can be arterial in origin are most often caused by the tearing of bridging veins. Acute SDH are hyperdense relative to the brain and become isodense to the brain in 1-3 weeks. EDH are biconvex (lenticular) in shape and are usually arterial in origin. An EDH does not cross intact skull sutures but can cross the tentorium and the midline.

❑❑ What is the test of choice for evaluating and staging renal trauma?

IV contrast-enhanced CT has replaced IVP for this purpose. CT is more accurate as IVP is not sensitive for renal injuries.

❑❑ What 2 studies can detect testicular torsion and differentiate it from epididymitis, orchitis, or torsion of the appendix testis?

Technetium 99m nuclear studies and, in some centers, duplex ultrasound.

❑❑ A laryngeal fracture is suggested by finding the hyoid bone elevated above what cervical level on X-ray?

C3.

❑❑ In children older than one year of age, where are foreign bodies in the airway usually located?

In the lower airway.

❑❑ In a child with malrotation, what is the most likely age of presentation, what is a common complication, and what signs and symptoms are usually present?

1) Malrotation usually occurs in children under 12 months of age.
2) Volvulus is a common complication.
3) Signs and symptoms usually include vomiting, blood streaked stools, and abdominal pain.

❑❑ Name two causes of Toxic Epidermal Necrolysis, (a.k.a., scalded skin syndrome).

1) Drug or Chemical: Occurs usually in adults. Cleavage at dermo-epidermal junction.
2) *Staphylococcal.* Occurs usually in children < 5 years. SSSS results in intraepidermal cleavage beneath stratum granulosum.

❑❑ Describe the presentation of SSSS.

Disease begins after URI or purulent conjunctivitis. First lesions are tender, erythematous and scarlatiniform, usually found on face, neck, axillae and groin. Skin peels off in sheets with lateral pressure and a + Nikolsky's sign.

❑❑ What is appropriate treatment for Toxic Epidermal Necrolysis?

Regardless of cause, treat skin loss similarly to partial thickness burns. Do not use silver sulfadiazine. Adults can have large fluid loss. Admit patients with >10% BSA to burn unit. For SSSS treat with IV penicillinase-resistant penicillin.

❑❑ What is a positive Chvostek's sign?

Twitch in the corner of the mouth occurring when the examiner taps over the facial nerve in front of the ear. It is present in approximately 10 to 30% of normal individuals. Eyelid muscle contraction with Chvostek's maneuver is generally considered to be diagnostic of hypocalcemia.

❑❑ What is Trousseau's sign and when is it seen?

Trousseau's sign is a carpal spasm-induced when a blood pressure cuff on the upper arm maintains a pressure above systolic for approximately three minutes. Fingers become spastically extended at the interphalangeal joints and flexed at the metacarpophalangeal joints. Trousseau's sign is generally a more reliable indicator of hypocalcemia than is Chvostek's sign. A positive Trousseau's sign may also be found in hypomagnesemia, severe alkalosis, and strychnine poisoning.

❑❑ Activated charcoal is not an effective treatment for which substances?

Alcohols, ions, and acids and bases.

❑❑ Describe the DeBakey classification of regions of aortic dissection?

(I) Ascending and descending aorta.
(II) Ascending aorta.
(III) Descending aorta distal to the left subclavian artery.

❑❑ What is the most common rhythm disturbance in a pediatric arrest?

Bradycardia.

❑❑ Describe the common features of a slipped femoral capital epiphysis?

Injury usually occurs in adolescence. The rupture typically presents with an insidious development of knee or thigh pain, and a painful limp. Frequently hip motion is limited, particularly that of internal rotation.

❑❑ What are the common concerns with anterior dislocation of the shoulder?

Axillary nerve injury, axillary artery injury in the elderly patients, compression fracture of the humeral head (Hillsack's deformity), a rotator cuff tear, fractures of the anterior glenoid lip, and fractures of the greater tuberosity.

❑❑ Describe a Monteggia fracture/dislocation?

A fracture of the proximal ulna with dislocation of the radial head.

Treatment usually requires open reduction and internal fixation. When a Monteggia fracture is suspected, X-rays should include the forearm, elbow and wrist.

❑❑ Describe a Galeazzi's fracture/dislocation?

A radial shaft fracture with dislocation of the distal radioulnar joint.

❑❑ Describe the clinical characteristics of carboxyhemoglobin concentrations, specifically for ranges of near 10%, 10 to 20%, near 30%, 40%, 50%, 60% and 70%.

Frontal headache usually becomes evident with CoHb levels of 10%.
At 10 to 20% CoHb may produce symptoms of headache and dyspnea.
30% causes nausea, dizziness, visual disturbance, fatigue, and impaired judgment.

40% leads to syncope and confusion.
Levels of 50% may produce coma and seizures.
60% causes respiratory failure and hypotension.
70% level may be lethal.

❑❑ What is the appropriate treatment for cyanide poisoning?

Amyl nitrite, sodium nitrite IV, followed by sodium thiosulfate IV.

❑❑ Organisms which produce focal nervous system pathology via an exotoxin include?

C. diphtheria, C. botulinum, C. tetani, Wood and dog tick (*Dermacentor A&B*), and *S. aureus.*

❑❑ Describe botulism intoxication.

Botulism exotoxin is elaborated by *C. botulinum.* It affects the myoneural junction and prevents the release of acetylcholine. In the United States, it is caused principally by ingestion of foods that have been inadequately prepared.
The most common neurologic complaints are related to the bulbar musculature. Neurologic symptoms usually occur within 24 to 48 hours of ingestion of contaminated foods. Muscle paralysis and weakness usually spread rapidly to involve all muscles of the trunk and extremities. It is important to distinguish between botulism poisoning and myasthenia gravis. This distinction can be made by using the edrophonium (Tensilon) test, usually performed by a neurologist.

❑❑ In a patient who is either less than 10 or greater than 50 years of age, with both deep partial thickness and full thickness burns, what percentage of total body surface area must be burned before referral to the burn center is indicated?

10%.

❑❑ In a patient who is <u>between</u> the ages of 10 and 50 years, with both deep partial thickness and full thickness burns, what percentage of total body surface area must be burned before referral to the burn center is indicated?

20%.

❑❑ In a patient who has full thickness burns, what percentage of total body surface area must be burned before referral to the burn center is indicated?

5%: Independent of age.
NB.: Above are guidelines from one text, burns to hand, face and perineum require extra caution and burn center referral may be appropriate.

❑❑ Poor prognostic signs <u>on admission</u> of a patient with pancreatitis include . . . . ?

Age over 55 years.
Glucose level greater than 200 mg/dL.
LDH level greater than 350 IU/L.
WBC count greater than 16,000.
SGOT level greater than 250 U/L.

NOTICE - NO AMYLASE INVOLVEMENT!

❑❑ Which pain medicine is theoretically contraindicated in the treatment of pain from acute diverticulitis?

Codeine and morphine are contraindicated because their use may increase intraluminal colonic pressure. Meperidine (Demerol) is a good substitute as it inhibits segmental contraction of the colon.

❑❑ What test is best to confirm the diagnosis of Boerhaave's syndrome?

An esophagram using a water soluble contrast medium should be used in place of barium to confirm the diagnosis.

❑❑ What are the signs and symptoms of a patient with Boerhaave's syndrome?

Substernal and left sided chest pain with a history of forceful vomiting leading to spontaneous esophageal rupture.

❑❑ What are Kanavel's four cardinal signs of infectious digital flexor tenosynovitis?

Tenderness along the tendon sheath, finger held in flexion, pain on passive extension of the finger, and finger swelling.

❑❑ What symptoms are associated with the presentation of regional enteritis (Crohn's disease, granulomatous ileocolitis)?

Patients with regional enteritis may present with fever, abdominal pain, weight loss, and diarrhea. Fistulas, fissures, and abscesses may be noted.
Ulcerative colitis, on the other hand, usually presents with bloody diarrhea.

❑❑ A patient presents to your emergency department after being bitten by a wild raccoon. What treatment would you provide?

Wound care, tetanus prophylaxis, RIG, 20 IU/kg, (1/2 at bite site and 1/2 IM), and HDCV, 1 cc IM.

❑❑ Which animals are the most common vectors of rabies in the world? In the U.S.?

Worldwide, the dog is the most common carrier of rabies.
In the United States, the skUnk has become the most common source of disease. Bats, raccoons, cows, dogs, foxes and cats (descending order) are also sources.
Recall, parenthetically, that your rodents (Rocky (the flying squirrel), Dale (the chipmunk), Micky and Ratfink) and your lagomorphs (wild wangy wabbits), are NOT carriers of rabies.

❑❑ A septic appearing adult has multiple 1 cm diameter skin lesions with a necrotic, ulcerated center and an erythematous surrounding region. What is the likely pathogen?

Pseudomonas aeruginosa.

❑❑ Describe the signs and symptoms of spinal shock.

Spinal shock represents complete loss of spinal cord function below the level of injury. Patients have flaccid paralysis, complete sensory loss, areflexia and loss of autonomic function. Such patients are usually bradycardic, hypotensive, hypothermic and vasodilated.

❑❑ Positive birefringent crystals in synovial fluid analysis is suggestive of . . . . ?

Pseudogout. If you are POSITIVE, it must be PSEUDOgout - of course!.

❑❑ Describe the chest X-ray of Mycoplasma pneumonia.

Patchy densities involving the entire lobe are most common. Pneumatoceles, cavities, abscesses and pleural effusions can occur, but are uncommon. Erythromycin.

❑❑ Where is the most likely location of a Boerhaave's tear?

Left posterolateral region of the mid-thoracic esophagus.

❑❑ How does a coin appear on AP view of the trachea?

On its side.

❑❑ How does a coin in the esophagus appear on AP?

Like a solid circle.

❑❑ What are the principal signs and symptoms of ulcerative colitis?

Fever, weight loss, tachycardia, pancolitis, and six bloody bowel movements per day.

❑❑ What are two fairly common conditions in pediatrics that produce cardiac syncope?

Aortic stenosis, which is not cyanotic, and tetralogy of Fallot, which is cyanotic.

❑❑ What are two unique clinical findings of tetralogy of Fallot?

A boot shaped heart on X-ray and exercise intolerance which is relieved by squatting. TOF is treated by placing the patient in the knee chest position and giving morphine.

❑❑ What would be the signs and symptoms of aortic stenosis in a child?

Exercise intolerance, chest pain, and a systolic ejection click with a crescendo, decrescendo murmur, radiating to the neck with a suprasternal thrill. No cyanosis.

❑❑ What are the signs of left sided heart failure in an infant?

Increased respiratory rate, shortness of breath, and sweating during feeding.

❑❑ **What is the single most common cause of CHF in the second week of life?**

Coarctation of the aorta.

❑❑ **What are the signs and symptoms of Reye's syndrome:**

Irritable, combative, and lethargic, right upper quadrant tenderness, history of influenzae B or recent chicken pox, papilledema, hypoglycemia, and seizures. Lab findings will include hypoglycemia, and an elevated ammonia level greater than 20 times the normal. The bilirubin level is NORMAL.

❑❑ **What are the first, second, and third drugs of choice for the treatment of seizures in children?**

The first is phenobarbital, the second is phenytoin, and the third is carbamazepine.

❑❑ **Which is the drug of choice for treating a febrile seizure?**

Benzodiazepines are used acutely, followed by phenobarbital for supression.

❑❑ **What is the most common cause of painless lower GI bleeding in an infant or child?**

Meckel's diverticulum.

❑❑ **A 16 month old presents with bilious vomiting, a distended abdomen, and blood in the stool. What is the diagnosis?**

Malrotation of the mid-gut.

❑❑ **What are some possible complications of sodium bicarbonate therapy?**

Hypokalemia, paradoxical CSF acidosis, impaired O_2 dissociation, and sodium overload.

❑❑ **Differentiate between non-ketotic hyperosmolar coma and DKA.**

In non-ketotic hyperosmolar coma, glucose is very high, often > 800. The serum osmolality is also very high, with average about 380. A nitroprusside test is negative.
In DKA, glucose is more often in the range of 600, the serum osmolality is approximately 350, and the nitroprusside test is positive.

❑❑ **What focal signs may be present in a patient with non-ketotic hyperosmolar coma?**

These patients may have hemisensory deficits or perhaps hemiparesis. Ten to fifteen percent of these patients have a seizure.

❑❑ **What is the most common cause of hyperthyroidism?**

Grave's disease (toxic diffuse goiter).

❑❑ **What is the most common precipitating cause of thyroid storm?**

Pulmonary infection.

❑❑ **What is another name for life threatening hypothyroidism?**

Myxedema coma. Commonly occurs in elderly women during the winter months and is stimulated by infection and stress.

❑❑ **What is the most common cause of hypothyroidism?**

Overtreatment of Grave's disease with iodine or subtotal thyroidectomy.

❑❑ **What is the second most common cause of hypothyroidism?**

Autoimmune Hashimoto's thyroiditis.

❑❑ **How may primary hypothyroidism be distinguished from secondary?**

In primary hypothyroidism the TSH levels are high, patients often have a history of thyroid surgery and may have a goiter; in secondary the TSH levels are low or normal, no hx of surgery and no goiter.

❑❑ **What ECG finding would you expect in myxedema coma?**

Bradycardia.

❑❑ **What is a common "surgical problem" in myxedema that should be treated conservatively?**

Acquired megacolon.

❑❑ **What is primary adrenal insufficiency?**

Addison's disease, that is, failure of the adrenal cortex.

❑❑ **What is Waterhouse-Fredrickson syndrome?**

Septicemia secondary to meningococcemia with associated bilateral adrenal gland hemorrhage. The patient will have a petechial rash, purpura, shaking chills, and severe headache.

❑❑ **What effect does Addison's disease have on cortisol and aldosterone levels?**

Cortisol and aldosterone levels are low. Low cortisol levels lead to nausea, vomiting, anorexia, lethargy, hypoglycemia, water intoxication, and inability to withstand even minor stress without shock. Low aldosterone levels means sodium depletion, dehydration, hypotension, and syncope.

❑❑ **What are the principal signs and symptoms in adrenal crisis?**

Abdominal pain, hypotension and shock. The common cause is withdrawal of steroids. Treatment of adrenal crisis is hydrocortisone (Solu-Cortef), 100 mg IV bolus, and 100 mg added to the first liter of D_5 0.9 NS.

❑❑ **In the pediatric esophagus, where is the most common site of a foreign body?**

Cricopharyngeal narrowing.

❑❑ **Thyrotoxicosis may be treated with . . . ?**

Support and hydration, IV propylthiouracil, 1 g, sodium iodine, IV 1 g q 12 hour, or IV propanolol, 1 mg/minute up to 10 mg.

❑❑ **A fracture of the proximal fibular shaft is commonly associated with . . . . ?**

Medial ankle fracture or sprain. This is a Maisonneuve fx, it may be present with a widened mortise and no fx seen in the ankle.

❑❑ **What is the best X-ray view for diagnosing lunate and perilunate dislocations?**

Lateral X-ray views of the wrist.

❑❑ **What is the most common cause of periorbital cellulitis in a two year old child?**

The most common cause is *H. influenzae*. The second most common cause is *S. aureus*.

❑❑ **Which is the most appropriate drug for a patient with low cardiac output and pulmonary congestion?**

Dobutamine.

❑❑ **In a humeral shaft fracture, which nerve is most commonly injured?**

Radial nerve.

❑❑ **What is the most common dysrhythmia in a child?**

Paroxysmal atrial tachycardia.

❑❑ **What are some common causes of increased anion gap?**

Aspirin, methanol, uremia, diabetes, idiopathic (lactic), ethylene glycol, and alcohol are reasonably common.

Numerous etiologies may produce the entity above listed demurely as "lactic." Lactic acidosis may be the result of shock, seizures, acute hypoxemia, INH, cyanide, ritodrine, inhaled acetylene, carbon monoxide, and ethanol. Sodium nitroprusside, povidone-iodine ointment, sorbitol, and xylitol can cause an anion gap acidosis.

Other causes of anion gap acidosis include toluene intoxication, iron intoxication, sulfuric acidosis, short bowel syndrome (D-lactic acidosis), formaldehyde, nalidixic acid, methenamine, and rhubarb (oxalic acid). Inborn errors of metabolism, such as methylmalonic acidemia and isovaleric acidemia may also cause a gap acidosis.

Recall some pearls for sorting out the differential diagnosis:

Methanol: Visual disturbances and headache common. Can produce quite wide gaps as each 2.6 mg/dL of methanol contributes 1 mOsm/L to gap. Compare this with alcohol, each 4.3 mg/dL adds 1 mOsm/L to gap.

Uremia: Is quite advanced before it causes an anion gap.
Diabetic Ketoacidosis: Usually has both hyperglycemia and glucosuria; alcoholic ketoacidosis (AKA) often has a lower blood sugar and mild or absent glucosuria.

Salicylates: High levels contribute to gap.

Lactic Acidosis: Can check serum level. Itself has broad differential as above.

Ethylene glycol: Causes calcium oxalate or hippurate crystals in urine. Each 5.0 mg/dL contributes 1 mOsm/L to gap.

A reasonably comprehensive mnemonic device for recalling causes of anion gap acidosis is A MUDPILE CAT.

A MUDPILE CAT

A = alcohol,

M = methanol,
U = uremia,
D = DKA,
P = paraldehyde,
I = iron and isoniazid,
L = lactic acidosis,
E = ethylene glycol,

C = carbon monoxide,
A = ASA (aspirin),
T = toluene.

❑❑ What are the causes of <u>normal</u> anion gap metabolic acidosis?

Causes include diarrhea, ammonium chloride, renal tubular acidosis, renal interstitial disease, hypoadrenalism, ureterosigmoidostomy, and acetazolamide.

❑❑ What are some common causes of respiratory alkalosis?

Respiratory alkalosis is defined as a pH above 7.45, and a pCO_2 less than 35. Common causes of respiratory alkalosis include any process that may cause hyperventilation, such as shock, sepsis, trauma, asthma, PE, anemia, hepatic failure, heat stroke and exhaustion, emotion, salicylate poisoning, hypoxemia, pregnancy, and inappropriate mechanical ventilation. Alkalosis shifts the O_2 disassociation curve to the left. It also causes cerebrovascular constriction. Kidneys compensate for respiratory alkalosis by excreting HCO_3^-.

❑❑ How should a patient with hypertrophic cardiomyopathy be treated who presents with chest pain and normal vital signs except for a heart rate of 140?

ß-antagonists are the primary treatment for hypertrophic cardiomyopathy. ß-antagonists are first-line treatment for any symptomatic patient even without tachycardia present. Calcium channel blocking drugs are second-line therapeutics.

❑❑ **What is the preferred management of neurogenic shock?**

Neurogenic shock is treated with replacement of volume deficit followed by vasopressors.

❑❑ **An elderly male presents to your emergency department with ataxia, confusion, amnesia and ocular paralysis. The patient is apathetic to his situation and has an otherwise normal neurologic exam. What is the likely cause of the patient's problem?**

Vitamin B deficiency associated with Wernicke-Korsakoff's syndrome.

❑❑ **What are the classic ECG findings of a patient with a posterior MI.**

A large R-wave and ST depression in V1 and V2.

❑❑ **What is the classic ECG finding in Wolff-Parkinson-White syndrome?**

A change in the upstroke of QRS, the delta wave.

❑❑ **What is the best treatment for an unstable patient with Wolff-Parkinson-White syndrome presenting with rapid atrial fibrillation?**

Shock.

❑❑ **What is the best treatment for a verapamil-induced bradycardia?**

Calcium chloride 10%, 10-20 mL IV. (This is about 10-20 mg/kg, use 10-30 mg/kg in children).

❑❑ **What is the <u>most common</u> cause of valvular-induced syncope in the elderly?**

Aortic stenosis is the most common valvular cause of syncope in the elderly.
Vasovagal mechanisms are the most common mechanism overall.

❑❑ **Describe the signs, symptoms, and ECG finding associated with lithium toxicity.**

Tremor, weakness, and flattening of the T-waves.

❑❑ **A patient has an orbital floor fracture. What are associated symptoms and signs?**

The most common symptom would be diplopia due to entrapment of the inferior rectus and inferior oblique muscles, and resultant paralysis of upward gaze. In addition, one would worry that the inferior orbital nerve could be damaged with paresthesia resulting to the lower lid, infraorbital area and side of the nose.

❑❑ **What are the signs of an upper motor neuron lesion?**

Upper motor neuron lesion involves the corticospinal tract. The lesion usually gives paralysis with:

1) initial loss of muscle tone and then increased tone, resulting in spasticity;
2) Babinski sign;
3) loss of superficial reflexes;
4) increased deep tendon reflexes.

A lower motor neuron lesion is associated with the anterior horn cells' axons. The lesion gives paralysis with decreased muscle tone and prompt atrophy.

❑❑ Which condition commonly presents with ocular bulbar deficits?

Botulism poisoning. Patients with myasthenia gravis may present similarly. Diphtheria toxin may rarely produce similar deficits.

❑❑ Describe the symptoms and signs of myasthenia gravis.

Weakness and fatigability with ptosis, diplopia and blurred vision are the initial symptoms in 40% to 70% of patients. Bulbar muscle weakness is also common with dysarthria and dysphagia.

❑❑ Describe the key features of vertebrobasilar insufficiency.

Vertigo is nearly always positional, provoked by certain head positions. Nystagmus usually accompanies the vertigo. Other signs of arteriosclerosis may be found.
Vertebrobasilar insufficiency is usually seen in older persons and may occur with other symptoms of brainstem ischemia, visual symptoms being the most common.

❑❑ What disease would you expect in a patient with a two week history of lower limb weakness?

Guillain-Barré is usually an ascending weakness which begins in the lower extremity.
With botulism poisoning, the weakness is descending. Cranial nerves are typically affected first with myasthenia gravis.

❑❑ What is the mortality rate of Wernicke's encephalopathy?

10-20%. Treat with thiamine IV. Symptoms include ocular palsies, nystagmus, confusion, and ataxia.

❑❑ What therapy should be used for a patient with hemophilia A who suffers a head injury?

Treat this patient with cryoprecipitate. Keep total volume as low as possible. Cryoprecipitate has an increased concentration of factor VIII complex and has less volume than fresh frozen plasma.

❑❑ Describe a patient with sigmoid volvulus.

Patients with sigmoid volvulus are typically either psychiatric patients or elderly who suffer from severe chronic constipation. Symptoms include intermittent cramping, lower abdominal pain, and progressive abdominal distention.

❑❑ Describe a typical patient with intussusception.

Intussusception typically occurs in children of ages 3 months to 2 years. The majority are in the 5 to 10 month age group. It is more common in boys. The area of the ileocecal valve is usually the source of the problem.

❑❑ What are the common symptoms and signs of hyperthyroidism?

Symptoms include weight loss, palpitations, dyspnea, edema, chest pain, nervousness, weakness, tremor, psychosis, diarrhea, hyperdefecation, abdominal pain, myalgias, and disorientation. Signs include fever, tachycardia, wide pulse pressure, CHF, shock, thyromegaly, tremor, weakness, liver tenderness, jaundice, and stare. Mental status changes include somnolence, obtundation, coma, or psychosis. Pretibial myxedema may be found (a true misnomer!)

❑❑ **What are radiological and laboratory findings of duodenal injury?**

Retroperitoneal air and increased serum amylase.

❑❑ **What is the current therapeutic regimen for treatment of meningitis in a neonate?**

Initially, ampicillin and aminoglycoside were favored for treating the neonate with meningitis. However, today recommendations include ampicillin and cefotaxime.
A combination used in infants up to 2 months of age will cover coliform, Group B *Streptococci*, *Listeria*, and *Enterococcus*. Over 2 months of age up to 6 years, cefotaxime alone is indicated.

❑❑ **What is the formula for calculating a change in potassium with changes in pH?**

For each pH increase of 0.1, expect the potassium to drop by 0.5 mmol/L.

❑❑ **A patient has alcoholic ketoacidosis (a.k.a., AKA), what is the appropriate treatment?**

Alcoholic ketoacidosis usually presents with nausea, vomiting and abdominal pain occurring 24 to 72 hours after cessation of drinking. No specific physical findings are typically evident, though abdominal pain is a common complaint/finding. AKA is thought to be secondary to increased mobilization of free fatty acids with lipolysis to acetoacetate and ß-hydroxybutyrate.

Treatment usually includes normal saline and glucose. As acidosis is corrected, K^+ may drop. Sodium bicarbonate should not be given unless pH drops below 7.1.

❑❑ **Describe the symptoms of optic neuritis.**

The patient suffers a variable loss of central visual acuity with a central scotoma and change in color perception. The patient also has eye pain. The disk margins are blurred from hemorrhage and the blind spot is increased.

❑❑ **What is the antidote for ethylene glycol?**

Ethanol. dialysis and fomepizole (Antizol).

❑❑ **What is the antidote for iron?**

Deferoxamine.

❑❑ **What are the signs and symptoms of acute pericardial tamponade?**

Triad of hypotension, elevated CVP, and tachycardia is usually indicative of either acute pericardial tamponade, or a tension pneumothorax in a traumatized patient. Muffled heart tones may be auscultated.

❑❑ **What ECG finding is pathognomonic of pericardial tamponade?**

Total electrical alternans. Pulsus paradoxus is nonspecific. Muffled heart tones are subjective findings and are difficult to appreciate.

❑❑ How does a chronic pericardial effusion appear on chest X-ray?

Gradual pericardial sac distention results in a "water bottle" appearance of the heart.

❑❑ The treatment for myxedema coma includes . . . . ?

IV thyroid replacement with thyroxine, IV glucose, hydrocortisone, and consideration of water restriction.

❑❑ What are the symptoms and signs of thyrotoxicosis?

Weight loss and weakness may be reported. Tachycardia and fever are common abnormal vital signs with hypotension and shock occurring less frequently. Mental status changes of decreased consciousness or psychosis may be present. Signs of CHF, thyromegaly, tremor, eye signs including lid lag, and proptosis should also be sought.

❑❑ Describe a patient with acute narrow angle closure glaucoma.

Symptoms include nausea, headache, vomiting and abdominal pain. Visual acuity is markedly diminished. The pupil is semi-dilated and nonreactive. There is usually a glassy haze over the cornea and the eye is red and very painful. Intraocular pressure may be as high as 50 or 60 mm Hg.

❑❑ Describe the treatment of acute narrow angle glaucoma.

1) Mannitol to decrease intraocular pressure.
2) Miotics, such as pilocarpine, to open the angle.
3) Carbonic anhydrase inhibitor to minimize aqueous humor production.
4) An iridectomy is eventually performed to provide aqueous outflow.

❑❑ What is the appropriate treatment for a hyphema?

Elevate the head. Other treatments are controversial; however, most ophthalmologists believe patients should be hospitalized. Treatment <u>may</u> include double eye patch, topical cortisone, and cycloplegics. Visual acuity is often decreased.

❑❑ Describe the classic symptoms and signs of retinal detachment.

The patient is typically myopic and will complain of seeing a curtain coming down across his or her eye. This is usually accompanied by flashes of light but no discomfort. The patient may also see flashing lights, black dots, or a sudden change in vision. On funduscopic exam, the detached areas will appear gray in comparison to the normal pink retina. Treatment includes bilateral eye patch, strict bedrest, and a consultation with an ophthalmologist for laser photocoagulation of the retinal detachment.

❑❑ What is the standard dose of atropine in a child?

0.02 mg/kg.

❑❑ What is the <u>most common</u> cause of bacterial meningitis in a child more than one month of age?

Hemophilus influenzae. *S. pneumoniae* is second most common. *N. meningitis* is third. This condition is treated with ampicillin and chloramphenicol. A single agent treatment with a third generation cephalosporin may also be used.

❑❑ **What is the initial dose of sodium bicarbonate for children during a cardiopulmonary arrest?**

1 mEq/kg.

❑❑ **How is the expected normal systolic blood pressure for a pediatric patient, toddlers and up, calculated?**

Multiply the age by 2 and add 90 to the result to determine expected systolic BP.

Average SBP (mm Hg) = (Age x 2) + 90

Low normal limit SBP (mm Hg) = (Age x 2) + 70.

SBP for a term newborn is about 60 mm Hg.

❑❑ **What is the correct dose of epinephrine and atropine during a pediatric code?**

Epinephrine, 0.01 mg/kg/dose. Atropine, 0.02 mg/kg/dose.

❑❑ **What are the signs and symptoms of Kawasaki's disease?**

Kawasaki's initial presentation is with a high spiking fever, conjunctivitis, morbilliform rash, strawberry tongue, and erythema of the distal extremities with cervical adenopathy. It is a disease of the mucocutaneous lymph nodes. Patients should be hospitalized to rule out myocarditis, pericarditis, and coronary aneurysms. Aspirin is therapeutic.

❑❑ **Which is the initial antibiotic treatment for a child with epiglottitis?**

The most likely cause is *H. influenzae*. The child should be treated with a second or third generation cephalosporin.

❑❑ **What are the characteristics of a posterior hip dislocation?**

Posterior hip dislocations are typically caused by posteriorly directed force applied to the flexed knee. The extremity is shortened, internally rotated and adducted. Acetabular fractures are associated with this injury. Ninety percent of hip dislocations are posterior.

❑❑ **Describe the key features of central cord syndrome.**

Central cord syndrome typically occurs with hyperextension injuries in older patients with spondylosis, degenerative changes, or stenosis in the cervical spine. Symptoms include weakness that is more pronounced in the arms than the legs.

❑❑ **What are the key features of anterior spinal cord syndrome?**

The anterior cord syndrome involves compression of the anterior cord causing complete motor paralysis and loss of pain and temperature sensation distal to the lesion. Posterior columns are spared - light touch and proprioception are preserved.

❑❑ **How does myasthenia gravis typically present?**

Weakness of voluntary muscles, usually the extraocular muscles.

Diagnostic confirmation relies on the edrophonium (Tensilon) test that we don't do.
Treatment includes neurologic consultation, anticholinesterases, steroids, and thymectomy.

❑❑ **What are the signs and symptoms of posterior inferior cerebellar artery syndrome?**

Cerebellar dysfunction, such as vertigo, ataxia, and dizziness.

❑❑ **Describe the signs and symptoms of neuroleptic malignant syndrome.**

Patients present with muscle rigidity, autonomic disturbances, and acute organic brain syndrome. Blood pressure and pulse fluctuate wildly and temperature may reach as high as 42° C (108° F). Muscle necrosis may occur with resultant myoglobinuria.
Mortality ranges as high as 20%.

❑❑ **Describe the presentation of placenta previa.**

Placenta previa typically presents with painless bright red vaginal bleeding.

❑❑ **Describe the presentation of abruptio placentae.**

Dark red, painful, vaginal bleeding.

❑❑ **Signs of tension pneumothorax on physical exam include . . . . ?**

Tachypnea, unilateral absent breath sounds, tachycardia, pallor, diaphoresis, cyanosis, tracheal deviation, hypotension, and neck vein distention.

❑❑ **Which medications should be used to treat preeclampsia and eclampsia?**

Magnesium and hydralazine.

❑❑ **How much fluid is needed in the pericardial sac to increase the cardiac silhouette on chest X-ray?**

About 250 mL.

❑❑ **What is the most common dysrhythmia associated with Wolff-Parkinson-White syndrome?**

Paroxysmal atrial tachycardia.

❑❑ **What are the symptoms and signs of aortic stenosis?**

Exertional dyspnea, angina and syncope.
Narrowed pulse pressure with decreased SBP.
Slow carotid upstroke.
Prominent S_4.

❑❑ **What is the best method to open an airway while maintaining c-spine precautions?**

Jaw thrust.

❑❑ **How should hypercalcemia be treated?**

Furosemide and normal saline. Mithramycin may be used, especially in hypercalcemia secondary to bone cancer. Other treatments include calcitonin, hydrocortisone, and indomethacin.

❑❑ **What is the treatment for multifocal atrial tachycardia?**

Treat underlying disorder. Administer magnesium sulfate, 2 g over 60 seconds with supplemental potassium to maintain serum K^+ above 4 mEq/L.
A second treatment is verapamil, 10 mg IV.

❑❑ **What is the treatment for ectopic SVT due to digitalis toxicity?**

Stop digitalis, correct hypokalemia, consider digoxin specific Fab, magnesium IV, lidocaine IV, or phenytoin IV.

❑❑ **What is the treatment for ectopic SVT not due to digitalis toxicity?**

Digitalis, verapamil, or ß-blocker to slow rate.
Quinidine, procainamide, or magnesium to decrease ectopy.

❑❑ **What is the treatment for verapamil-induced hypotension?**

Calcium gluconate, 1 g IV over several minutes.

❑❑ **Which drugs are contraindicated in the treatment of Le Torsade de pointes?**

A drug which prolongs repolarization (QT interval). For example, class Ia antiarrhythmics, such as quinidine and procainamide. Other drugs that share this effect include TCAs, disopyramide, and phenothiazines.

❑❑ **What is the treatment for Le Torsade de pointes?**

1) Magnesium sulfate, 2 g IV.
2) Pacemaker cranked to 90-120 bpm to "overdrive" pace.
3) Isoproterenol.

The goal is to accelerate the heart rate and shorten ventricular repolarization. (If it's me, start with the mag, SHP & JNA).

❑❑ **Discuss the treatment for digitalis toxicity.**

1) Charcoal.
2) Phenytoin (Dilantin) for ventricular arrhythmias (it increases AV node conduction) or lidocaine.
3) Atropine or pace for bradyarrthymias.
4) Digoxin specific Fab (Digibind).

❑❑ **Which drug should be used to treat a patient in cardiac arrest secondary to hyperkalemia?**

Calcium chloride IV acts the fastest. Also provide $NaHCO_3$ and hyperventilate (elevate pH by 0.1 and lower K by 0.5).

❑❑ Which is the drug of choice for digitalis toxicity resulting in a ventricular arrhythmia?

Phenytoin and digoxin specific Fab (Dilantin and Digibind).

❑❑ For each 100 increase in glucose, what is the effect on serum sodium?

Each 100 increase in glucose decreases the serum sodium by 1.6 to 1.8 mEq/L.

❑❑ In a patient with tachycardia from cocaine abuse, which medications are appropriate?

Sedation with benzodiazepines may calm the patient and decrease tachycardia. Nitroprusside may be used to treat hypertension. Caution must be used with ß-adrenergic antagonist agents alone as they may leave a-adrenergic stimulation unopposed, increasing the patient's risk for intracranial hemorrhage or aortic dissection.

❑❑ What traditional anti-arrhythmic agents may be used to treat digitalis-induced ventricular arrhythmias in addition to phenytoin?

Lidocaine and bretylium. Procainamide and quinidine are contraindicated in digitalis toxicity.

❑❑ In a trauma patient receiving multiple units of transfused blood, when should the blood products be supplemented with fresh frozen plasma?

For each five units of transfused blood, fresh frozen plasma is usually given.

❑❑ What are the common presentations of a transfusion reaction?

Myalgia, dyspnea, fever associated with hypocalcemia, hemolysis, allergic reactions, hyperkalemia, citrate toxicity, hypothermia, coagulopathies, and altered hemoglobin function.

❑❑ What are the signs of the Cushing reflex?

Increased systolic blood pressure and bradycardia.

❑❑ In testing a patient's oculovestibular reflex, what is the direction of nystagmus anticipated in response to cold-water irrigation; toward or away from the irrigated ear?

Recall that nystagmus is defined as the direction of the fast component of saccadic eye movement. Emergency physicians will commonly perform a crude but secure test of the oculovestibular reflex using ice water. After irrigation, nystagmus should be away from the irrigated ear. Try the mnemonic COWS - Cold Opposite, Warm Same.

❑❑ Signs and symptoms of an uncal herniation include . . . . ?

Coma, ipsilateral pupillary dilation and either ipsilateral or contralateral hemiparesis. Blunting of corneal reflex may occur. Oculovestibular response may be lost.

❑❑ What is the antidote for organophosphates?

Atropine and pralidoxime (2-PAM).

❑❑ What is a common finding on sinus X-ray suggesting basilar skull fracture?

Blood in the sphenoid sinus.

❑❑ What three toxicologic emergencies require immediate dialysis?

Ethylene glycol, methyl alcohol, and Amanita phalloides.

❑❑ For which drugs may hemoperfusion be indicated?

Salicylates, theophylline, and long-acting barbiturates.

❑❑ For which drugs may dialysis be indicated?

Salicylates, theophylline, and long-acting barbiturates.
Also - Methyl alcohol, ethylene glycol, amphetamine, lithium, and thiocyanate.

❑❑ What are the four stages of acetaminophen toxicity?

I (within an hour): Anorexia, nausea, vomiting and diaphoresis.

II (24-48 hours): Liver function test abnormalities and right upper quadrant pain.

III (72-96 hours): Jaundice, return of GI symptoms, peak of liver function abnormalities, coagulation defects.

IV (4 days -2 weeks): Get better or die.

❑❑ When does acetaminophen become toxic?

When there is no glutathione to detoxify its toxic intermediate.

❑❑ How does N-acetylcysteine act to interrupt acetaminophen toxicity?

Exact mechanism unknown, however, likely that NAC enters cells, and is metabolized to cysteine which is a precursor for glutathione. Thus it may increase glutathione stores.

❑❑ What is the early acid base disturbance seen in salicylate overdose?

Respiratory alkalosis. Approximately 12 hours later, one might see an anion gap metabolic acidosis or mixed acid base picture.

❑❑ What are common symptoms and signs of chronic salicylism?

Fever, tachypnea, CNS alterations, acid base abnormalities, electrolyte abnormalities, chronic pain, ketonuria, and noncardiogenic pulmonary edema.

❑❑ What is the treatment of salicylate overdose?

Decontaminate, lavage and charcoal, fluid replacement, potassium supplementation, alkalize the urine with use of bicarbonate, cooling for hyperthermia, glucose for hypoglycemia, oxygen and PEEP for pulmonary edema, multiple dose activated charcoal, and dialysis.

❑❑ A patient presents with vomiting, hematemesis, diarrhea, lethargy, coma and shock. What cause is suspected?

Iron intoxication. Order a flat plate of the abdomen to look for concretions.

❑❑ What is the treatment for iron ingestion?

If patient has no symptoms for 6 hours and is completely normal on exam, discharge home.

If patient has minimal symptoms and appears fine and has iron level close to maximum normal level (150 μg/dL) measured 4 hours after ingestion, discharge home.

Cathartics for patients without diarrhea (controversial).
Hydration and treat GI hemorrhage.

Deferoxamine if:
- Moderate or severely symptomatic,
- Serum iron level > TIBC,
- Serum iron level > 350 μg/dL.

Deferoxamine is a specific agent for iron and will not chelate other metals. The IV dose of deferoxamine is 10 to 15 mg/kg/hour IV.

❑❑ What are the symptoms and signs of cyanide overdose?

Dryness and burning in the throat, air hunger, and hyperventilation. If not removed from the toxic environment, loss of consciousness, seizures, bradycardia, and apnea follow prior to asystole.

❑❑ What is the treatment for cyanide overdose?

1) Oxygen, CPR prn.
2) Amyl nitrite perle inhaled.
3) Sodium nitrite, 10 cc of 3% solution in an adult which is 300 mg, or 0.2-0.33 mL/kg.
4) Sodium thiosulfate, 12.5 mg, in an adult which is 50 cc of a 25% solution or 1.0-1.5 mL/kg in a child (five times the volume of sodium nitrite).

Excess nitrites may require treatment with methylene blue for very, very rare case of dangerous methemoglobinemia..

❑❑ Where do endoscopic perforations of the esophagus typically occur?

They usually occur near the distal esophagus or at the site of pre-existing disease, such as a caustic burn.

❑❑ How may a posterior urethral tear be diagnosed in a male?

A high riding, boggy prostate suggests this injury.

❑❑ Describe the mechanism of injury and signs & symptoms associated with an anterior urethral tear?

Straddle or crush injury mechanism, severe perineal pain with blood usually found at the meatus, and good urinary stream is maintained.

❑❑ **What is the mechanism of a posterior urethral tear?**

Associated with pelvic fracture.
Urethral stricture, impotence, and incontinence.

❑❑ **A patient has a pelvic fracture with suspected bladder or ureteral injury. Which test should be performed first, a cystogram or an IVP?**

When a pelvic fracture is present or suspected, the cystogram is usually performed first so that distal ureteral dye from the IVP will not mimic extravasation from the bladder.

❑❑ **What is the most common cause of immediate postpartum hemorrhage?**

Uterine atony, followed by vaginal/cervical lacerations, and retained placenta or placental fragments.

❑❑ **How is an acute hemorrhagic overdose of Coumadin best treated?**

Fresh frozen plasma, Vit K IM will help prevent subsequent hemorrhage.

❑❑ **Describe a patient with tick paralysis.**

A rapid progressive ascending paralysis that develops over 1-2 days. First systems occur in the extremities and trunk and move to bulbar musculature. It is almost identical to Guillain-Barré Syndrome.

❑❑ **What is the pathophysiology of myasthenia gravis?**

Circulatory antibody against ACh receptor which binds at the motor end plate. In myasthenics, ACh receptors are in short supply resulting in fatigable weakness.

❑❑ **What are some factors commonly associated with meningitis?**

Age less than 5 years or greater than 60 years; low socioeconomic status; male sex; crowding; black race; sickle cell disease; splenectomy; alcoholism; diabetes and cirrhosis; immunologic defects; dural defect from congenital, surgical or traumatic source; contiguous infections, such as sinusitis, household contacts, malignancy, bacterial endocarditis, intravenous drug abuse; and thalassemia major.

❑❑ **Explain how methylene blue functions as an antidote for methemoglobinemia.**

A normal level of 3% methemoglobin is usually maintained by a NADPH - dependent enzyme. This enzyme capacity can be exceeded with oxidant poisoning. Methylene blue enhances NADPH - dependent hemoglobin reduction by acting as a cofactor.
Methylene blue is usually only needed for metHb levels > 30%; its dose is 1-2 mg/kg IV over 5 minutes.

❑❑ **How much elemental iron will 100 mg of deferoxamine bind?**

About 8.5 mg of elemental iron is bound by 100 mg of deferoxamine.

❑❑ **Which drug will most rapidly decrease K^+?**

Calcium chloride IV, 1-3 minutes.

❑❑ What is a potential side effect of the use of Kayexalate?

Kayexalate exchanges sodium for K^+. As a result, sodium overload and CHF may occur.

❑❑ ECG changes associated with tricyclic antidepressant overdose?

Prolongation of the PR, QRS and QT interval, as well as conduction defects such as bundle branch block, typically on the right.

❑❑ What dose of ASA will cause mild to moderate toxicity?

200-300 mg/kg. Greater than 500 mg/kg is potentially lethal.

❑❑ What is the treatment for lithium overdose?

Saline diuresis and hemodialysis.

❑❑ Which electrolyte abnormality commonly occurs with salicylate toxicity?

Hypokalemia.

❑❑ How does a patient present with Boerhaave's syndrome?

Boerhaave's syndrome is spontaneous esophageal perforation. It usually occurs after forceful vomiting. The patient suffers an acute collapse, chest and abdominal pain. A left pleural effusion is seen in 90% of patients on chest X-ray and most have mediastinal emphysema.

❑❑ What are the classic findings of shaken baby syndrome?

Failure to thrive, lethargy, seizures, and retinal hemorrhages. A CT may show subarachnoid hemorrhage or subdural hematoma from torn bridging veins.

❑❑ What is the immediate treatment for cord prolapse?

Displace the head cephalad.

❑❑ Which nerve may be injured in a distal femoral fracture?

Peroneal nerve.

❑❑ Describe the signs and symptoms and X-ray tests for diagnosing a slipped capital femoral epiphysis.

Gradual onset of hip pain and stiffness with restriction of internal rotation. Patient may walk with a limp. X-ray analysis should include both the anterior-posterior and lateral views of both hips. The slip of the epiphyseal plate posteriorly is best seen on the lateral view.

❑❑ How does a patient present with a retropharyngeal abscess?

Patients typically prefer a supine position. Retropharyngeal abscesses are common under 3 years of age. On examination, the uvula and tonsil are displaced away from the abscess. Soft tissue swelling and forward displacement of the larynx are present. Soft tissue X-ray films of the neck may assist in the diagnosis.

❑❑ How does an adult with epiglottitis present?

Pharyngitis and dysphagia are prominent symptoms. Adenopathy is uncommon. The patient may have a muffled voice and speak softly. However, hoarseness is rare. Pharyngitis is present and pain is out of proportion to objective findings.

❑❑ Describe a patient with intussusception.

Patients with intussusception are most likely very young. Seventy percent occur within the first year of life. In children, the cause is thought to be secondary to lymphoid tissue at the ileocecal valve, whereas in adults, it is thought to be caused by local lesions, Meckel's diverticulum, or tumor. On exam, bowel sounds are usually normal. Intussusception typically involves the terminal ileum. Meckel's diverticulum is the single most common intrinsic bowel lesion involved.

❑❑ In a patient with acute testicular pain, relief of pain with elevation of the scrotum (Prehn's sign) is classically associated with . . . . ?

Epididymitis.

❑❑ How much protamine is required to neutralize 100 units of heparin?

One mg of protamine will neutralize ~ 100 units of heparin. The maximum dose of protamine is 100 mg.

❑❑ Which test is most sensitive for evaluating a PE?

Perfusion scan is the <u>most</u> <u>sensitive</u> test, even more so than a pulmonary angiogram. Unfortunately, it is not a specific test, as 5% of normal volunteers will have an abnormal scan, and virtually any pulmonary pathology will produce an abnormal scan.

❑❑ You see a patient with a severe high concentration burn of hydrofluoric acid burn. How do you treat this patient?

In addition to topical jelly and cutaneous injections of calcium gluconate, provide IV treatment with 10 cc of 10% calcium gluconate, not calcium chloride, diluted in 50 cc of D_5W. This is given via a pump over 4 hours.

❑❑ How should an ocular burn secondary to hydrofluoric acid be treated?

Use calcium gluconate in a 1% solution mixed with saline and irrigate the eyes with this solution. The solution is made by diluting one part of standard 10% calcium gluconate solution with ten parts of saline which produces a 1% solution.

❑❑ Which electrolyte is depleted when a victim is burned by hydrofluoric acid?

Hydrofluoric acid results in <u>hypocalcemia</u>. Patients may require calcium replacement. Keep in mind that normal signs and symptoms of hypocalcemia, such as Chvostek's sign do not typically appear with hypocalcemia secondary to HF.

❑❑ How should a patient with neuroleptic malignant syndrome be treated?

1) Ice packs to the groin and axilla.
2) Cooling blankets.
3) Fan.
4) Water mist evaporation.

5) Dantrolene at an IV rate of 0.8 to 3 mg/kg IV q 6 hours to a total of 10 mg/kg.

❑❑ A patient presents with back pain and complaints of incontinence. On exam, loss of anal reflex, and decreased sphincter tone is noted. What is the diagnosis?

Cauda equina syndrome. The most consistent finding with cauda equina syndrome is urinary retention. On physical exam, expect saddle anesthesia, that is, numbness over the posterior superior thighs as well as numbness of the buttocks and perineum.

❑❑ A trauma patient has a closed head injury with suspected elevated intracranial pressure. What treatments should be considered?

1) Paralyze the patient and hyperventilate.
2) Maintain hypovolemia (fluid restrict).
3) Elevate the head of the bed to 30 degrees after the c-spine has been cleared.
4) Consider mannitol, 500 mL of a 20% solution over 20 minutes for a 70 kg adult.

Use of diuretics like furosemide is controversial. Steroids are no longer recommended. Barbiturate use is also not recommended. Mannitol use is also losing favor.

❑❑ When monitoring a pregnant female trauma victim, which vital signs are more appropriate to follow - the mother's or those of the fetus?

It is probably best to consider monitoring the fetal heart rate because it is more sensitive to inadequate resuscitation. Remember that the mother may lose 10 to 20% of her blood volume without change in vital signs whereas the baby's heart rate may increase or decrease above 160 or below 120 indicating significant fetal distress.

❑❑ What two findings on physical exam are indicative of uterine rupture?

Loss of uterine contour and palpable fetal part.

❑❑ What physical exam findings may be discovered in abruptio placenta?

Rapidly increasing fundal height secondary to bleeding into the uterus or a higher than expected fundal height.

❑❑ What are the indications for administering digitalis specific Fab?

Ventricular arrhythmias, $K^+ > 5.5$ mEq/L, and unresponsive bradyarrhythmias.

Some authors refer to an ingestion of more than 0.3 mg/kg as requiring Fab (Digibind).
The dose of Fab is:

vials required = 1.33 x mg ingested,

or use formula to determine the dose based on serum digoxin level,
or give 10 vials, 40 mg Fab each, if the amount ingested is not known.

Adolescents and children have an even higher sensitivity to the serious complications of digoxin overdose and may need Fab therapy with ingestion of less than the recommended level of 0.3 mg. per kilogram.

Remember, in an acute overdose situation, the serum level of digitalis is unreliable in evaluating toxicity. Digitalis levels typically only become accurate after 4 to 6 hours; this is too long to wait for treatment.

❑❑ What distinguishes heat stroke from heat exhaustion?

Heat exhaustion is progressive loss of electrolytes and body fluid depletion. Therapy is rehydration.

Heat stroke occurs when temperatures are above 42° C and enzyme systems cease to function normally. As a result, there is necrosis, denaturing, and organ failure. Heat stroke requires much more aggressive treatment as compared to simple fluid rehydration.

Remember, in patients with an altered sensorium and a core temperature above 42° C, always suspect heat stroke. Half of patients will be diaphoretic.

❑❑ How should a patient with heat stroke be treated?

1) Cool the patient with lukewarm water and fans.
2) Pack the axillae, neck and groin with ice.
3) Give fluids cautiously as large boluses of fluids may precipitate pulmonary edema.
4) Treat shivering with chlorpromazine (Thorazine), 25 to 50 mg IV.

❑❑ What complications can result from heat stroke?

Renal failure, rhabdomyolysis, DIC, and seizures. Remember antipyretics will not help.

❑❑ Describe the appearance of a black widow spider bite?

Two tiny red marks with surrounding erythematous patch. The initial bite may be painless. If a "pinprick" type bite is followed by abdominal cramps, think of a black widow spider. Exam reveals abdominal rigidity without true tenderness. Patients are restless and move about the gurney. An antivenin should probably be given to patients who are pregnant, younger than 16 and older than 65, and symptomatic. It also should be given to patients with underlying cardiac disease. Other treatments include calcium, diazepam (Valium), or methocarbamol (Robaxin). Traditional treatment also includes calcium gluconate.

❑❑ An elderly patient presents with sudden onset of severe abdominal pain followed by a forceful bowel movement. What is the diagnosis?

Acute mesenteric ischemia. Keep in mind that abdominal series may be normal early in acute mesenteric ischemia. Possible late X-ray findings include absent bowel gas, ileus, gas in the intestinal wall and thumb-printing of the intestinal mucosa. In most cases, films are normal or not specifically suggestive. Expect heme-positive stools. Patients who are especially prone to mesenteric ischemia include those with CHF and chronic heart disease.

❑❑ How may hyperglycemic, hyperosmolar, non-ketotic coma be differentiated from DKA?

The serum osmolality is higher in NKHC. $NaHCO_3$ is normal in NKHC and depleted in DKA and the pH is usually maintained at > 7.2 in NKHC.

❑❑ For which types of overdoses is activated charcoal <u>not</u> indicated?

Alcohol ingestion, electrolytes, heavy metals, lithium, hydrocarbons and caustic ingestions.

❑❑ Which type of blood test is used to determine if a patient needs RhoGAM therapy?

A Kleihauer-Betke checks for fetomaternal bleeding.

❑❑ A young patient has a threatened abortion in the first trimester. Laboratory studies reveal she is Rh negative and her husband is Rh positive. What is the treatment?

The patient will need 50 mcg of Rh immunoglobulin (RhoGAM) IM. After the first trimester, the dose is increased to 300 mcg IM.

❑❑ What are the signs and symptoms of preeclampsia?

Upper abdominal pain, headache, visual complaints, cardiac decompensation, creatinine greater than 2, proteinuria greater than 100 mg/dL, and a blood pressure of greater than 160 mm Hg systolic or 110 mm Hg diastolic.

Preeclampsia is most common in nulliparous women late in pregnancy, typically after 20 weeks gestation. Look for edema, hypertension, and proteinuria to diagnose these patients.

The ED treatment for preeclampsia is IV hydralazine titrated to a blood pressure of 90 to 110 diastolic using 5 mg boluses q 20 to 30 minutes. Blood pressure must be lowered slowly to avoid compromising the uteroplacental blood flow. Patients with moderate to severe preeclampsia need IV magnesium, although its true utility is not well demonstrated.

❑❑ Which type of rattlesnake bite causes most deaths?

Diamond Back rattlesnake is the cause of nearly all lethal snake bites in the United States. However, the Diamond Back accounts for only 3% of the total incidences of snake bites. Treat with 10 to 20 vials of antivenin.

❑❑ What is the only absolute contraindication to IVP?

Profound hypotension - the kidneys won't be perfused. Two relative contraindications are renal insufficiency with a creatinine greater than 1.6 and a history of allergic reactions.

❑❑ What are the National Institutes of Health treatment recommendations for spinal cord injury?

Administer high dose methylprednisolone, (Solu-Medrol) 30 mg/kg bolus over 15 minutes, followed by 45 minutes normal saline drip. Over the subsequent 23 hours, the patient should receive an infusion of 5.4 mg/kg/hour of methylprednisolone.

❑❑ How is a retropharyngeal abscess diagnosed on plain films of a one year old child?

Look for prevertebral thickening of the soft tissues. More than 3 mm suggests the possibility of a retropharyngeal abscess. Air/fluid level may be present.

If still unsure, order a CT of the neck. On CT scan, retropharyngeal abscesses are just anterior to the vertebral column, will appear in only a few cuts, and appear as a gray area of about the same density as the spinal canal on CT.

❑❑ How is a laryngeal fracture diagnosed on plain films?

On a lateral soft tissue X-ray of the c-spine, check for retropharyngeal air, and elevation of the hyoid bone. The hyoid bone is usually at the level of C3 if there is no evidence of a laryngeal fracture. Elevation of the hyoid bone above C3 suggests a laryngeal fracture.

❑❑ **What is the Parkland formula for treating a pediatric burn victim?**

Ringer's lactate 4 mL x %BSA x wgt kg over 24 hours with 1/2 given in first 8 hours.

❑❑ **A trauma patient presents with a complaint of severe burning pain in the upper extremities and associated neck pain. On physical exam, the patient has good strength in his upper extremities and no obvious neurologic deficits in the lower extremities. Although the c-spine series is negative, what problem is still suspected?**

Central cord syndrome. This injury is due to hyperextension of the spinal cord. Diagnostic findings include upper extremity neurologic symptoms and minimal or no lower extremity symptoms. Tingling, paresthesias, burning pain, and severe weakness or paralysis in the upper extremities with little or no symptoms in the lower extremities.

❑❑ **Differentiate between a hypertensive emergency and a hypertensive urgency.**

Elevated BP + end organ damage = hypertensive emergency.
Elevated BP + no symptoms or signs of end organ damage = hypertensive urgency; usually DBP > 115 mm Hg. Requires acute treatment.

❑❑ **A patient presents with fever, neck pain or neck stiffness and trismus. Exam reveals pharyngeal edema with tonsil displacement and edema of the parotid area. What is the diagnosis?**

Parapharyngeal Abscess.

❑❑ **A patient presents with hearing loss, nystagmus, complaint of facial weakness, and diplopia. Vertigo is provoked with sudden movement. A lumbar puncture reveals elevated CNS protein. What diagnosis is suspected?**

An acoustic neuroma.

❑❑ **What are the key features of Stevens-Johnson Syndrome?**

It is a bullous form of erythema multiforme with involvement of mucous membranes. It may cause corneal ulcerations, anterior uveitis and blindness.

❑❑ **Which drugs most commonly induce toxic epidermal necrolysis?**

Phenylbutazone, barbiturates, sulfa drugs, anti-epileptics, and antibiotics.

❑❑ **How is erysipelas treated?**

Penicillin. Administer erythromycin for penicillin allergic patients.

❑❑ **What are some of the common causes of prerenal acute renal failure?**

Volume depletion and decreased effective volume (CHF, sepsis, cirrhosis).

❑❑ **What are the causes of acute renal failure which are renal in nature?**

Acute Tubular Necrosis, acute interstitial nephritis, acute glomerulonephritis, and vascular disease.

❑❑ **What arrhythmia is frequently encountered during renal dialysis.**

Hypokalemia-induced ventricular fibrillation.

❑❑ **Painful third trimester vaginal bleeding likely represents . . . .?**

Abruptio placenta.

❑❑ **When can one auscultate the fetal heart?**

1) Ultrasound: 6 weeks.
2) Doppler: 10-12 weeks.
3) Stethoscope: 18-20 weeks.

❑❑ **Describe a Brudzinski sign.**

Flexion of the neck produces flexion of the knees.

❑❑ **Describe Kernig's sign.**

Extension of the knees from the flexed thigh position results in strong passive resistance.

❑❑ **What opening pressure and protein levels are expected with bacterial meningitis?**

Opening pressure of near 30 cm H_2O and protein level of greater than 150 mg/dL. Glucose level will drop with bacterial meningitis, with TB and with fungal infections.

❑❑ **A heroin addict presents with pulmonary edema. What is the best treatment?**

Naloxone, O_2 and ventilatory support. Don't bother using diuretics. This seems like a good test question.

❑❑ **An alcoholic patient presents with complaints of abdominal pain and blurred vision. The patient is very photophobic and blood gases reveal a metabolic acidosis. What is the diagnosis?**

Methanol poisoning. These patients may describe seeing something resembling a snowstorm.

❑❑ **What alcohol poisoning is suggested by a plasma bicarbonate level of zero (cipher, null, empty set, zip, Ø)?**

Methanol. It also produces a large osmolar gap and large anion gap. Methanol poisoning is treated with IV ethanol and hemodialysis.

❑❑ **What are the signs and symptoms of ethylene glycol poisoning?**

Hallucinations, nystagmus, ataxia, papilledema, and a large anion gap.

❑❑ **How should ethylene glycol poisoning be treated?**

Gastric lavage, sodium bicarbonate, thiamine and pyridoxine, IV ethanol and hemodialysis.

❑❑ **What are the major lab findings in a patient with isopropanol poisoning?**

Elevated osmolal gap, acetonemia and acetonuria., acetone, and Ø acidosis.

❑❑ **What are the signs and symptoms of isopropanol poisoning?**

Sweet odor of breath (acetone), hypotension and hemorrhagic gastritis, CNS depression from isopropanol and from its metabolite, acetone.

❑❑ **What is the treatment for cocaine toxicity?**

Sedate with benzodiazepine. Treat unresponsive hypertension with nitroprusside or phentolamine. Return to text book to re-read discussion of worsening symptoms with ß-adrenergic antagonists.

❑❑ **For which drugs will alkalinization of the urine increase excretion?**

TCA's, salicylates, and long-acting barbiturates. *May* be of some use to enhance lithium excretion.

❑❑ **What laboratory test can aid in the evaluation of a possible toxic iron ingestion?**

Total iron binding capacity measured 3 to 5 hours after ingestion. If serum iron level is significantly less than the total iron binding capacity, a toxic iron ingestion is less likely.

❑❑ **Deferoxamine should be given for what ratio of serum iron to total iron binding capacity?**

Administer deferoxamine if serum iron is > total iron binding capacity.

❑❑ **When do CK levels first begin to rise and when do they peak in an MI?**

CK - MB earliest rise is in 6-8 hours, th peak is in 24-30 hours, the levels normalize within 48 hours.

❑❑ **Inferior wall MIs commonly lead to which two types of heart block (via mechanism of damage to autonomic fibers in the atrial septum giving increased vagal tone impairing AV node conduction)?**

1) First degree AV block.
2) Mobitz Type I (Wenckebach) second-degree AV block.
3) Sinus bradycardia can also occur.

Progression to complete AV block is not common.

❑❑ **Anterior wall MIs may directly damage intracardiac conduction. This may lead to which type of arrhythmias?**

The dangerous type! Mobitz II second-degree AV block that can suddenly progress to complete AV block.

❑❑ **What is the initial drug of choice to treat SVT in a pediatric patient.**

Adenosine, 0.1 mg/kg is drug of choice. Digoxin, 0.02 mg/kg may take ~ 4 hours for conversion. Verapamil may be used in children > 2 years of age. It is contraindicated in younger children due to several deaths. Perform synchronized cardioversion at 0.5-1.0 J/kg.

❑❑ After the first month of life, what is the number one cause of meningitis and of pneumonia in children?

Most common cause of meningitis after the first month of life is *H. influenza*.
Most common cause of pneumonia after the first month of life is *S. pneumoniae* and *H. influenza* is the second most common cause. For bacteremia in children greater than one month, the most common causes are *S. pneumoniae,* (70%). and *H. influenza,* (20%).

❑❑ Which type of alcohol ingestion is associated with hypocalcemia?

Ethylene glycol.

❑❑ For what disorder is vigorous digital massage of the orbit indicated?

Central retinal artery occlusion. DO NOT do this in central vein occlusion!

❑❑ What is the initial dose of blood to be given in children?

10 mL/kg of packed RBCs.

❑❑ Who should receive prophylaxis after exposure to *Neisseria meningitidis*?

People living with the patient or having close intimate contact.

❑❑ What is the difference between carbamates and organophosphates?

Carbamates produce similar symptoms as organophosphates, however, the bonds in carbamate toxicity are reversible.

❑❑ What are key signs and symptoms of organophosphate poisoning?

Ataxia, abdominal pain and cramping, blurred vision, seizures, diarrhea, diaphoresis, vomitting, sweating and miosis.

❑❑ A patient presents with miotic pupils, muscle fasciculations, diaphoresis and diffuse oral and bronchial secretions. The patient has an odor of garlic on his breath. What is the diagnosis?

Organophosphate poisoning.

❑❑ What ECG changes may be associated with organophosphate poisoning?

Prolongation of the QT interval, and ST and T wave abnormalities.

❑❑ What is the key laboratory finding in the diagnosis of organophosphate poisoning?

Decreased red blood cell cholinesterase activity. The serum cholinesterase level (pseudocholinesterase) is more sensitive but less specific. RBC cholinesterase is regenerated slowly and can take months to approach normal levels.

❑❑ What is the treatment for organophosphate poisoning?

Decontaminate, charcoal, large doses ofatropine and pralidoxime prn.

❑❑ **Describe the wound resulting from AC.**

AC produces an entrance and exit wound of similar size. The damage from AC is usually worse than that from DC.

❑❑ **Describe a DC wound.**

Small entrance wound, large exit wound.

❑❑ **Which type of arrhythmia does lightning produce?**

It is a DC and produces asystole.

❑❑ **Which type of arrhythmia does AC tend to produce?**

Ventricular fibrillation.

❑❑ **What is a frequent complication of ethmoid sinusitis?**

Orbital cellulitis.

❑❑ **What is the most accurate X-ray finding in traumatic rupture of the aorta?**

Rightward deviation of the esophagus more than 1-2 cm.

❑❑ **A person with a history of a motor vehicle accident has X-ray findings of retroperitoneal air seen on a flat plate of the abdomen. What is a probable diagnosis?**

Duodenal injury. Tentative test is a contrast study. Extravasation confirms a duodenal injury.

❑❑ **What ECG change is associated with hypocalcemia?**

Prolonged T waves.

❑❑ **A patient is digitalis toxic. Which electrolytes will need to be replaced?**

It is important to replace potassium and magnesium.

❑❑ **What is the most common complication of verapamil and how should it be treated?**

Hypotension. Treat with calcium gluconate IV over several minutes, glucagon can follow.

❑❑ **Third degree heart block is often seen in which type of myocardial infarction?**

Acute anterior wall myocardial infarction.

❑❑ **Which is the most common arrhythmia associated with Wolff-Parkinson-White syndrome?**

PAT. The patient presents with angina, syncope, and shortness of breath.

❑❑ **How can mydriasis caused by mydriatics and anticholinergic drugs be distinguished from those caused third cranial nerve compression?**

Pilocarpine. Pilocarpine will reverse cranial nerve compression but will have no effect on anticholinergic drugs or mydriatics.

❑❑ **Which drugs should never be used in atrial fibrillation with Wolff-Parkinson-White?**

Digitalis, verapamil, and phenytoin. Atrial fibrillation with Wolff-Parkinson-White should be treated with cardioversion or procainamide. SVT with Wolff-Parkinson-White should be treated with verapamil or adenosine.

❑❑ **Name the drug of choice for Wolff-Parkinson-White with atrial flutter or fibrillation?**

Procainamide.

❑❑ **What laboratory findings are expected in a child with pyloric stenosis?**

Hypokalemia, hypochloremia and metabolic alkalosis.

❑❑ **What is the most common cause of tricuspid regurgitation?**

Right heart failure secondary to left heart failure, typically caused by mitral stenosis.

❑❑ **What is the treatment for a propranolol overdose?**

Glucagon.

❑❑ **What are the X-ray findings in ischemic bowel disease?**

"Thumb" printing on the plain film and a ground glass appearance with absence of bowel gas.

❑❑ **A patient with currant jelly sputum is likely to have which type of pneumonia?**

Klebsiella or Type 3 Pneumococcus.

❑❑ **How do patients present with Babesia infection?**

Intermittent fever, splenomegaly, jaundice, and hemolysis. The disease may be fatal in patients without spleens. The disease can simulate rickettsial diseases like Rocky Mountain spotted fever. Treatment is with clindamycin and quinine.

❑❑ **Which is the most frequently transmitted tick-borne disease?**

Lyme's disease. The causative agent is spirochete *Borrelia burgdorferi*. The vector is *Ixodes dammini* (deer tick) also *I. pacificus, Amblyomma americanum*, and *Dermacentor variabilis*.

❑❑ **What side effect is expected with too rapid an infusion of procainamide?**

Hypotension. Other side effects include: QRS/QT prolongation, V-fib, and Torsade de pointe.

❑❑ When is dobutamine used in CHF?

Potent inotrope with some vasodilation activity, used when heart failure is not accompanied by severe hypotension.

❑❑ How is atrial flutter treated?

Initiate A-V nodal blockade with ß-adrenergic or calcium channel blockers or with digoxin. If necessary, in a stable patient, attempt chemical cardioversion with a class IA agent such as procainamide or quinidine after digitalization. If such treatment fails, or if patient is unstable and requires immediate electrocardioversion, do so with 25-50 J.

❑❑ What are the causes of atrial fibrillation?

Hypertension, rheumatic heart disease, pneumonia, thyrotoxicosis, and ischemic heart disease are common causes. Pericarditis, ethanol intoxication, PE, CHF, and COPD are other causes.

❑❑ How is atrial fibrillation treated?

Control rate with ß-blockade or verapamil then convert with procainamide, quinidine, or verapamil. Digoxin may be considered, although its effect will be delayed. Synchronized cardioversion at 100 to 200 J in an unstable patient requiring cardioversion. In a stable patient with a-fib of unclear duration, anticoagulation for 2-3 weeks should be considered prior to chemical or electrical cardioversion.

❑❑ What are the causes of SVT?

Ectopic SVT may be due to digitalis toxicity (25% of digitalis induced arrhythmias), pericarditis, MI, COPD, preexcitation syndromes, mitral valve prolapse, rheumatic heart disease, pneumonia, and ethanol.

❑❑ How is SVT caused by digitalis toxicity treated?

Stop digitalis, treat hypokalemia. Administer Mg or phenytoin. Provide digoxin-specific antibodies in the unstable patient. Avoid cardioversion.

❑❑ What is the treatment for stable SVT not caused by dig toxicity or by WPW syndrome?

Adenosine, vagal maneuvers, verapamil, ß-blockers, and Mg.

❑❑ Describe the key features of Mobitz I (Wenckebach) 2° AV block.

Progressive prolongation of the PR interval until atrial impulse is not conducted. If symptomatic, administer atropine and transcutaneous/transvenous pacing.

❑❑ Describe the features and treatment of Mobitz II 2° AV block.

Constant PR interval. One or more beats fail to conduct. Treat with atropine and transcutaneous/transvenous pacing.

❑❑ Name 5 causes of mesenteric ischemia.

Arterial thrombosis at sites of atherosclerotic plaques, emboli from left atrium in patients with a-fib or rheumatic heart disease who are not anticoagulated, arterial embolism most commonly to the superior mesenteric artery, insufficient arterial flow, and venous thrombosis.

❑❑ **What lab abnormalities are expected in a patient with mesenteric ischemia?**

Leukocytosis >15,000, metabolic acidosis, hemoconcentration, and elevation of phosphate and amylase.

❑❑ **What are the contraindications to ß-blockers?**

CHF, variant angina, AV block, COPD, asthma (relative), bradycardia, hypotension, and IDDM.

❑❑ **What can a new systolic murmur indicate in a patient with an AMI?**

Ventriculoseptal rupture or mitral regurgitation as a result of papillary muscle rupture or dysfunction.

❑❑ **Why do T waves invert in an AMI?**

Infarction or ischemia causes a reversal of the sequence of repolarization (endocardial-to-epicardial as opposed to normal epicardial-to-endocardial).

❑❑ **What ECG changes are seen in a true posterior infarction?**

Large R-wave and ST depression in V1 and V2.

❑❑ **What conduction defects are commonly seen in an anterior MI?**

The dangerous kind. Damage to the conducting system results in a Mobitz II 2° or in a 3° AVB.

❑❑ **What conduction defects are commonly seen in an inferior MI?**

Inferior MI affects the autonomic fibers in the atrial septum which increases vagal tone and impairs AV nodal conduction; 1° AV block and Mobitz type I 2° (Wenckebach) AV block are common.

❑❑ **How should PSVT be treated during an AMI?**

Vagal maneuvers, adenosine, or cardioversion. Stable patients may be able to tolerate verapamil or even ß-adrenergic blockers which are negative inotropes.

❑❑ **A patient presents 1 day after discharge for an AMI with a new harsh systolic murmur along the left sternal border and pulmonary edema. What is the diagnosis?**

Ventricular septal rupture. Diagnosis is confirmed with Swan-Ganz catheterization or echo. Treatment includes nitroprusside for afterload reduction and possible intra-aortic balloon pump followed by surgical repair.

❑❑ **Which type of infarct commonly leads to papillary muscle dysfunction?**

Inferior MI. Signs and symptoms include a mild transient systolic murmur and pulmonary edema.

❑❑ **A patient presents 2 week post AMI with chest pain, fever, and pleuropericarditis. A pleural effusion is detected by CXR. What is the diagnosis?**

Dressler's (postmyocardial infarction) syndrome which is caused by an immunologic reaction to myocardial antigens.

❑❑ What is the most common symptom of acute pericarditis?

Sharp or stabbing retrosternal or precordial chest pain. Pain increases when supine and decreases when sitting-up and leaning forward. Pain may be increased with movement and deep breaths. Other symptoms include fever, dyspnea described as pain with inspiration, and dysphagia.

❑❑ What physical findings are associated with acute pericarditis?

Pericardial friction rub is the most common. Rub is best heard at the left sternal border or apex in a sitting leaning forward position. Other findings include fever and tachycardia.

❑❑ What ECG changes occur with acute pericarditis?

ST segment elevation in the precordial leads, especially V5 and V6 and in lead I. PR depression occurs in leads II, aVF, V4-V6.

❑❑ What are the most common symptoms and signs of PE?

CP, (88%), tachypnea, (92%), dyspnea (84%), anxiety, (59%), fever (43%), tachycardia, (44%), DVT, (32%), hypotension, (25%), and syncope, (13%).

❑❑ What is the most common CXR finding in PE?

Elevated dome of one hemidiaphragm as a result of decreased lung volume observed in 50% of PEs. Other common findings include pleural effusions, atelectasis, and pulmonary infiltrates.

❑❑ What are two relatively specific findings in PE on CXR?

1) Hampton's Hump: Area of lung consolidation with a rounded border facing the hilus.
2) Westermark's sign: Dilated pulmonary outflow tract ipsilateral to the emboli with decreased perfusion distal to the lesion.

❑❑ What does a normal perfusion scan rule out?

Rules out a PE. An abnormal scan can be caused by PE, asthma, emphysema, bronchitis, pneumonia, pleural effusion, carcinoma, CHF, and atelectasis.

❑❑ What does normal ventilation with decreased perfusion suggest?

PE.

❑❑ What are some of the indications for pulmonary angiography in a patient thought to have a PE?

1) Patients at high risk for bleeding complications with anticoagulation.
2) Negative test for DVT and low or medium probability lung scans.
3) Unstable patients for whom fibrinolytic therapy is being considered.

❑❑ What physical findings may be found with mitral stenosis?

Prominent a-wave, early-systolic left parasternal lift, 1st heart sound is loud and snapping, and early-diastolic opening snap with a low-pitched, mid-diastolic rumble that crescendos into S1.

❑❑ What triad of symptoms is characteristic of aortic stenosis?

Syncope, angina, and left heart failure. As the disease progresses, systolic BP decreases and pulse pressure narrows.

❑❑ What are the signs and symptoms of acute aortic regurgitation?

Dyspnea, tachycardia, tachypnea, and chest pain. Causes include infectious endocarditis, acute rheumatic fever, trauma, spontaneous rupture of valve leaflets, or aortic dissection.

❑❑ Define a hypertensive emergency.

Increased BP with associated end-organ dysfunction or damage. A controlled drop in BP over one hours should be attempted.

❑❑ What are the signs and symptoms of hypertensive encephalopathy?

Nausea, vomiting, headache, lethargy, coma, blindness, nerve palsies, hemiparesis, aphasia, retinal hemorrhage, cotton wool spots, exudates, sausage linking, and papilledema. Treat with labetalol or sodium nitroprusside, lower the mean arterial pressure to approximately 120 mm Hg.

❑❑ Which two drugs are used to treat eclampsia?

Magnesium sulfate, 4 to 6 g bolus IV followed by a 2 g/hour infusion, as well as hydralazine, 10 to 20 mg IV. Labetalol may also be used.

❑❑ What physical findings are suspicious for acute aortic dissection?

BP differences between arms, cardiac tamponade, and aortic insufficiency murmur.
An abnormal ECG may also be present.

❑❑ What CXR findings occur with a thoracic aortic aneurysm?

Change in appearance of aorta, mediastinal widening, hump in the aortic arch, pleural effusion (most common on the left), and extension of the aortic shadow.

❑❑ How are Stanford type A and B aortic dissections defined and treated?

Type A: Ascending, proximal to left subclavian (DeBakey I & II) - surgery.
Type B: Descending, distal to left subclavian (DeBakey III) - usually medical treatment.

❑❑ What historical findings suggest an embolus vs. a thrombosis in a lower extremity?

1) Embolus: Arrhythmia, valvular disease, MI, no skin changes of chronic arterial insufficiency, and no symptoms in the opposite extremity.
2) Thrombosis: Opposite extremity shows evidence of chronic arterial occlusive disease with history of rest pain claudication, etc.

❑❑ What is the initial fluid bolus that should be given to children in shock?

20 mL/kg.

❑❑ **What is the initial treatment of tension pneumothorax?**

Large bore IV catheter placed in the 2nd intercostal space but not a chest tube.

❑❑ **What is the most important cause of hypoxia in a patient with flail chest?**

The underlying lung contusion.

❑❑ **What is Hamman's sign?**

Also called Hamman's crunch. Crunching sound over the heart during systole secondary to pneumomediastinum.

❑❑ **What is the most common complaint in a patient with traumatic aortic injury?**

Retrosternal or intrascapular pain.

❑❑ **Name five clinical signs of basilar skull fracture.**

Periorbital ecchymosis (raccoon's eyes), retroauricular ecchymosis (Battle's sign), otorrhea or rhinorrhea, hemotympanum or bloody ear discharge, and 1st, 2nd, 7th, and 8th CN deficits.

❑❑ **What is the most common cause of shock in patients with blunt chest trauma?**

Pelvic or extremity fractures.

❑❑ **What is the differential diagnosis of distended neck veins in a trauma patient?**

Tension pneumothorax, pericardial tamponade, air embolism, and cardiac failure. Neck vein distention may not be present until hypovolemia has been treated.

❑❑ **A trauma patient presents with a "rocking-horse" type of ventilation. What is the diagnosis?**

Probable high spinal cord injury with intercostal muscle paralysis.

❑❑ **A trauma patient presents with subcutaneous emphysema. What is the differential diagnosis?**

Pneumothorax, laryngeal injury or pneumomediastinum; if emphysema is severe, consider a major bronchial injury.

❑❑ **A pneumothorax is suspected but does not show up on PA and Lat CXR. What other X-rays should be considered?**

Expiratory films. A pneumothorax is usually best seen on expiratory films.

❑❑ **Which rib fracture has the worst prognosis?**

The first rib. First and second rib fractures are associated with bronchial tears, vascular injury, and myocardial contusions.

❑❑ **What cardiovascular injury is commonly associated with sternal fractures?**

Myocardial contusions (blunt myocardial injury).

❑❑ **How much fluid needs to collect in the chest to be seen on decubitus or upright chest X-rays?**

200 to 300 mL; if supine, greater than 1 L may be necessary to be detected on AP CXR.

❑❑ **Describe Beck's triad.**

Muffled heart tones, hypotension, and distended neck veins. Causes include: myocardial contusion, AMI, pericardial tamponade, and tension pneumothorax. Tamponade may also cause pulsus paradoxus and distention of neck veins during inspiration. Total electrical alternans is highly specific for pericardial tamponade.

❑❑ **What is the most likely cause of a new systolic murmur and ECG infarct pattern observed in a patient with chest trauma?**

Ventricular septal defect.

❑❑ **What is the most accurate plain film X-ray finding indicating traumatic rupture of the aorta?**

Deviation of the esophagus > 2 cm right of the spinous process of T4.

❑❑ **What is the basic disorder contributing to the pathophysiology of compartment syndrome?**

Increased pressure within closed tissue spaces compromising blood flow to muscle & nerve tissue. There are three prerequisites to the development of compartment syndrome:

1) Limiting space.
2) Increased tissue pressure.
3) Decreased tissue perfusion.

❑❑ **What are the two basic mechanisms for elevated compartment pressure?**

1) External compression: By burn eschar, circumferential casts, dressings, or pneumatic pressure garments.
2) Volume increase within the compartment: Hemorrhage into the compartment, IV infiltration, or edema secondary to direct injury or post-ischemic reperfussion.

❑❑ **What are the early general signs & symptoms of compartment syndrome?**

Early findings: 1) Tenderness and pain out of proportion to the injury, 2) pain with active and passive motion, and 3) hypesthesia (paresthesia) -- abnormal 2-point discrimination. Late findings: 1) Compartment tense, indurated, and erythematous, 2) slow capillary refill, and 3) pallor and pulselessness.

❑❑ **What intracompartmental pressure raises concern?**

Normal pressure is less than 10 mm Hg. It is generally agreed that > 30 mm Hg mandates emergent fasciotomy. The treatment for compartment pressures between 20 and 30 mm Hg is controversial and may require surgical consultation especially if the patient is unreliable, i.e., with altered level of consciousness.

❑❑ **Define increased intracranial pressure.**

ICP > than 15 mm Hg.

❑❑ **Where is the most common site of a basilar skull fracture?**

Petrous portion of the temporal bone.

❑❑ **Which is the most common artery involved with an epidural hematoma?**

The meningeal artery, specifically the middle.

❑❑ **Where are epidural hematomas located?**

Between the dura and inner table of the skull.

❑❑ **Where are subdural hematomas located?**

Beneath the dura and over the brain and arachnoid. Caused by tears of pial arteries or of bridging veins. Subdurals typically become symptomatic within 24 hours to 2 weeks after injury.

❑❑ **For a trauma victim, which test is most helpful for evaluating retroperitoneal organs?**

A CT.

❑❑ **How should a DPL be performed in a trauma victim with a fractured pelvis?**

Supraumbilical incision to avoid pelvic hematoma.

❑❑ **Absolute contraindication to DPL?**

None. Relative contraindications are clear indication for laparotomy, previous abdominal surgery, and gravid uterus, (use the open technique).

❑❑ **What clues are evident with duodenal injury?**

Increased serum amylase and retroperitoneal free air.

❑❑ **Which organ is the most frequently injured with a blunt trauma?**

Spleen.

❑❑ **What is Kehr's sign?**

Left shoulder pain with splenic rupture.

❑❑ **Which type of injury most commonly damages the pancreas?**

Penetrating.

❑❑ **Inability to pass a nasogastric tube in a trauma victim suggests damage to which organ?**

Diaphragm, usually on the left.

❑❑ **Which type of contrast medium should be used to evaluate the esophagus if traumatic injury is suspected?**

Gastrografin.

❑❑ **Describe the 3 zones of the neck and their evaluation?**

I: Below the cricoid cartilage - Arteriogram.
II: Between the cricoid and the mandible - Surgery. "2 surgery!"
III: Above the angle of the mandible - Arteriogram.

❑❑ **What percent of fractures are detected on lateral, odontoid, AP films of the neck?**

Lateral, (90%), Odontoid, (10%), and AP, (just a few).

❑❑ **On lateral C-spine, how much soft tissue prevertebral swelling is normal from C1-4?**

Up to 4 mm is normal; > 5 mm suggests fracture.

❑❑ **How much anterior subluxation is normal on an adult lateral C-spine?**

3.5 mm.

❑❑ **On lateral C-spine, what does "fanning" of the spinous processes suggest?**

Posterior ligamentous disruption.

❑❑ **What are the three most unstable cervical spine injuries?**

1) Transverse atlantal ligament rupture.
2) Dens fracture.
3) Burst fracture with posterior ligament disruption.

❑❑ **Describe a Jefferson fracture.**

Burst of ring of C1, usually from vertical compression force. Best detected on an odontoid view.

❑❑ **Describe a Hangman's fracture.**

C2 bilateral pedicle fracture. This fracture is usually caused by hyperextension.

❑❑ **What is a clay-shoveler's fracture?**

In order of frequency, C7, C6, or T1 avulsion fracture of the spinous process, flexion, or direct blow.

❑❑ **Describe the key features of spinal shock.**

Sudden areflexia which is transient and distal which lasts hours to weeks. Blood pressure is usually 80 to 100 mm Hg with paradoxical bradycardia.

❑❑ **A trauma patient has blood at the urinary meatus. What test should be ordered?**

A retrograde urethrogram. Ten millileters of radiocontrast solution is injected into the urinary meatus.

❑❑ **Which are the two most commonly injured genitourinary organs?**

Kidney and bladder, associated with pelvic fracture.

❑❑ **Describe the leg position in a patient with a femoral neck fracture.**

Shortened, abducted, and slightly externally rotated.

❑❑ **Describe the leg position in a patient with an anterior dislocation.**

Hip is abducted and externally rotated. Mechanism is forced abduction. If anterior superior, hip is extended. If anterior inferior, hip is flexed.

❑❑ **Describe the leg position in a patient with a posterior hip dislocation.**

Shortened, adducted, and internally rotated. Force is applied to a flexed knee directed posteriorly. Associated with sciatic nerve injury, (10%), and avascular necrosis of the femoral head.

❑❑ **What factors increase the probability of a wound infection?**

Dirty or contaminated wounds, stellate or crushing wounds, wounds longer than 5 cm, wounds older than 6 hours, and infection prone anatomic sites.

❑❑ **Which has greater resistance to infection, sutures or staples?**

Staples.

❑❑ **Which types of wounds result in the majority of tetanus cases?**

Lacerations, punctures, & crush injuries.

❑❑ **What is the risk associated with not treating a septal hematoma of the nose?**

Aseptic necrosis, followed by absorption of the septal cartilage resulting in septal perforation.

❑❑ **Which are the three most common carpal fractures?**

The scaphoid, dorsal chip (triquetrum), and the lunate. All may be 2° falls on an outstretched hand. Radiographs may initially be normal. <u>The scaphoid is the most common</u>.

❑❑ **What is Kienbock's disease?**

Avascular necrosis of the lunate with collapse of the lunate secondary to fracture. As with a navicular (scaphoid) fracture, initial wrist X-rays may not demonstrate the fracture. Therefore, tenderness over the lunate warrants immobilization.

❑❑ **Which tarsal bone is most commonly fractured?**

Calcaneus, (60%). Calcaneal fractures are commonly associated with lumbar compression injuries, (10%).

❑❑ **The second metatarsal is the locking mechanism of the mid-part of the foot. A fracture at the base of the second metatarsal should raise suspicion of what?**

A disrupted joint - treatment may require ORIF.

❑❑ **Which patellar fracture requires orthopedic consultation?**

Displaced transverse fracture, comminuted fractures, and open fractures.

❑❑ **What is the most common mechanism for fractures of the femoral condyles?**

Direct trauma, fall or blow to the distal femur.

❑❑ **Of tibial plateau fractures, where is the most common site?**

Lateral, more common in the older population, usually presenting with swollen painful knee and limited range of motion.

❑❑ **With complete rupture of medial or collateral ligaments, how much laxity is expected on exam?**

> 1 cm without endpoint as compared to uninjured knee.

❑❑ **Which ligamentous injury to the knee is most common?**

Anterior cruciate ligament, usually from non-contact injury.

❑❑ **Why 'tap' a knee with an acute hemarthrosis?**

To relieve pressure and pain and to determine whether fat globules are present indicating a fracture.

❑❑ **How is a 'locked" knee un-locked'?**

Hang leg over table at 90 degree flexion, allow relaxation, and apply a longitudinal traction with internal and external rotation.

❑❑ **Where is the most common site of compartment syndrome?**

Anterior compartment of the leg - contains tibialis anteriorus, extensor digitorum longus, extensor hallucis longus, and peroneus muscles, as well as anterior tibial artery and deep peroneal nerve.

❑❑ **Where is the most common site for a palpable defect of Achilles' tendon?**

2-6 cm proximal to its insertion.

❑❑ What are the most common lower extremity fractures in children?

Tibial and fibular shaft fractures, usually secondary to twist forces.

❑❑ What is a toddler fracture?

Common cause of limp or refusal to walk in this age group is a spiral fracture of the tibia without fibular involvement.

❑❑ What is the most common cause of a painful hip joint in infants?

Septic arthritis. *Staphylococcus* is the most common cause in infancy. The hip usually abducted, flexed, and externally rotated.

❑❑ What is the most common cause of painful hip in older children?

Transient synovitis. It can be difficult to distinguish from septic arthritis.

❑❑ An 8 year old male presents with a limp. On exam, hip range of motion is decreased. What rare disease should be considered?

Children, 5-9 years, may acquire idiopathic avascular necrosis of the femoral heal, i.e., Legg-Calvé-Perthes Disease.

❑❑ Describe a common patient with a slipped capital femoral epiphysis.

Obese boy, age 10 to 16 years. Groin or knee discomfort increases with activity; may have a limp. Often bilateral. The slip is best detected by a lateral view.

❑❑ What is the most important complication of a proximal tibial metaphyseal fracture?

Arterial involvement, especially when there is a valgus deformity.

❑❑ What is unique about avulsion fractures at the base of the fifth metatarsal?

It is one of the most commonly missed fractures. Patient probably has a history is of ankle injury from plantar flexion and inversion.

❑❑ A 21 year old female complains of pain and 'clicking' sound located at the posterior lateral malleolus. You sense a 'fullness' beneath the lateral malleolus. What is the diagnosis?

Peroneal tendon subluxation, with associated tenosynovitis.

❑❑ A patient cannot actively abduct her shoulder. Which injury does this suggest?

Rotator cuff tear. The cuff is comprised of the supraspinatus, infraspinatus, subscapularis, and the teres minor muscles and tendons.

❑❑ Why is the displaced supracondylar fracture (of distal humerus) in a child considered a true emergency?

The injury often results in injury to brachial artery or median nerve. It can also cause compartment syndrome.

❑❑ **What signs and symptoms develop from a compartment syndrome involving the anterior compartment of the leg?**

Pain on active and passive dorsi-flexion, plantar-flexion of the foot, and hypesthesia of the first web space of the foot.

❑❑ **How is a scaphoid fracture diagnosed?**

Frequently, the initial radiograph will appear normal. Therefore, if the patient has tenderness in the anatomical snuff box, a scaphoid (navicular) fracture is presumed and the hand splinted. A follow-up radiograph, 10-14 days following the injury, may then reveal the fracture.

❑❑ **What metatarsal fracture is highly associated with a disrupted tarsal-metatarsal joint.**

Fracture to the base of the 2nd metatarsal. Treatment may require open reduction and internal fixation.

❑❑ **What fracture is frequently missed when the patient complains of an ankle injury?**

Fracture at the base of the fifth metatarsal caused by plantar flexion and inversion. Radiographs of the ankle may not include the fifth metatarsal.

❑❑ **What life-threatening injury is associated with pelvic fractures?**

Severe hemorrhage. It is usually retroperitoneal. Up to 6 L of blood can be accommodated in this space.

❑❑ **Which fracture is associated with avascular necrosis of the femoral head?**

Femoral neck fractures. Avascular necrosis occurs with 15% of non-displaced femoral neck fractures and with near 90% of displaced femoral neck fractures.

❑❑ **A child presents after falling and knocking out his front tooth. How would the management differ if the child was 3 versus 13?**

With primary teeth, no reimplantation should be attempted because of the risk of ankylosis or fusion to the bone. However, with permanent teeth, reimplantation should occur as soon as possible. Remaining periodontal fibers are a key to success. Thus, the tooth should not be wiped dry because this may disrupt the periodontal ligament fibers still attached.

❑❑ **Why shouldn't topical analgesics be used for Ellis Class III tooth fractures?**

Severe tissue irritation or sterile abscesses may occur with their use. Treatment includes application of tinfoil, analgesics and immediate dental referral.

❑❑ **A patient presents 3 days after tooth extraction with severe pain and a foul mouth odor and taste. What is the diagnosis? What is the treatment?**

Alveolar osteitis (dry socket) results from loss of the blood clot and local osteomyelitis. Treat by irrigation of the socket and application of a medicated dental packing or iodoform gauze moistened with Campho-Phenique or eugenol.

❑❑ **A patient presents with gingival pain and a foul mouth odor and taste. On exam, fever and lymphadenopathy are present. The gingiva is bright red and the papillae are**

ulcerated and covered with a gray membrane. What is the diagnosis? What is the treatment?

Acute necrotizing ulcerative gingivitis. Antibiotics, such as tetracycline or penicillin, and topical anesthetic. A possible complication of this disease is the destruction of alveolar bone.

❑❑ **What is the most common oral manifestation of AIDS?**

Oropharyngeal thrush. Some other AIDS-related oropharyngeal diseases are Kaposi's sarcoma, hairy leukoplakia, and non-Hodgkin's lymphoma.

❑❑ **A 47 year old female presents to the ED with a complaint of excruciating waxing and waning "electric shock type" pain in the right cheek. What is the diagnosis? What is the treatment?**

Tic douloureux. The most significant finding is that the pain follows the distribution of the trigeminal nerve. Often minor trigger zone stimulation can consistently reproduce the pain. Administer carbamazepine, 100 mg bid starting dose and increasing to 1200 mg daily if needed. Refer to a neurologist and a dentist to rule out cerebellopontine angle tumors, MS, nasopharyngeal carcinoma, cluster headaches, polymyalgia rheumatica, temporal arteritis, and oral pathology.

❑❑ **A three year old child presents with a unilateral purulent rhinorrhea. What is the probable diagnosis?**

Nasal foreign body.

❑❑ **What potential complications of nasal fractures should always be considered on physical examination?**

Septal hematoma and cribriform plate fractures. A septal hematoma appears as a bluish mass on the nasal septum and, if not drained, aseptic necrosis of the septal cartilage and septal abnormalities may occur. A cribriform plate fracture should be considered in a patient who has a clear rhinorrhea after trauma.

❑❑ **What physical exam findings suggest the diagnosis of posterior epistaxis rather than anterior epistaxis?**

1) Inability to see the site of bleeding. Anterior nosebleeds usually originate at Kiesselbach's plexus, an area easily visualized on the nasal septum.
2) Blood from both sides of the nose. In a posterior nosebleed the blood can more easily pass to the other side because of the proximity of the choanae.
3) Blood trickling down the oropharynx.
4) Inability to control bleeding by direct pressure.

❑❑ **A patient returns to the emergency department with fever, nausea, vomiting and hypotension 2 days after having nasal packing placed for an anterior nosebleed. What potential complication of nasal packing should be considered?**

Toxic shock syndrome.

❑❑ **A child with a sinus infection presents with proptosis, a red swollen eyelid, and a inferiolaterally displaced globe. What is the diagnosis?**

Orbital cellulitis and abscess associated with ethmoid sinusitis.

❑❑ An ill-appearing patient presents with a fever of 103° F, bilateral chemosis, 3rd nerve palsies, and untreated sinusitis. What is the diagnosis?

Cavernous sinus thrombosis. This life-threatening complication occurs from direct extension through the valveless veins. Complication of sinusitis may be local, (osteomyetitis), orbital, (cellulitis), or within the central nervous system, (meningitis or brain abscess).

❑❑ Retropharyngeal abscess is most common in which age group? Why?

Six months to three years. This is because the retropharyngeal lymph nodes regress in size after the age of three.

❑❑ How do patients with retropharyngeal abscesses appear?

These children are often ill appearing, febrile, stridorous, drooling, and in an opisthotonic position Patients may complain of difficulty swallowing or may refuse to feed.

❑❑ What radiographic sign can be used to make the diagnosis of a retropharyngeal abscess?

A widening of the retropharyngeal space that is normal 3-4 mm or less than half the width of the vertebral bodies. False widening may occur if the X-ray is not obtained during inspiration with the patient's neck extended. Occasionally, an air fluid level may be noted in the retropharyngeal space.

❑❑ A 48 year old male presents with a high fever, trismus, dysphagia, and swelling inferior to the mandible in the lateral neck. What is the diagnosis?

Parapharyngeal abscess.

❑❑ Peritonsillar abscesses are <u>most common</u> in which age group?

Adolescents and young adults. Symptoms may include ear pain, trismus, drooling, and alteration of the voice.

❑❑ What is the <u>most common</u> origin of Ludwig's angina?

Lower 2nd and 3rd molar. It is a swelling in the region of the submandibular, sublingual, and submental spaces. This soft tissue swelling may cause displacement of the tongue upward and posteriorly. The most common organisms are hemolytic *Streptococci*, *Staphylococcus*, and mixed anaerobe and aerobes.

❑❑ Why is needle aspiration preferred over incision and drainage for a fluctuant acute cervical lymphadenitis?

Development of a fistula tract is possible if the patient has atypical mycobacterium or cat scratch fever rather than a bacterial lymphadenitis.

❑❑ What are the signs and symptoms of a mandibular fracture?

Malocclusion, pain, opening deviation or abnormal movement, decreased range of motion, bony deformity, swelling, ecchymosis, and lower lip (mental nerve) anesthesia.

❑❑ Bilateral mental fractures may cause what acute complication?

The tongue may cause acute airway obstruction because of loss of anterior support.

❑❑ What are the two most common findings with an orbital floor fracture?

Diplopia and globe lowering.

❑❑ What radiographic finding might be seen with an orbital blowout fracture?

1) Fracture lines or bony fragments in the maxillary sinus.
2) Subcutaneous or orbital emphysema.
3) Air-fluid level in the maxillary sinus.
4) A "teardrop" sign where a soft tissue mass may protrude into the maxillary sinus.

❑❑ Define a Le Fort I fracture.

Fracture line runs from the nasal opening along the wall of the maxillary sinuses bilaterally, across the pterygomaxillary tissue to the lateral pterygoid plates. Also called a horizontal maxillary fracture. X-rays often do not detect this fracture. Mobility of the maxilla without movement at the nasal bridge or zygoma is noted on physical examination.

❑❑ Describe a Le Fort II fracture.

Fracture involves facial aspects of the maxillae extending to the nasal and ethmoid bones. The fracture also involves the maxillary sinuses and infraorbital rims bilaterally and cross the nasal bridge. This is also called a pyramidal fracture. Swelling of the nose, lips and midface may be noted. Subconjunctival hemorrhage may present with blood in the nares. Suspect cerebrospinal involvement and check for CSF rhinorrhea. Diagnosis can be made clinically by crepitation or movement at the nasal bridge when the maxilla is moved.

❑❑ Describe a Le Fort III fracture.

The fracture line runs through the frontozygomatic suture lines bilaterally extending through the orbits, the base of the nose and the ethmoid region. Movement of the zygoma and midface is suggestive. This is also called a "Dishface" fracture or complete craniofacial dysjunction.

❑❑ In which Le Fort fracture is CSF rhinorrhea most common?

III.

❑❑ A 16 year old boxer presents with right ear pain and swelling after receiving a blow to the ear. What is the treatment?

The ear should be aseptically drained by incision or aspiration and a mastoid conforming dressing should be applied. An ENT follow-up is mandatory. If the ear is not treated appropriately, a cauliflower deformity may result.

❑❑ A patient presents with a swollen, tender, red left auricle. What is the diagnosis?

Perichondritis caused by *Pseudomonas.*

❑❑ What would the physical finding be in unilateral sensory hearing loss?

The patient will lateralize, have air conduction greater than bone conduction, i.e., normal Rinne test indicating no conductive loss. The Weber test will lateralize to the normal ear. The most common cause of this is viral neuronitis.

❑❑ **If a patient has bilateral sensory hearing loss, what causes should be suspected?**

Noise or ototoxins such as certain antibiotics, loop diuretics, antineoplastics as well as others.

❑❑ **What is the most common neuropathy associated with acoustic neuroma?**

Due to trigeminal nucleus involvement the corneal reflex may be lost.

❑❑ **Name some causes of tympanic membrane perforation.**

Blast injuries, (water or air), foreign bodies in the ear, (particularly Q-tips), lightning strikes, otitis media, and associated temporal bone fractures.

❑❑ **What is the most common cause of laryngeal trauma?**

Blunt trauma secondary to motor vehicle accidents.

❑❑ **A patient presents with well demarcated swelling of the lips and tongue. She had been started on an antihypertensive agent three weeks ago. Which agent is most likely?**

Angiotensin converting enzyme inhibitor. Although, angioneurotic edema may occur anytime during therapy with an ACE inhibitor it is most likely in the first month of treatment.

❑❑ **A lower airway foreign body is suspected. What will plain films show?**

Plain films may show air trapping on the affected side. Inspiration and expiration views demonstrate mediastinal shift away from the affected side.

❑❑ **Which two conditions are true ophthalmologic emergencies?**

Chemical burns requiring immediate irrigation and central retinal artery occlusion requiring re-establishment of blood flow within 90 minutes.

❑❑ **How is a Schiotz tonometer interpreted?**

Low scale readings suggest high pressure and high scale readings suggest low pressure. With a 5.5 g weight a scale of 4 or greater is equal to 20 mm Hg or less (normal).

❑❑ **A patient presents with the sensation of a foreign body in the eye. Slit-lamp reveals a dendritic figure which has a Christmas tree pattern. What is the treatment?**

Antiviral agents and cycloplegics are used to treat herpes simplex keratitis. Steroids spell disaster.

❑❑ **A patient presents with sudden vision loss in one eye which returns quickly. What is the diagnosis?**

Amaurosis fugax. This condition usually is caused by central retinal artery emboli from extracranial atherosclerosis.

❑❑ When and where do retinal detachments occur after a blunt traumatic injury?

Frequently there is a delay between the incident and detachment. Half occur in the first eight months. Two years following the accident 80% will be noted. The detachment most commonly occurs in the inferotemporal quadrant.

❑❑ A patient was hit in the eye during a fight last night while intoxicated. He presents eight hours after the incident with proptosis and visual loss? The examination reveals an intact globe and an afferent pupillary defect. What is the problem?

Retro orbital hematoma with ischemia of the optic nerve or retina. The pressure of the blood in the orbit exceeds the profusion pressure causing lack of blood flow and loss of function. Treatment is to release the pressure by lateral canthotomy. A similar situation can occur with orbital emphysema.

❑❑ What are complications of a hyphema?

The 4 S's -

1) Secondary rebleeds which usually occur between the second and fifth day post injury since t his is the time of clot retraction. Rebleeds tend to be worse than the initial bleed.
2) Significantly increased intraocular pressure which can lead to acute glaucoma, chronic late glaucoma, and optic atrophy.
3) Staining of the cornea due to hemosiderin deposits.
4) Synechiae which interfere with iris function.

❑❑ Why do patients with sickle cell anemia and a hyphema require special consideration when presenting with ophthalmologic concerns?

Increased intraocular pressure can occur if the cells sickle in the trabecular network prevent aqueous humor from leaving the anterior chamber. Medication, such as hyperosmotics and Diamox, which increase the likelihood of sickling must be avoided

❑❑ What are causes of a subluxed or dislocated lens?

Trauma, Marfan's syndrome, homocystinuria, and Weill-Marchesani syndrome.

❑❑ Which is worse, acid or alkali burns of the cornea?

Alkali because of deeper penetration than acid burns. A barrier is formed from precipitated proteins with acid burns. The exception is hydrofluoric acid and heavy metal containing acids which can penetrate the cornea.

❑❑ When shouldn't an eye be dilated?

With known narrow angle glaucoma and with an iris-supported intraocular lens.

❑❑ Three hours ago, a patient experienced sudden, painless visual loss in her right eye. Central retinal artery occlusion is suspected. What would be the expected finding on eye examination? What is the prognosis?

Afferent pupillary defect, pale gray retina and a small pink dot near the fovea. This cherry red spot is the choroidal vaculature being seen at the macular where the retina is the thinnest. After two hours the prognosis is extremely poor for visual recovery. Digital massage or anterior chamber paracentesis may dislodge the clot.

❑❑ What conditions have been associated with central retinal vein occlusion?

Hyperviscosity syndromes, diabetes, and hypertension. Funduscopic exam shows a chaotically streaked retina with congested dilated veins. There are superficial and deep retinal hemorrhages, cotton wool spots, and macular edema.

❑❑ A patient presents with atraumatic pain behind the left eye, a left pupil afferent defect, central visual loss, and a left swollen disc? What are the diagnosis and potential causes?

Optic neuritis. This may be idiopathic or may be associated with multiple sclerosis, Lyme's disease, neurosyphilis, lupus, sarcoid, alcoholism, toxins, or drug abuse.

❑❑ After entering a dark bar a patient developed eye pain, nausea, vomiting, blurred vision and sees "halos" around lights. Why would this patient be given mannitol, pilocarpine, and acetazolamide?

This patient has acute narrow angle glaucoma. The goal of treatment is to decrease intraocular pressure. This can be done by:

1) decreasing the production of aqueous (carbonic anhydrase inhibitor),
2) decreasing the intraocular volume by making the plasma hypertonic to the aqueous humor (as with glycerol or mannitol) and to
3) constrict the pupil (as with pilocereine) allowing increased flow of the aqueous out through the previously blocked canals of Schlemm.

❑❑ A patient felt something fly into his eye while mowing the lawn. On examination, there is a brown foreign body on the cornea and a tear drop iris pointing towards the foreign body. What is the diagnosis?

Perforated cornea with extruded iris. A similar foreign body may appear black on the sclera with scleral perforation.

❑❑ A patient presents with the sensation of painless loss of vision in one eye described as a wall slowly developing in the visual field. What findings are expected on exam?

Gray detached retina. Patient may also complain of flashing lights in the peripheral visual field or "spider webs" in the visual field. Inferior detachment is treated with the patient sitting up. Superior detachment is treated with the patient lying flat.

❑❑ What is the risk of placing a patient with COPD on a high FiO_2?

Suppression of the hypoxic ventilatory drive.

❑❑ Which therapies for asthma should be avoided in the pregnant patient?

Parenteral ß-adrenergic agonists and epinephrine.

❑❑ If a patient has a patchy infiltrate on a chest X-ray and bullous myringitis, which antibiotic should be given?

Erythromycin for Mycoplasma.

❑❑ **An older patient with GI symptoms, hyponatremia, and a relative bradycardia most likely has what type of pneumonia?**

Legionella.

❑❑ **What is the treatment for Legionella pneumonia?**

IV erythromycin.

❑❑ **Describe the classic chest X-ray findings in Legionella pneumonia.**

Dense consolidation and bulging fissures. Expect elevated liver enzymes and hypophosphatemia.

❑❑ **What are the classic signs and symptoms of TB?**

Night sweats, fever, weight loss, malaise, cough, and a green/yellow sputum most commonly seen in the mornings.

❑❑ **Where are some common extrapulmonary TB sites?**

Lymph node, bone, GI tract, GU tract, meninges, liver, and the pericardium.

❑❑ **Right upper lobe cavitation with parenchymal involvement is classic for:**

TB. Lower lung infiltrates, hilar adenopathy, atelectasis, and pleural effusion are also common.

❑❑ **What accessory X-rays may be obtained to diagnose a pneumothorax?**

1) Expiratory film.
2) Lateral decubitus film on the affected side.

❑❑ **Which kind of pneumonias are commonly associated with a pneumothorax?**

Staphylococcus, TB, Klebsiella, and PCP.

❑❑ **Which diagnostic test is helpful in sub-clinical PCP infection?**

Exertional pulse oximetry is positive for PCP if after 3 minutes of exercise the 02 saturation decreases by 3% or the A-a gradient increases by 10 mm Hg from rest.

❑❑ **Which laboratory tests aid in the diagnosis of PCP?**

A rising LDH or LDH > 450 and an ESR > 50. A low albumin implies a worse prognosis.

❑❑ **The initial therapy for PCP includes which antibiotics?**

TMP-SMZ or pentamidine.

❑❑ **When are corticosteroids recommended for severe PCP?**

pO_2 < 70 mm Hg or an A-a gradient > 35 mm Hg.

❑❑ **List two drugs that can cause ARDS.**

Heroin and aspirin.

❑❑ **How is the A-a gradient calculated for a patient breathing room air?**

A - a = 150 - Pa_{O2} - (Pa_{CO2} x 1.25) or 4 + age/4 or 140 - (Pa_{O2} + Pa_{CO2}) Normal ≅ 2-10.

❑❑ **After a week, an ill-appearing patient says her sore throat worsened and she complains of spiking fevers and central chest burning. What is the concern?**

Retro- or parapharyngeal abscess with extension to superior mediastinitis.

❑❑ **A child presents with odynophagia and drooling. What is expected on examination of the oropharynx?**

Trouble, if you look with a tongue blade! A patient with suspected epiglottitis is at high risk for upper airway compromise; therefore, intubation with direct visualization, typically in the OR, is best. This dogma may be evolving secondary to a decrease in H influenza.

❑❑ **A patient says food gets stuck in his mid-chest, then is regurgitated as a putrid, undigested mess. A barium study shows a dilated esophagus with a distal "beak." What is the diagnosis?**

Achalasia.

❑❑ **A woman with telangiectasias, "tight knuckles," and "acid indigestion" might have what findings on an upper GI series?**

Aperistalsis, characteristic of scleroderma.

❑❑ **A patient with an "acid stomach" develops melena and vomits bright red blood. Is esophagitis a probable cause?**

No. Capillary bleeding rarely causes impressive acute blood loss. Arterial bleeding, from a complicated ulcer, foreign body, or Mallory-Weiss tear, or variceal bleeding are much more likely.

❑❑ **A cirrhotic patient vomits bright red blood. He has a systolic blood pressure of 90 mm Hg. After an aggressive fluid resuscitation, 4 units of PRBC, and gastric lavage, his pressure is 90 mm Hg. What's next?**

Assume a coagulopathy and transfuse fresh frozen plasma, start a vasopressin drip, and arrange for an emergent endoscopic intervention for sclerotherapy or banding.

❑❑ **Repeated, violent bouts of vomiting can result in both Mallory-Weiss tears and Boerhaave's syndrome. Differentiate the two.**

Mallory-Weiss tears involve the submucosa and mucosa, typically in the right posterolateral wall of the GE junction. Boerhaave's is a full-thickness tear, usually in the unsupported left posterolateral wall of the abdominal esophagus.

❑❑ **After a high-speed MVA, an unrestrained driver develops abdominal and chest pain radiating to the neck. An upper chest film shows left pleural fluid. What**

gastroesophageal catastrophe might have occurred?

Impact against a steering wheel can result in Boerhaave's syndrome with esophageal perforation and mediastinitis.

❑❑ **You suspect a perforated esophagus. Which test should be ordered next?**

A water-soluble contrast study. In the mean time, start broad-spectrum antibiotics and call the surgeons ASAP.

❑❑ **Pediatric foreign bodies lodge at which esophageal levels?**

Typically at levels of the cricopharyngeus muscles (most usual), thoracic inlet, aortic arch, tracheal bifurcation, and lower esophageal sphincter.

❑❑ **When is removing a button battery lodged in the esophagus indicated?**

Always. If this corrosive foreign body was swallowed less than 2 hours ago and endoscopy is not available, consider attempting Foley balloon removal. More wisely, find a scope Doc for immediate endoscopic removal.

❑❑ **X-rays are crucial in the search for a suspected swallowed foreign body. In kids, what physical findings can tip you off?**

Besides a child's distress, you may also find a red or scratched oropharynx, dysphagia, a high fever, or peritoneal signs. Subcutaneous air suggests perforation.

❑❑ **An obstructing meat bolus should be removed within 12 hours. What's the best approach?**

Endoscopy, through a trial of IV glucagon given as 1 mg push after a small test dose, then repeated as a 2 mg dose at 20 minutes if there is no relief, or sublingual nifedipine, 10 mg, may work. Both relax esophageal smooth muscle. Meat tenderizer is best avoided, since perforation has occurred.

❑❑ **After fluid and blood resuscitation for a bleeding ulcer, what is the most useful diagnostic test?**

Endoscopy, which can also be therapeutic, with cryo- or electrocautery of an arterial bleeder.

❑❑ **Are "stress ulcers" a surgical problem?**

Not usually. The diffuse gastric bleeding that results from CNS tumors, head trauma, burns, sepsis, shock, steroids, aspirin, or alcohol is usually mucosal, can be life-threatening, and can most often be managed medically. Endoscopic diagnosis is key.

❑❑ **Burning epigastric pain shooting to the back, hypovolemic shock, and a high amylase suggests . . .?**

Posterior perforation of a duodenal ulcer.

❑❑ **Who gets acalculous cholecystitis?**

Dehydrated post-op, post-trauma, and burn patients, as well as those with transfusion related hemolysis or narcotic use (illicit or prescribed).

❑❑ **What is the most common cause of lower GI perforation?**

Diverticulitis, followed by tumor, colitis, foreign bodies, and instrumentation.

❑❑ **A pregnant woman with right upper quadrant pain should be assumed to have what intraabdominal pathology until proven otherwise?**

Acute appendicitis.

❑❑ **What does ultrasound show in an acute appendicitis?**

A fixed, tender, non-compressible mass, but only in 75 to 90% of cases.

❑❑ **What is the most common cause of small bowel obstruction?**

Adhesions are the most common causes of extraluminal obstruction, followed by incarcerated hernia, while gallstones and bezoars are the most common causes of intraluminal obstruction.

❑❑ **Recurrent small bowel obstruction in an elderly woman associated with unilateral pain into one thigh suggests what occult process?**

Obturator hernia incarceration. May often present with pain down medial thigh to knee.

❑❑ **What are the most common causes of colonic obstruction?**

Cancer, then diverticulitis followed by volvulus.

❑❑ **A KUB is suspicious for a large bowel obstruction. What are the next step(s) in evaluation?**

Unprepped sigmoidoscopy to confirm obstruction, then a barium study to determine the cause. If you suspect pseudo-obstruction (typically due to medications), don't order a barium study for fear of concretion and obstruction. Colonoscopy can be diagnostic and therapeutic.

❑❑ **A patient tells you that 2 days ago his groin bulged and he developed severe pain with progressive nausea and vomiting. He has a tender mass in his groin. What shouldn't you do?**

Don't try to reduce a long-standing, tender incarcerated hernia! The abdomen is no place for dead bowel.

❑❑ **How does the pathology of Crohn's disease differ from that of ulcerative colitis?**

Crohn's is a trans-mucosal, segmental, granulomatous process, while ulcerative colitis is a mucosal, juxtapositional, ulcerative process.

❑❑ **A young man with atraumatic chronic back pain, eye trouble, and painful red lumps on his shins develops bloody diarrhea. What is the point of this question?**

To remind you of extraintestinal manifestations of inflammatory bowel disease, such as ankylosing spondylitis, uveitis, and erythema nodosum, not to mention kidney stones.

❑❑ **At least a third of patients with Crohn's disease have kidney stones. Why?**

Dietary oxalate is usually bound to calcium and excreted. When terminal ileal disease leads to decreased bile salt absorption, the resulting fattier intestinal contents bind calcium by saponification. Free oxalate is "hyper-absorbed" in the colon, resulting in hyperoxaluria and calcium oxalate nephrolithiasis.

❑❑ **A patient with chronic, occasionally bloody diarrhea develops severe diarrhea and abdominal pain with marked distention. What "can't-miss" diagnosis does this suggest?**

Toxic megacolon, a life-threatening complication of ulcerative colitis.

❑❑ **A patient with new diarrhea and abdominal pain tells you she took antibiotics for sinusitis two weeks ago. Sigmoidoscopy might reveal what?**

Yellowish superficial plaques suggestive of pseudomembranous colitis. Stool studies would show *C. difficile* toxin.

❑❑ **What's the treatment?**

Oral vancomycin, 125 mg qid or oral metronidazole, 500 mg qid. Either regimen should be given for 7 to 10 days. Cholestyramine, which binds the toxin, can help limit the diarrhea. Follow-up stool studies should confirm clearance of the toxin.

❑❑ **What barium findings distinguish colonic obstruction due to acute diverticulitis from that due to colon cancer?**

Diverticulitis is extraluminal, so the mucosa appears intact and involved bowel segments are longer. Adenocarcinoma distorts the mucosa, involves a short segment of bowel, and has overhanging edges.

❑❑ **Which is more sensitive for locating the source of GI bleeding, a radioactive Tc-labeled red cell scan, or angiography?**

A bleeding scan can find a site bleeding at a rate as low as 0.12 mL/minute, while angiography requires rapid bleeding greater than 0.5 mL/minute.

❑❑ **A post-surgical patient develops right upper quadrant pain, nausea, and low-grade fevers. According to his surgeon, the gallbladder was normal intraoperatively. What's a probable diagnosis?**

Acalculous cholecystitis.

❑❑ **Eight years after her cholecystectomy, a woman develops right upper quadrant pain and jaundice. What's the chance of developing recurrent biliary tract stones after cholecystectomy?**

At least 10%, due either to retained stones or *in-situ* formation by biliary epithelium.

❑❑ **List the ultrasound findings suggestive of acute cholecystitis.**

Presence of gall stones (or sludge, in acalculous cholecystitis), ultrasonographic Murphy's sign, gall bladder wall thickening > 5 mm, and pericholecystic fluid. A dilated common bile duct (> 10 mm) suggests common duct obstruction.

❑❑ **Name two findings in acute cholecystitis that mandate emergent laparotomy.**

Emphysematous cholecystitis and perforation. Otherwise, timing of surgery is somewhat institution- and surgeon-dependent.

❑❑ **A high fever and leukocytosis accompanying acute alcoholic hepatitis is worrisome. Why?**

Alcohol is marrow toxic, so leukocytosis often reflects serious associated infection. Obtain a chest X-ray, obtain blood cultures, a urinalysis, and an ascitic fluid for cell count and culture.

❑❑ **What is the best diuretic of choice for most cirrhotics with ascites?**

Potassium-sparing agents. Treat the hyperaldosterone state specifically.

❑❑ **A confused cirrhotic presents to the ED. She is afebrile and has asterixis. What should your exam consist of as you look for the precipitant of hepatic encephalopathy?**

Administer thiamine and folate. Assess her mental status and search for localizing neurologic signs, such as an occult head injury; exam for dry mucous membranes and a low jugular venous pressure, including hypovolemia and azotemia; and check a stool Guaiac to determine GI bleeding. Focused lab testing can pinpoint other causes, such as diuretic overuse and hypokalemia, hypoglycemia, anemia, hypoxia, and infection.

❑❑ **An ascitic patient presents with fever but no localizing signs or symptoms of infection, and a normal WBC. Because you know that spontaneous bacterial peritonitis can be an occult disease, you perform an abdominal paracentesis. What WBC in ascitic fluid suggests SBP?**

Greater than $250/mm^3$. You should also Gram stain the fluid and send at least 10 cc in blood culture bottles for aerobic and anaerobic culture.

❑❑ **Which two therapies can reduce the risk of recurrent SBP?**

Diuretics decrease ascitic fluid and nonabsorbable oral antibiotics decrease the gut bacterial load, limiting bacterial translocation. Both treatments have cut the risk of recurrence in compliant patients.

❑❑ **Which is a more sensitive test for pancreatitis, serum amylase or lipase?**

Amylase elevation is 70-90% sensitive for pancreatitis; lipase is 75-100% sensitive; the combination is up to 95-97% sensitive. Remember that up to 10% of patients with severe acute pancreatitis may have a normal amylase. In chronic pancreatitis, up to 30% may have a normal amylase.

❑❑ **What are Ranson's five predictors of complications from acute pancreatitis <u>upon admission</u>?**

Age over 55, blood glucose > 200 mg/dL, WBC > $16,000/mm^3$, SGOT (AST) > 250 U/L, and LDH > 350 IU/L.

❑❑ **<u>Symptoms</u> that last longer than a week or the presence of an abdominal mass, hyperamylasemia, and leukocytosis suggest what potentially disastrous complications of pancreatitis?**

Pancreatic abscess or pseudocyst.

❑❑ Distinguish, by location, the following: anal cryptitis, anal fissure, anorectal abscess, and fistula in ano.

Cryptitis, fissures and perianal abscess typically occur in the posterior midline; deep abscesses can point to areas far from the anus. Goodsall's rule on fistulas: those that open anteriorly go straight to the anal canal, while those that open posteriorly may follow a circuitous route.

❑❑ T/F: Antibiotics are unnecessary after an uncomplicated perirectal abscess is incised and drained.

True, assuming the patient has no underlying immunoincompetence, such as HIV, diabetes, malignancy. Sitz baths beginning the next day are the primary after-care.

❑❑ Procidentia in adults mandates what intervention?

Rectal prolapse can be manually reduced in children with good results. Adults typically require proctosigmoidoscopy and surgical repair.

❑❑ The most common causes of dysphagia in the elderly population include what?

Hiatal hernia, reflux esophagitis, webs/rings, and cancer.

❑❑ Radiographs should be performed in all patients suspected of swallowing coins to determine the presence and location of the FB. How will the coin appear on the X-ray in the AP view?

Coins in the esophagus lie in the frontal plane. Coins in the trachea lie in the sagittal plane.

❑❑ What is the management of button batteries that have passed the esophagus?

In the asymptomatic patient - repeat radiographs. The symptomatic patient and those patients where the battery has not passed the pylorus after 48 hours require endoscopic retrieval.

❑❑ What medical conditions are associated with an increase incidence of PUD?

COPD, cirrhosis, and chronic renal failure.

❑❑ Where is the most common location of a perforated peptic ulcer?

Anterior surface of the duodenum or pylorus and the lesser curvature of the stomach.

❑❑ Which types of patients are at risk for gallbladder perforation?

Elderly, diabetics, and those with recurrent cholecystitis.

❑❑ What percentage of patients with a perforated viscus have radiographic evidence of a pneumoperitoneum?

60-70%. Therefore, one-third of patients will not have this sign. Keep the patient in either the upright or left lateral decubitus position for at least 10 minutes prior to performing X-rays.

❑❑ **What are the indications for the surgical removal of a GI foreign body?**

GI obstruction, GI perforation, toxic properties of the material, and length, size and shape that will prevent the object from passing safely.

❑❑ **What size objects rarely pass the stomach?**

Objects longer than 5 cm and wider than 2 cm.

❑❑ **Are gastric and duodenal perforations more common in malignant or benign ulcers?**

Benign ulcerations.

❑❑ **What are the most common causes of non-traumatic perforations of the lower GI tract?**

Diverticulitis, carcinoma, colitis, foreign bodies, barium enemas, and endoscopy.

❑❑ **The hallmark of a perforated viscus is . . .?**

Abdominal pain.

❑❑ **Which is one of the earliest signs of sepsis?**

Respiratory alkalosis on an ABG.

❑❑ **What conditions are associated with an atypical presentation of acute appendicitis?**

Situs inversus viscerum, malrotation, hypermobile cecum, long pelvic appendix, and pregnancy, (1/2200).

❑❑ **What are the most frequent symptoms of acute appendicitis?**

Anorexia and pain. Anorexia and periumbilical pain with progression to constant RLQ pain is present in only 60% of cases.

❑❑ **What percentage of acute appendicitis cases have an elevated WBC count?**

An elevated leukocyte count and an elevated absolute neutrophil count are present in 86% and 89% respectively.

❑❑ **What are the causes of factitious hyponatremia?**

Hyperglycemia, hyperlipidemia, or hyperproteinemia.

❑❑ **How does hyperglycemia lead to hyponatremia?**

Because glucose stays in the extracellular fluid, hyperglycemia draws water out of the cell into the extracellular fluid. Each 100 mg/dL increase in plasma glucose decreases the serum sodium by 1.6 to 1.8 mEq/L.

❑❑ **What are the ECG findings in a patient with hypokalemia?**

Flattened T-waves, depressed ST segments, prominent P and U waves, and prolonged QT and PR intervals.

❑❑ **What is the first ECG finding in a patient with hyperkalemia?**

At levels of 5.6 to 6.0 mEq/L, the development of tall, peaked T waves, best seen in the precordial leads, occur first.

❑❑ **What is the quickest way to treat hyperkalemia?**

Give calcium gluconate (10%), 10-20 mL IV with an onset of action of 1-3 minutes.

❑❑ **What are the causes of hyperkalemia?**

Acidosis, tissue necrosis, hemolysis, blood transfusions, GI bleed, renal failure, Addison's disease, primary hypoaldosteronism, excess po K+ intake, RTA IV, medication (succinylcholine, b-blockers, captopril, spironolactone, triamterene, amiloride, and high dose penicillin).

❑❑ **What are the causes of hypocalcemia?**

Shock, sepsis, multiple blood transfusions, hypoparathyroidism, vitamin D deficiency, pancreatitis, hypomagnesemia, alkalosis, fat embolism syndrome, phosphate overload, chronic renal failure, loop diuretics, hypoalbuminemia, tumor lysis syndrome, and medication (Dilantin, phenobarbital, heparin, theophylline, cimetidine, and gentamicin).

❑❑ **What are the most common causes of hypercalcemia?**

1) Malignancy.
2) Primary hyperparathyroidism.
3) Thiazide diuretics.

❑❑ **What are the signs and symptoms of hypercalcemia?**

A classic mnemonic can be used to remember these:

Stones	renal calculi
Bones	osteolysis
Abdominal groans	peptic ulcer disease and pancreatitis
Psychic overtones	psychiatric disorders

The most common gastrointestinal symptoms are anorexia and constipation.

❑❑ **What is the initial treatment for hypercalcemia?**

Patients with hypercalcemia are dehydrated because high calcium levels interfere with ADH and the ability of the kidney to concentrate urine. Therefore, the initial treatment is restoration of the extracellular fluid with 5 to 10 L of normal saline in 24 hours. Once the patient is rehydrated, give furosemide in doses of 1 to 3 mg/kg.

❑❑ **What are the two primary causes of primary adrenal insufficiency?**

Tuberculosis and autoimmune destruction account for 90% of cases.

❑❑ **What are the signs and symptoms of primary adrenal insufficiency?**

Fatigue, weakness, weight loss, anorexia, hyperpigmentation, nausea, vomiting, abdominal pain, diarrhea, and orthostatic hypotension.

❑❑ **What are the characteristic lab findings associated with primary adrenal insufficiency?**

Hyperkalemia, hyponatremia, hypoglycemia, azotemia, (if volume depletion is present), and a mild metabolic acidosis.

❑❑ **How should acute adrenal insufficiency be treated?**

Hydrocortisone, 100 mg IV, and crystalloid fluids containing dextrose.

❑❑ **What are the main causes of death during an adrenal crisis?**

Circulatory collapse and hyperkalemia-induced arrhythmias.

❑❑ **What are the causes of acute adrenal crisis?**

It occurs secondary to a major stress such as surgery, severe injury, myocardial infarction, or any other illness in a patient with primary or secondary adrenal insufficiency.

❑❑ **What is thyrotoxicosis and what are the causes?**

A hypermetabolic state that occurs secondary to excess circulating thyroid hormone caused by thyroid hormone overdose, thyroid hyperfunction, or thyroid inflammation.

❑❑ **What are the hallmark clinical features of myxedema coma?**

Hypothermia, (75%), and coma.

❑❑ **What is the role of phosphate replacement during the treatment of DKA?**

Phosphate supplementation is not indicated until a serum concentration is below 1.0 mEq/dL.

❑❑ **What is the most important initial step in the treatment of DKA?**

Rapid fluid administration with the first liter given over 30 minutes to 1 hour followed by 3 to 5 L over the next 3 hours.

❑❑ **Why would the nitroprusside test be negative in a patient with alcoholic ketoacidosis?**

This test is used to detect the presence of ketones in the urine and serum. It does not detect ß-hydroxybutyrate , which may be the predominant ketone in a patient with alcoholic ketoacidosis.

❑❑ **In the first two years of life, what is the most common cause of <u>drug-induced</u> hypoglycemia?**

Salicylates. In the 2-8 year old group, alcohol is the most likely cause, and in the 11 to 30 year old group, insulin and sulfonylureas are the most probable culprits.

❑❑ **How is sulfonylurea-induced hypoglycemia treated?**

IV glucose alone may be insufficient. It may require diazoxide, 300 mg slow IV over 30 minutes repeated every four hours.

❑❑ What is the most common cause of hypoglycemia in a child?

Ketotic hypoglycemia. Attacks usually occur when the child is stressed with caloric deprivation. It is most common in boys typically between 18 months and 5 years of age. Attacks may be episodic, vomiting may occur, and are more frequent in the morning or during periods of illness.

❑❑ What are the neurologic signs and symptoms of hypoglycemia?

Hypoglycemia may produce mental and neurologic dysfunction. Neurologic manifestations may include paresthesias, cranial nerve palsies, transient hemiplegia, diplopia, decerebrate posturing, and clonus.

❑❑ What lab findings are expected with diabetic ketoacidosis?

Elevated ß-hydroxybutyrate, acetoacetate, acetone, and glucose. Ketonuria and glucosuria are present. Serum bicarbonate level, pCO_2, and pH are decreased. Potassium may be initially elevated but falls if the acidosis is corrected.

❑❑ What is the treatment for DKA?

1) Fluids, approximately 5-10 L of normal saline alternating with 1/2 normal saline.
2) Potassium, 100-200 mEq in the first 12-24 hours.
3) Insulin, 20 unit bolus, followed by 0.1 U/kg/hour.
4) Add glucose to the IV fluid when glucose levels fall below 250 mg/dL.
5) Phosphate supplement when level drops below 1.0 mg/dL.
6) For peds, NS, 20 mL/kg/hour for 1-2 hours, and insulin, 0.1 U/kg bolus, followed by 0.1 U/kg/hour drip.

❑❑ What are the key features of nonketotic hyperosmolar coma?

Hyperosmolality, hyperglycemia, and dehydration. Blood sugar should be greater than 800 mg/dL, serum osmolality should be greater than 350 mOsm/kg, and serum ketones should be negative.

❑❑ What is the treatment for nonketotic hyperosmolar coma?

Fluids (normal saline), potassium, 10-20 mEq/hour, insulin, 5-10 U/hour, and glucose should be added to the IV when the blood sugar drops below 250 mg/dL.

❑❑ What are the pathognomonic findings as well as confirmatory lab tests diagnostic of thyroid storm?

Trick question. Thyroid storm is based on clinical impression. There are no findings or confirmatory tests available.

❑❑ What is the most common precipitant of thyroid storm?

Infections, typically pulmonary infections, are the most common precipitating event.

❑❑ What clinical clues might help in the diagnosis of thyroid storm?

Eye signs of Graves' disease, a history of hyperthyroidism, widened pulse pressure, and a palpable goiter.

❑❑ **What are the signs and symptoms of thyroid storm?**

Tachycardia, fever, diaphoresis, increased CNS activity, emotional lability, heart failure, coma, and death.

❑❑ **What are the diagnostic criteria for thyroid storm?**

Tachycardia, CNS dysfunction, cardiovascular dysfunction, GI system dysfunction, and a temperature greater than 37.8° C (100° F).

❑❑ **What are the complications of bicarbonate therapy in DKA?**

Paradoxical CSF acidosis, hypokalemia, cardiac arrhythmias, decreased oxygen delivery to tissue, and fluid and sodium overload.

❑❑ **What is the <u>most</u> <u>common</u> cause of hypothyroidism?**

Primary thyroid failure. The most common etiology of hypothyroidism in adults is the use of radioactive iodine or subtotal thyroidectomy in the treatment of Graves' disease. The second most common cause is autoimmune thyroid disorders.

❑❑ **In a patient receiving anticoagulation therapy with heparin, when is adrenal hemorrhage most likely to strike?**

Typically between the 3rd and 18th day of anticoagulation. Patients present with sudden hypotension and flank or epigastric pain. Nausea, vomiting, fever, and a change in sensorium may be associated.

❑❑ **What is the most common cause of secondary adrenal insufficiency and adrenal crisis?**

Iatrogenic adrenal suppression from prolonged steroid use. Rapid withdrawal of steroids may lead to collapse and death.

❑❑ **How is the anion gap calculated from electrolyte values?**

Anion gap = Na - Cl - CO_2 The normal gap is 12 $^+/-$ 4 mEq/L.

❑❑ **What are the two primary causes of metabolic alkalosis?**

1) Loss of hydrogen and chloride from the stomach.
2) Overzealous diuresis with loss of hydrogen, potassium and chloride.

❑❑ **What is central pontine myelinolysis, a.k.a., osmotic demyelination syndrome?**

The complication of brain dehydration following too rapid correction of severe hyponatremia. Correct hyponatremia slowly, less than 12 mEq/day in chronic hyponatremia.

❑❑ **Tetralogy of Fallot (TOF) consists of VSD, an "overriding" aorta, pulmonary stenosis and right ventricular hypertrophy. Which type of intracardiac shunting occurs?**

Right-to-left shunting whose severity is related to the degree of pulmonary stenosis.

❑❑ Describe the murmurs of TOF.

1) Holosystolic of VSD - 3rd ICS @ LSB.
2) Crescendo-decrescendo murmur of pulmonary stenosis - 2nd ICS @ LSB.

❑❑ What common physical diagnostic sign can be detected in a childhood atrial septal defect?

A fixed split of S-2 on deep inspiration.

❑❑ What do X-ray findings often reveal in coarctation of the aorta?

The "3" sign made up of the aortic knob and the dilated post coarctation segment of the descending aorta. The "E" sign is the same thing seen in a negative image on barium esophagram.

❑❑ Verapamil should not be used to treat infants of less than what age?

Do not use verapamil in infants less than two years of age. It can lead to asystole.

❑❑ If cardioversion is necessary to treat an infant with unstable SVT, what is the appropriate energy to use?

0.25-1 J/kg.

❑❑ What is the most common cause of neonatal stridor?

Laryngotracheomalacia.

❑❑ Can the type of stridor localize the level of the obstruction?

Yes, Inspiratory stridor points to a site of obstruction above the vocal folds while expiratory stridor points to obstruction below the vocal folds.

❑❑ Define apnea.

No respiration for > 20 s.

❑❑ A neonate presents with a history of poor feeding, vomiting, and respiratory distress. He also has abdominal distention and is found to have hyperbilirubinemia. What is the probable cause of this complex?

This neonate is septic!

❑❑ Jaundice due to breast feeding occurs after 7 days and can reach very high levels over weeks; how high?

Levels of bilirubin near 25 mg/dL can be reached.

❑❑ Which type of jaundice causes some of the highest levels of bilirubin elevation?

A-O incompatibility.

❑❑ **A septic pediatric patient is in shock. An initial bolus of normal saline at 20 mL/kg has been given. What urine output should be maintained by delivery of appropriate fluid?**

1-2 mL/kg/hour.

❑❑ **Why is albuterol the usual agent of choice?**

Of nebulized ß-adrenergic agonists, it has the longest duration of action and the greatest degree of $ß_2$-adrenergic selectivity.

❑❑ **If mechanical ventilation is required for such a patient, what is an appropriate setting for initial tidal volume?**

10 mL/kg.

❑❑ **Neonatal seizures have a broad range of presentations. What are the two frequent causes of myoclonic seizures?**

Metabolic disorders and hypoxia.

❑❑ **The spectrum of likely etiology of a pneumonia changes with patient age. Which are probable pneumonia-causing agents in neonates?**

Bacterial -

Group B *Streptococci* (Lancefield Group B, mostly *S. agalactiae*).
Listeria monocytogenes.
Enteric Gram negative bacilli.
Chlamydia.

Viral:

Rubella, CMV, Herpes

❑❑ **SIDS is the <u>most common</u> cause of death of infants between 1 month and 1 year of age. The incidence is 2 per 1000 = 10,000/year. What are the four risk factors that increase an infant's risk of SIDS?**

1) Prematurity with low birth weight.
2) Previous episode of apnea or apparent life threatening event (ALTE).
3) Mother is a substance abuser.
4) Sibling of infant who died of SIDS.

❑❑ **Among pediatric emergency patients, what is the <u>most common</u> skin infection?**

Nonbullous Impetigo caused by Group A, b-*hemolytic Streptococcus*. Impetigo is a bacterial infection of the dermis, most commonly caused by group A ß-*hemolytic Streptococcus*. It comes in two flavors - impetigo contagiosa and the bullous form.

❑❑ **"Strawberry tongue" is a physical finding associated with what systemic bacterial infection also caused primarily by Group A, *ß-hemolytic Streptococci*?**

Scarlet fever. Also seek characteristic Pastia's lines found in the antecubital area.
Recall the scarlet rash that spares the perioral area usually has onset 1-2 days after high fever, sore throat, headache and occasional vomiting and abdominal pain. Mucocutaneous lymph node syndrome (Kawasaki disease), a disorder of unclear etiology, may also present with this finding.

❑❑ Speaking of rashes...Dermacentor andersoni is a vector for *Rickettsia rickettsii* which causes Rocky Mountain Spotted Fever. The rash of RMSF usually begins on the wrists and ankles and spreads centripetally. What is the underlying pathologic lesion that induces the serious sequelae of this disease, as well as the hemorrhagic rash?

Vasculitis 2° to rickettsial invasion of endothelial cells in small blood vessels, including arterioles.

❑❑ What are the characteristic findings in measles?

The three "C's", cough, coryza and conjunctivitis in addition to the characteristic morbilliform rash that begins on the head and spreads downward.

❑❑ A child presents in DKA. On average, how dehydrated is this patient likely to be, in mL/kg?

125 mL/kg average fluid volume deficit.

❑❑ What is the dose of insulin to be used for low-dose continuous infusion therapy?

0.1 unit/kg/hour of regular insulin.

❑❑ Is intestinal intussusception associated with GI bleeding?

Yes, though the classic history of sudden onset of severe pain that often is relieved as quickly as it arose and is recurrent is more sensitive. The currant jelly stool associated with this disorder is present in about half of cases.

❑❑ About how old is the average patient presenting with intussusception?

One year, +/- 6 months.

❑❑ Pyloric stenosis usually presents at about what age?

4 weeks.

❑❑ What is the eponym for congenital aganglionic megacolon. (Remember, this disease involves a portion of the distal colon that lacks ganglion cells thereby impairing the normal inhibitory innervation in the myenteric plexus. As a result, coordinated relaxation is also impaired which can in turn causes clinical symptoms of obstruction. Eighty five percent of the time, this condition presents <u>after</u> the newborn period)?

Hirschsprung's disease.

❑❑ Acute enterocolitis with development of "toxic" megacolon is the life-threatening complication of Hirschsprung's disease. Between what range of ages does this complication most frequently present?

2-3 months.

❑❑ What is the most concerning aspect of the definition of Reye's syndrome provided by the CDC?

Two of the criteria required may be determined at autopsy. The mortality is about 25% or less overall and varies with age of patient and clinical stage. The underlying abnormality is one of mitochondrial morphology and function, affecting primarily brain and liver.

❑❑ Describe stage I and stage II of Reye's syndrome.

Stage I: Vomiting, lethargy and liver dysfunction.
Stage II: Disorientation, combativeness, delirium, hyperventilation, increased deep tendon reflexes, liver dysfunction, hyperexcitable, tachypnea, fever, tachycardia, sweating and papillary dilatation.

❑❑ What is the treatment for stages I and II?

Supportive.

❑❑ Describe Stages III, IV, and V of Reye's syndrome.

Stage III: Coma, decorticate rigidity, increased respiratory rate, mortality rate of 50%.
Stage IV: Coma, decerebrate posturing, no ocular reflexes, loss of corneal reflexes, and liver damage.
Stage V: Loss of DTRs, seizures, flaccid, respiratory arrest, 95% mortality.

❑❑ What is the treatment for advanced stages of Reye's syndrome?

Manage ICP - elevate HOB, paralyze, intubate and hyperventilate, furosemide, mannitol, dexamethasone, pentobarbital coma. Also consider hypertonic glucose and bowel sterilization.

❑❑ Which motor deficit occurs with an anterior cerebral artery infarct?

Leg weakness greater than arm weakness on the contralateral side.

❑❑ What signs develop with a middle cerebral artery stroke?

1) Contralateral sensory/motor deficits.
2) Arm/ face weakness greater than leg weakness.

❑❑ What is the most common neurologic findings in adult botulism?

Eye and bulbar muscle deficit.

❑❑ What is the typical presentation of Guillain-Barre syndrome?

Ascending motor neuron involvement.

❑❑ What is the most common medication associated with Neuroleptic Malignant Syndrome?

Haloperidol. Other drugs antipsychotic medications are also causative.

❑❑ What is the hallmark motor finding in Neuroleptic Malignant Syndrome?

"Lead-pipe" rigidity.

❑❑ What neoplastic process is most commonly associated with myasthenia gravis?

Thymoma.

❑❑ **What is the definition for status epilepticus?**

Continuous seizure activity for greater than 30 minutes or two or more seizures which occur without full recovery of consciousness between attacks.

❑❑ **What is the significance of bilateral nystagmus with cold caloric testing?**

It signifies that an intact cortex, midbrain, and brainstem are present.

❑❑ **How can upper motor neuron (UMN) lesions of CN VII (facial nerve) be distinguished from peripheral lesions?**

1) UMN: Unilateral weakness of the lower half of the face.
2) Peripheral: Involve entire half of the face.

❑❑ **A patient presents with facial droop on the left and weakness of the right leg. Where is the most likely site of the lesion?**

Brainstem, specifically the left pons.

❑❑ **A 30 year old presents with progressively severe intermittent vertigo for six months and progressive unilateral hearing loss for 3 months. What is the diagnosis?**

Cerebellopontine angle tumor. Confirm diagnosis with MRI scan.

❑❑ **A 29 year old drunken male presents after having his head pounded into the concrete by his wife. The patient had a brief episode of LOC, but was then ambulatory and alert. Now he appears drowsy and just threw up on you. What is the diagnosis?**

Epidural hematoma.

❑❑ **A 64 year old presents with a bilateral "burning" headache. She describes jabs of pain which are worse at night. What is the treatment?**

Temporal arteritis is treated with long-term steroids. Treatment should begin immediately, do not wait for biopsy confirmation. ESR over 50 mm/hour is highly suggestive.

❑❑ **A 53 year old female presents with unilateral right sided sudden-onset lancinating pain in the distribution of the second and third branches of the fifth cranial nerve. What is treatment?**

Carbamazepine treats trigeminal neuralgia. An MRI to rule out a brainstem process (tumor) is indicated.

❑❑ **A 50 year old female presents with acute vertigo, nausea, and vomiting. She reports similar episodes over the last 20 years, sometimes but not always associated with hearing change and/or hearing loss and tinnitus. She has permanent right > left sensorineural hearing loss. What is the diagnosis?**

Ménière's Disease.

❑❑ The Nylen-Barany maneuver is performed as follows: the patient is rapidly brought from the sitting to supine position and the head is turned 45°. Match the findings with peripheral and central vertigo:

1) Nystagmus is multi-directional, nonfatiguing, has no latent period, and lasts over a minute.
2) Vertigo increased. Nystagmus is unidirectional, fatiguing, latent period is 2-20 seconds, with duration less than a minute.

1 - Central.
2 - Peripheral.

❑❑ What is the dangerous diagnosis of a purpuric, petechial rash?

Think meningococcemia. Other causes include *Hemophilus influenzae, Streptococcus pneumoniae,* and *Staphylococcus aureus.*

❑❑ On LP, opening pressure is markedly elevated. What should be done?

Close 3-way stopcock, remove only a small amount of fluid from manometer, abort LP, and initiate measures to decrease intracranial pressure.

❑❑ A patient presents with acute meningitis; when should antibiotics be initiated?

Immediately. Do not wait. Patients should receive a CT prior to LP only if papilledema or focal deficit is present.

❑❑ What is the most common presenting symptom of MS?

Optic neuritis, (about 25%).

❑❑ Which three bacterial illnesses present with peripheral neurologic findings?

Botulism, tetanus, and diphtheria.

❑❑ What is the appropriate treatment for QRS widening in a TCA poisoning?

$NaHCO_3$ is administered intravenously for patients with a QRS > 100 ms. One to two mEq/kg are initially administered and repeated until the blood pH is between 7.50 and 7.55. A continuous infusion of $NaHCO_3$, 3 Amps in 1 L of D_5W, may then be initiated and run in over 4-6 hours titrating to maintain appropriate pH. Potassium levels are closely monitored and supplementation may be required to prevent hypokalemia.

❑❑ What is the appropriate treatment of TCA-induced seizures?

Benzodiazepines and barbiturates are the agents of choice, phenytoin is not generally effective. Bicarbonate and alkalosis is mainstay of treatment.

❑❑ Which TCA may induce seizures without concomitant cardiac toxicity?

Amoxapine.

❑❑ What is the treatment for TCA-induced hypotension?

Isotonic saline is initially administered. If the patient is resistant to fluid resuscitation, a directly acting alpha agonist should be started such as norepinephrine. Dopamine and dobutamine administration are contraindicated as these agents may increase hypotension through b-adrenergic stimulation. Further, dopamine acts in part by releasing norepinephrine; this agent may already be depleted by the reuptake inhibition of the CA and by stress.

❑❑ **What is the clinical presentation of anticholinergic poisoning?**

Mydriasis, tachycardia, hypoactive bowel sounds, urinary retention, dry axilla, hyperthermia, and mental status changes.

❑❑ **An observation period of what time length is required prior to medically clearing a TCA overdose?**

6 hours.

❑❑ **What signs and symptoms are typical for the serotonin syndrome?**

Agitation, anxiety, sinus tachycardia, shivering, tremor, hyperreflexia, myoclonus, muscular rigidity, and diarrhea.

❑❑ **A 32 year old female is given meperidine (Demerol) for an open fracture. The patient is chronically on fluoxetine (Prozac). What is a potential complication?**

The serotonin syndrome.

❑❑ **A patient presents to the ED status post Thorazine poisoning. You expect her pupils to be...?**

Miotic. Thorazine is a potent alpha antagonist resulting in miosis in overdose.

❑❑ **What constellation of findings occur with the neuroleptic malignant syndrome?**

Altered mental status, muscular rigidity, autonomic instability, hyperthermia, and rhabdomyolysis.

❑❑ **What are the signs and symptoms of lithium toxicity?**

1) Neuro: Tremor, hyperreflexia, clonus, fasciculations, seizures, coma.
2) GI: Nausea, vomiting, diarrhea.
3) CV: ST-T wave changes, bradycardia, conduction defects and arrhythmias.

❑❑ **What is the treatment for lithium toxicity?**

Supportive care, normal saline diuresis, hemodialysis for patients with clinical signs of severe poisoning (seizures, arrhythmias etc.), renal failure, or decreasing urine output.

❑❑ **The administration of flumazenil to acutely poisoned patients has resulted in what adverse effect?**

Seizures. Flumazenil has induced seizures in patients status post ingestion of potential seizure-inducing agents particularly TCAs. Flumazenil may induce withdrawal seizures in patients chronically on benzodiazepines.

❑❑ **What is the pharmacological treatment for alcohol withdrawal?**

Benzodiazepines or barbiturates.

❑❑ **Isopropanol is metabolized via which enzyme to which metabolite?**

Isopropanol is metabolized by alcohol dehydrogenase in the liver to acetone.

❑❑ **What methanol level warrants dialysis?**

50 mg/dL. Other indications include visual impairment, severe metabolic acidosis, and ingestion of greater than 30 cc.

❑❑ **What two cofactors are administered to the patient with ethylene glycol poisoning?**

Thiamine and pyridoxine. These cofactors will aid in transforming glyoxylic acid to nontoxic metabolites. Both are administered intravenously in 100 mg increments.

❑❑ **Isopropanol, ethylene glycol, and methanol are all metabolized by alcohol dehydrogenase. Is an alcohol drip beneficial to all of these poisonings?**

No. Isopropanol is converted via alcohol dehydrogenase to the nontoxic acetone.

❑❑ **What are the three clinical phases of ethylene glycol poisoning?**

Stage I: Neurological symptomatology, i.e., inebriation.
Stage II: Metabolic acidosis and cardiovascular instability.
Stage III: Renal failure.

❑❑ **When should dialysis be initiated for ethylene glycol poisoning?**

At a serum level greater than 25 mg/dL, renal insufficiency, or severe metabolic acidosis.

❑❑ **What is the toxic dose of naloxone?**

There is none. Narcan is a safe drug and may be given in large quantities. The usual adult dosage is 2 mg IV and 0.01 mg/kg for a child. Narcan may precipitate acute withdrawal and may therefore be titrated to effect.

❑❑ **How does treatment for a cocaine induced MI differ from a typical MI?**

Both are treated the same with the exception that ß-blockers are not used in a cocaine induced MI secondary to unopposed alpha adrenergic activity. The tachycardia of a cocaine associated MI is first treated with benzodiazepine sedation.

❑❑ **Metabolic acidosis favors which form of salicylate, ionized or un-ionized?**

Un-ionized. Patients with salicylate poisoning should have arterial pH maintained at or greater than 7.4 so that salicylate is in the ionized form and therefore unable to cross the blood brain barrier. Urinary alkalinization promotes the formation of the ionized form of salicylate which is unable to be reabsorbed by the tubules thereby enhancing excretion.

❑❑ **What is the acid-base disturbance typical for salicylate poisoning?**

Mixed respiratory alkalosis (secondary to central respiratory center stimulation) and metabolic acidosis (secondary to uncoupling of oxidative phosphorylation).

❑❑ Arterial pH is 7.5 through alkalinization but urine pH is still low. Which electrolyte is probably responsible?

Potassium. When reabsorbing sodium, the renal tubules will preferentially excrete hydrogen ions into the tubular lumen rather than potassium ions thus, potassium should be maintained at 4.0 mmol/L.

❑❑ What is the treatment for a prolonged prothrombin time in salicylate poisoning?

Parenteral Vitamin K1 administration. Salicylates inhibit Vitamin K1 epoxide reductase in poisoning resulting in an ability for the inactive vitamin K1 epoxide to be regenerated into the active Vitamin K1.

❑❑ What are the indications for dialysis in salicylate poisoning?

1) Persistent CNS involvement.
2) ARDS.
3) Renal failure.
4) Severe acid-base disturbance despite appropriate care.
5) Acute salicylate level > 100 mg/dL.

❑❑ Can a patient present with salicylate poisoning and a therapeutic level?

Yes. Patients with chronic salicylate poisoning have a large Vd and thus may present with mental status changes and a therapeutic level.

❑❑ What are the four stages of acetaminophen (APAP) poisoning?

1) 1/2-24 hours: Nausea, vomiting.
2) 24-48 hours: Abdominal pain, elevated LFTs.
3) 72-96 hours: LFTs peak, nausea, vomiting.
4) 4 days-2 weeks: Resolution or fulminant hepatic failure.

❑❑ APAP poisoning produces which type of hepatic necrosis?

Centrilobular necrosis. The toxic metabolite of APAP is generated in the liver via the P450 system, located in the centrilobular region.

❑❑ Which is the toxic metabolite of APAP?

NAPQI. When the glucuronidation and sulfation pathways are saturated, APAP is metabolized by the P450 system to the toxic metabolite N-acetyl-para-benzoquinoneimine (NAPQI).

❑❑ What hepatic laboratory parameter is the first to become abnormal in APAP poisoning?

The prothrombin time (PT).

❑❑ An acutely intoxicated, nonalcoholic, otherwise healthy patient ingests APAP. Is this patient more or less likely to develop hepatotoxicity?

Less likely. An acute ingestion of alcohol will inhibit the P450 system thereby inhibiting the formation of NAPQI. A chronic alcoholic has an induced P450 system and will suffer greater APAP hepatic toxicity through increased NAPQI formation.

❑❑ What is the minimum dose of APAP in a child and an adult that is capable of causing hepatotoxicity?

Child: 140 mg/kg. Adult: 7.5 g.

❑❑ Per the Rumack-Matthew nomogram, which 4 hours APAP level requires treatment?

150 mg/mL.

❑❑ How is the nomogram utilized in a patient who ingests an Extended Relief formulation of APAP?

A four hour and an eight hour level are obtained. If either level is in the "Possible" hepatotoxic range, the patient should be treated.

❑❑ What is the appropriate initial treatment for theophylline-induced seizures?

Benzodiazepines and barbiturates. Theophylline-induced seizures warrant hemodialysis or hemoperfusion.

❑❑ What are absolute indications for hemodialysis or hemoperfusion in theophylline toxicity?

Seizures or arrhythmias that are unresponsive to conventional therapy.

❑❑ Why is multidose activated charcoal administration advocated for theophylline poisoning?

Theophylline undergoes enterohepatic circulation.

❑❑ What abnormal laboratory parameters are typical in the patient with acute theophylline poisoning?

Hypokalemia, hyperglycemia, and leukocytosis.

❑❑ What are absolute indications for Digibind administration in digoxin poisoning?

Ventricular arrhythmias, hemodynamically significant bradyarrhythmias unresponsive to standard therapy, and a potassium level greater than 5.0 mEq/L.

❑❑ Why is calcium chloride administration contraindicated in digoxin poisoning?

Digoxin inhibits the Na-K-ATPase, resulting in an increased intracellular concentration of sodium. The sodium-calcium exchange pump is then activated leading to high intracellular concentrations of calcium. Calcium chloride administration would further increase intracellular calcium leading to increased myocardial irritability.

❑❑ What is the appropriate treatment for hyperkalemia in digoxin poisoning?

1) Digibind.
2) Insulin and glucose.
3) Sodium bicarbonate.
4) Potassium resin binder (Kayexalate).
5) Hemodialysis.

❑❑ A patient on Digoxin presents bradycardic and hypotensive with significantly peaked T waves. What would be your initial line of treatment?

Administer 10 vials of Digibind intravenously and simultaneously treat the presumed hyperkalemia with insulin and glucose, sodium bicarbonate, and Kayexalate. Once the Digibind is administered, hyperkalemic-induced arrhythmias may be safely treated with calcium chloride.

❑❑ What is the antidote for b-blocker poisonings and what is the biochemical rational?

Glucagon. Glucagon receptors, located on myocardial cells, are G protein coupled receptors which activate adenylate cyclase leading to increased levels of intracellular cAMP. Thus, glucagon administration leads to the same intracellular effect as b-agonism.

❑❑ A child presents to the ED status post ingestion of a sustained release calcium channel blocker. What is the disposition?

Hospital admission to a monitored setting. Sustained release preparations have the capability of producing delayed toxicity.

❑❑ What are potential treatment modalities for a calcium channel blocker poisoning?

Symptomatic patients are admitted to an intensive care unit and treatment is best guided by Pulmonary Artery Catheter hemodynamic measurements. Therapeutic interventions include intravenous calcium, isoproterenol, glucagon, transvenous pacers, atropine, and vasopressors, such as norepinephrine, epinephrine, or dopamine.

❑❑ What are the four stages of iron poisoning?

1) (Initial hour) Gastrointestinal symptomatology. Abdominal pain, vomiting, and diarrhea secondary to the corrosive effects of iron.
2) (6 to 24 hours) Quiescent period during which iron is being absorbed.
3) (> 12 hours) Shock, metabolic acidosis, hepatic dysfunction, heart failure, cerebral dysfunction, and renal failure.
4) (Days to weeks) Gastric outlet or small bowel obstruction secondary to scarring.

❑❑ What dose of iron is expected to produce clinical toxicity?

20 mg/kg of elemental iron. A toddler ingests 10 tablets of 324 mg ferrous sulfate, 20% elemental iron. This equals 648 mg of elemental iron, which is a toxic dose of 32.4 mg/kg in a 20 kg child.

❑❑ What 4 hour iron level is generally considered toxic?

300-350 mg/dL.

❑❑ What are indications for deferoxamine therapy?

1) All symptomatic patients exhibiting more than merely transient symptomatology.
2) Patients with lethargy, significant abdominal pain, hypotension, or metabolic acidosis.
3) Patients with a positive KUB.
4) Any symptomatic patient with a level greater than 300 mg/dL.

❑❑ What is the standard dose of deferoxamine?

15 mg/kg/hr continuous intravenous infusion.

❑❑ When may a hydrocarbon ingestion be discharged safely to home?

After a six hour asymptomatic period patients with a normal chest X-ray and pulse ox may be discharged to home.

❑❑ Chronic solvent abusers develop what metabolic complication?

Renal tubular acidosis.

❑❑ Oral hydrofluoric acid exposure may result in which life threatening electrolyte abnormalities?

Hyperkalemia and hypocalcemia.

❑❑ What enzyme is inhibited by organophosphates?

Cholinesterase.

❑❑ What are the two principle antidotes used for organophosphate poisoning?

Atropine and Pralidoxime.

❑❑ Is pralidoxime administration beneficial in carbamate poisoning?

No. Carbamates bind reversibly to cholinesterases whereas organophosphates bind irreversibly. Pralidoxime is used to reactivate cholinesterase molecules phosphorylated by an organophosphate molecule. Pralidoxime should be administered prior to the onset of irreversible aging of the enzyme.

❑❑ What antihypertensive agent may induce cyanide poisoning?

Nitroprusside. One molecule of sodium nitroprusside contains 5 molecules of cyanide. In order to prevent toxicity, sodium thiosulfate should be infused with sodium nitroprusside at a ratio of 10:1 (thiosulfate:nitroprusside). Beware of thiocyanate toxicity.

❑❑ What order are the kinetics of elimination of ASA overdose?

Zero-order elimination with hepatic enzymatic clearance saturated and renal clearance becoming important.

❑❑ We all remember to think of ASA poisoning when a patient presents with mental status changes associated with respiratory alkalosis and metabolic acidosis. Many of us may recall that salicylate toxicity may be associated with elevated, normal, or decreased glucose levels. By what mechanisms are hyperglycemia and hypoglycemia caused?

Hyperglycemia is caused by salicylate-induced mobilization of glycogen.
Hypoglycemia is caused by salicylate inhibition of gluconeogenesis.

❑❑ Is ARDS more likely to be a complication of acute or chronic ASA poisoning?

Chronic.

❑❑ **What is the "magic number" for the dose of non-enteric coated ASA which must be exceeded to cause toxicity, in mg/kg?**

150 mg/kg.

❑❑ **Can a patient who is symptomatic with mental status changes from chronic salicylate poisoning have a level in the therapeutic range?**

Yes! Interestingly, patients taking acetazolamide are at particular risk for chronic salicylate poisoning because the carbonic anhydrase inhibitor results in acidified plasma (leading to increased V_d) and more alkalotic CSF, thereby encouraging salicylate concentration in the CNS.

❑❑ **Is hemodialysis used to treat salicylate toxicity?**

Yes, in severe poisoning (coma, ARDS, cardiac toxicity, serum level > 100 mg/dL), and for patients who are unresponsive to maximal therapy.

❑❑ **How does N-acetylcysteine (NAC, Mucomyst) work?**

Precise mechanism is still unknown. We know that NAC enters cells and is metabolized to cysteine ,which serves as a glutathione precursor.

❑❑ **Which measures of hepatic function are better indicators of prognosis, liver enzyme levels or bilirubin level and prothrombin time?**

Bilirubin level and prothrombin time.

❑❑ **Aromatic hydrocarbons, such as toluene present in glue, may be sniffed. Resulting effects most closely resemble those of which other class of compounds?**

Effects are similar to those of inhalational anesthetic agents. Initial excitatory response gives way to CNS depression.

❑❑ **Is degree of toxicity in CA overdose closely related to QRS duration?**

QRS > 100 ms has a specificity of 75% and a sensitivity of 60% for serious complications. A normal ECG will not rule out a serious overdose! Of those with QRS > 100 ms, 30% will seize; of those with QRS > 160 ms, 50% will develop arrhythmias.

❑❑ **What is the treatment for narcotic overdose?**

Naloxone, 0.4 to 2.0 mg in an adult, and 0.01 mg/kg in a child. Naloxone's half life is about 1 hour.

❑❑ **Describe the pathophysiologic features of HIV.**

HIV attacks the T4 helper cells. HIV genetic material consists of singlestranded RNA. HIV has been found in semen, vaginal secretions, blood and blood products, saliva, urine, cerebrospinal fluid, tears, alveolar fluid, synovial fluid, breast milk, transplanted tissue and amniotic fluid. There has not been documentation of infection from casual contact.

❑❑ **How quickly do patients infected with HIV become symptomatic?**

Five to ten percent develop symptoms within three years of seroconversion. Predictive characteristics include low T4 count and hematocrit less than 40. The mean incubation time is about 8.23 years for adults and 1.97 years for children less than 5 years. When AIDS develops, the survival rate is about 9 months. However, new treatments may improve survival.

❑❑ **Name the most common causes of fever in HIV-infected patients:**

HIV related fever, Mycobacterium aviumintracellular, CMV, nonHodgkin's and Hodgkin's lymphoma.

❑❑ **What is the <u>most common</u> cause of focal encephalitis in AIDS patients?**

Toxoplasmosis. Symptoms include focal neurologic deficits, headache, fever, altered mental status, and seizures. Ring enhancinglesions are seen on CT.

❑❑ **The differential diagnosis of ringenhancing lesions in AIDS patients is . . . . ?**

Lymphoma, cerebral tuberculosis, fungal infection, CMV, Kaposi's sarcoma, toxoplasmosis, and hemorrhage.

❑❑ **What are the signs and symptoms of CNS cryptococcal infection in an AIDS patient?**

Headache, depression, lightheadedness, seizures, and cranial nerve palsies. A diagnosis is made by India ink prep, fungal culture, or by the detection of the *Cryptococcal* antigen in the CSF.

❑❑ **On physical exam, what is the most common eye finding in AIDS patients?**

Cottonwool spots, which are thought to be associated with PCP. These may be hard to differentiate from fluffywhite, often perivascular retinal lesions that are associated with CMV.

❑❑ **An AIDS patient presents with complaints of decreased visual acuity, photophobia, redness, and eye pain. What is the diagnosis?**

Retinitis or malignant invasion of the periorbital tissue or eye.

❑❑ **What is the most common cause of retinitis in AIDS patients?**

Cytomegalovirus. Findings include photophobia, redness, scotoma, pain, or change in visual acuity. On exam, findings include fluffy white retinal lesions.

❑❑ **What is the most common opportunistic infection in AIDS patients?**

PCP. Symptoms may include nonproductive cough and dyspnea. A chest X-ray may show diffuse interstitial infiltrates or be negative. Gallium scanning is more sensitive but results in false positives. Initial treatment includes TMPSMX. Pentamidine is an alternative.

❑❑ **What is the incubation period in tetanus?**

Hours to over one month. The shorter the incubation the more severe the disease. Most patients in the U.S. who contract the disease are over 50 years old.

❑❑ What are the confirmatory tests for RMSF?

Immunofluorescent antibody staining of skin biopsy or serologic fluorescent antibody titer. The WeilFelix reaction and complement fixation tests are no longer recommended.

❑❑ What are the antibiotics for RMSF?

Tetracycline or chloramphenicol. Antibiotic therapy should not be withheld pending serologic confirmation.

❑❑ Which type of paralysis does tick paralysis cause?

Ascending paralysis. The venom which causes paralysis is probably a neurotoxin which causes a conduction block at the peripheral motor nerve branches. This prevents acetylcholine release at the neuromuscular junction. Forty three species of ticks are implicated as causative agents.

❑❑ What is the treatment of choice for a patient in anaphylactic shock?

Epinephrine, 0.3-0.5 mg IV of 1:10,000 solution. If no IV access, then inject into the venous plexus at base of the tongue.

❑❑ What is the most common cause of anaphylactoid reactions?

Radiographic contrast agents.

❑❑ What percentage of patients with relapsing polychondritis can be expected to have airway involvement?

Approximately 50% have airway involvement. They frequently present with acute onset of pain, oropharyngeal tenderness over cartilaginous structures, and hoarseness. Erythema and edema of the nose and oropharynx is also common.

❑❑ What is the appropriate treatment for a patient presenting with acute onset of relapsing polychondritis with airway involvement?

Admit for observation and high dose steroids. These patients may develop dyspnea, stridor, or cough. Repeated exacerbations may lead to asphyxiation .

❑❑ A RA patient presenting with painful speaking or swallowing, hoarseness, or stridor requires what type of diagnostic procedure?

Urgent laryngoscopy to evaluate involvement of the paired cricoarytenoid joints. These may become fixed in the closed position, resulting in airway compromise.

❑❑ Myocardial infarction can be related to which two rheumatic diseases?

Kawasaki disease and polyarteritis nodosa.

❑❑ A patient presents with fever, acute polyarthritis, or migratory arthritis a few weeks after a bout of Streptococcal pharyngitis, they should be evaluated for which disease?

Rheumatic fever. Approximately 30% will have subcutaneous nodules, erythema marginatum, or chorea.

❑❑ Name a common complication of SLE, RA, & JRA.

Pericarditis.

❑❑ What might a change in bladder or bowel function, limb paresthesias, or new weakness indicate in a patient with RA or ankylosing spondylosis?

Destruction of the c-spine ligamentous structures - this can lead to atlantoaxial subluxation.

❑❑ What is Lhermitte's sign, found in patients with RA or ankylosing spondylosis?

The sensation of an electric shock radiating down the back with neck flexion. A classic sign of c-spine instability.

❑❑ What disease entity should be investigated in a child with joint swelling following minor trauma?

JRA. Minor trauma may cause intra-articular bleeding. The joint should not be immobilized.

❑❑ What is the appropriate management for a child with normal X-rays and tenderness over the end of a long bone after trauma.

Immobilization and orthopedic evaluation for Salter-Harris type I fracture. These fractures may be occult.

❑❑ What pathologic process must be considered in a patient with painless progressive weakness in a c-spine distribution?

Cervical ventral root compromise by a degenerative disk. The dorsal and ventral nerve roots remain discrete in the c-spine in over half the population.

❑❑ What constitutes immediate admission criteria for a patient with acute low back pain?

Paraparesis, bowel or bladder incontinence, intractable L-S pain and spasticity, inability to sit or stand, upright sleeping position, metastatic cancer, 2nd ED visit, or X-ray film with defects.

❑❑ What are the two most common causes of fatal anaphylaxis?

#1 = Drug reactions, 95% to penicillin. Parenteral is the most dangerous with 300 deaths per year.
#2 = Hymenoptera stings with 100 deaths per year.

❑❑ What are characteristics of failure to thrive syndrome in infants?

Body mass index (BMI) < 5%, irritable, hard to console behavior, increased muscle tone in the lower extremities or hypotonia, and subsequent weight gain in the hospital.

❑❑ When considering failure to thrive syndrome, which historical features are important to assess?

History of prematurity, birth weight, maternal use of cigarettes, alcohol, and or drugs during the pregnancy, previous hospitalizations, and parental stature.

❑❑ **In the case of child sexual assault, which laboratory tests should be performed?**

As indicated, oral, rectal, vaginal, or urethral swabs for GC and Chlamydia. Serological tests for syphilis or HIV testing should be done if there is a history of, or clinical evidence of infection in the assailant or the victim. Urine or plasma ß-HCG should be checked in girls beyond age of menarche.

❑❑ **What is considered physical evidence of acute ano-genital trauma in the genital exam of a child?**

With acute sexual abuse you may see fissures, abrasions, hematomas, changes in tone (either dilation or spasm), or discharges, such as semen (fluoresces with a woods light), or examine under microscope. Erythema is a sign of inflammation, irritation, or manipulation, and is not specific for abuse.

❑❑ **What is considered physical evidence of chronic ano-genital trauma in the genital exam of a child?**

With chronic sexual abuse signs of an STD, such as vaginal or anal discharge, venereal warts or vesicles may be observed. Because injuries can heal without residual scarring, a lack of physical changes in no way rules out child sexual abuse.

❑❑ **In addition to the history, physical, laboratory tests and collection of physical evidence, what else needs to done in the case of child sexual abuse?**

File a report with child protective services and law enforcement agencies. Provide emotional support for the child and family. Arrange a return appointment for follow-up of STD cultures and testing for pregnancy, HIV, and syphilis as indicated. Assure follow up for psychological counseling by connecting the family/child to the appropriate services in your area.

❑❑ **In a patient with meningococcemia, what factors are associated with a poor prognosis?**

Petechia within 24 hours of admission, presence of purpura of ecchymosis, shock, coma, DIC, thrombocytopenia (<150,000), metabolic acidosis, and the absence of meningitis.

❑❑ **How soon does xanthochromia develope during a subarachnoïd hemorrhage?**

4-6 hours.

❑❑ **How can a tension PTX lead to death?**

As air progressively collects in the pleural space, intrapleural pressure increase causing a decrease in functional lung volume leading to a ventilation-perfusion mismatch subsequent hypoxia and acidosis.

The increasing intrapleural volume causes a mediastinal shift and a decreased systemic venous return due to a mechanical collapse of the venae cavae and increased intrathoracic pressure. The increased CO_2 and decreased O_2 leads to cardiovascular depression and collapse.

SAMPLE CASES

"Two roads diverged in a wood and
I took the one less traveled by,
And that has made all the difference."

Robert Frost

SAMPLE CASES

CASE 1 (Iron Overdose)

Examiner

A child has overdosed on iron. His mom states that the patient spent the entire day with the baby-sitter. When she picked him up, he seemed very sleepy. Upon questioning the 12 year old baby-sitter, via the phone, she noted that the child ate a few "harmless" vitamins while she was not looking. After the remaining pills were counted, 25 tablets of ferrous sulfate, 325 mg (20% elemental iron) are missing. The ingestion occurred 4 hours before arrival to the ED.

The candidate should be aggressive in rehydrating the patient. Vital signs will not normalize until packed RBCs are started. If therapy for iron toxicity is started prematurely, instruct nurse to try to push activated charcoal. The patient's mother will probably be concerned, inquisitive, and demanding. The physician should appropriately calm the mother.

1.1 Introduction:

A 3 year old male is brought to the ED by his mother with a complaint of weakness.

Vital signs are: BP 82/50, P 135, R 24, T 98.6 °F, Wt 18 kg.

1.2 Primary Survey:

- ❑ General impression: This is a well nourished, well developed (WN/WD) child who appears in distress. He is unable to provide a history but responds to verbal stimuli with appropriate motor response and speech.
- ❑ Airway: No pooling of secretions and the patient can speak.
- ❑ Breathing: Lungs are clear but the patient is tachypneic.
- ❑ Circulation: Tachycardia, decreased capillary refill, no petechiae, ecchymoses, or rash. Diaphoretic and cool to the touch.
- ❑ Disability: GCS 14, patient opens eyes to command, pupils are equal and reactive.
- ❑ Exposure: No signs of trauma, no medic alert tags.
- ❑ Finger: Heme positive stools.

1.3 Management:

- ❑ Intubation is not indicated at this time but ensure that the airway equipment is available.
- ❑ Start IV, O_2, and place on a cardiac monitor and a pulse oximeter.
- ❑ Administer two 20 mL/kg fluid boluses of NS.
- ❑ Insert a Foley catheter.
- ❑ Order appropriate X-rays and labs, including type and cross for packed RBCs.
- ❑ Consult Poison Control.

1.4 History:

- Allergies: None.
- Medications: None.
- PMH: No significant illnesses or injuries.
- Last meal: 2 hours ago.
- Amount of iron ingested per kg:

$$\frac{65 \text{ mg} \times 25 \text{ tablets}}{18} = 90 \text{ mg/kg}$$

- Family: Mother is present to answer questions. Family history is not applicable. The patient's pediatrician is available for more information if needed.
- Records: None.
- Immune: Up to date.
- Doctor: Dr. Pediatrician.

1.5 Secondary Survey:

- General: If appropriate rehydration has occurred, the patient will be more awake and alert.
- Skin: Diaphoretic, decreased capillary refill, no bruises, abrasions, or petechiae.
- HEENT: Normocephalic and atraumatic, pupils equal, round, and reactive to light and accommodation (PERRLA), conjunctiva normal, extraocular muscles intact (EOM-I), fundi normal, oropharynx moist, gag reflex is intact.
- Neck: Supple, no nodes.
- Chest: Normal.
- Lungs: Clear to auscultation.
- Heart: Tachycardia, no murmur.
- Abdomen: Diffusely tender with generalized guarding. No masses or organomegaly, bowel sounds are hyperactive.
- Perineum/GU: Normal male genitalia, Tanner stage I, both testis descended.
- Rectal: Loose stool, positive for occult blood.
- Back: Normal.
- Extremities: Normal and equal pulses without edema.
- Neuro: Moves all extremities, normal strength and sensation, symmetric deep-tendon reflexes. Cranial nerves intact.

1.6 Laboratory:

- CBC: WBC 20,000, Hgb 10, Hct 30%, Plt 178,000.
- Chemistry: Na 143, K 4, Cl 100, CO_2 17.
- BUN/Cr: 26/0.8.
- Glucose: 160.
- Ca/Mg: Normal.
- LFTs: Normal.
- PT/PTT: 14/24.
- ABG: pH 7.30, pO_2 95, pCO_2 40, HCO_3 23.
- U/A: Normal.
- Iron studies: Iron levels and TIBC are not available.

1.7 X-rays:

- ❑ KUB: Retained pills are present in the stomach.

1.8 Special Tests:

- ❑ ECG: Sinus tachycardia.

1.9 Critical Actions:

- ❑ Protect the airway and have intubation equipment present.
- ❑ No activated charcoal or cathartic. Consider gastric lavage with bicarbonate.
- ❑ Monitor cardiac responses.
- ❑ Start IV fluids.
- ❑ Monitor urine output with a Foley catheter.
- ❑ Transfuse PRBCs.
- ❑ Contact Poison Control.
- ❑ Admit to the pediatric ICU.
- ❑ Start deferoxamine therapy.

1.10 Pearls:

❑❑ When should deferoxamine therapy be instituted?

Patients who present with or develop multiple episodes of emesis or diarrhea or have evidence of hypovolemia or exhibit lethargy require deferoxamine and fluids regardless of the serum iron concentration.

❑❑ What are the stages of iron poisoning?

Stage 1: Initial period (1/2 to 6 hours): Nausea, vomiting, abdominal pain hematemesis, diarrhea, melena, and lethargy.
Stage 2: Latent period (6 to 24 hours): Improvement is seen but patient may be lethargic and hypotensive.
Stage 3: Systemic toxicity (4 to 40 hours): Cyanosis, lethargy, restlessness, disorientation, convulsions, coma, shock, coagulopathy.
Stage 4: Late complications (2 to 8 wks): Gastric outlet or small bowel obstruction.

CASE 2 (Abdominal Aortic Aneurysm)

Examiner

The patient falls due to an abdominal aortic aneurysm. The pain is a "dull ache" which is located in the mid-back and right inguinal region. It started suddenly 3 days ago and has progressively worsened. There are no GI or GU symptoms. Just prior to arrival, he was working in his shop when he became light-headed, passed out, and fell.

It is important for the physician to make this conclusion after obtaining a history and performing a physical exam. If the candidate continues to pursue the orthopedic problems, allow the patient's VS worsen. If an angiogram or CT scan is ordered, do not make the results available. Have the candidate convince the vascular surgeon to come in to treat the patient.

2.1 Introduction:

A 68 year old man presents, via paramedics, complaining of pain in the mid-back and right groin secondary to a fall. The patient is accompanied by his wife.

Vital Signs are: BP 100/70, P 100, R 20, T 99.0 °F.

2.2 Primary Survey:

- ❑ General: The patient is an obese white male lying supine, holding a hand near his right groin. He is awake but pale, anxious, and in obvious discomfort.
- ❑ Airway: Intact.
- ❑ Breathing: Normal.
- ❑ Circulation: Normal.
- ❑ Disability: Negative.
- ❑ Exposure: No obvious injuries.
- ❑ Finger: Normal rectal, heme negative.

2.3 Management:

- ❑ Determine that the fall was due to a syncopal episode.
- ❑ Start two large bore IVs with a NS or LR bolus.
- ❑ Place on O_2, pulse oximeter, and cardiac monitor.
- ❑ Perform frequent VS and mental status checks.
- ❑ Consider an ultrasound of the abdomen if it can be obtained quickly, but do not delay an early vascular consultation.
- ❑ Order screening labs and ECG.

2.4 History:

- ❑ Allergies: None.
- ❑ Medications: Furosemide, 80 mg po bid, and Methyldopa, 250 mg po qid.
- ❑ PMH: Hypertension, coronary artery disease, cholecystectomy, renal stone 10 years ago.
- ❑ Last meal: 1 hour ago.
- ❑ Family: Wife is present for information. Family doctor is available. Both of the patient's parents died from heart attacks in their 60's.
- ❑ Records: Available upon request.
- ❑ Immune: Up to date.
- ❑ Narcotics: No illicit drug use.
- ❑ Doctor: Consultants are available.
- ❑ Social history: No alcohol or tobacco use. Lives with his wife. Occupation an accountant.

2.5 Secondary Survey:

- ❑ General: Continues to be anxious, uncomfortable, with VS unchanged.
- ❑ Skin: Pale, dry, no bruising.
- ❑ HEENT: Normal.
- ❑ Neck: Normal.
- ❑ Chest: Nontender.

- ❑ Lungs: Clear.
- ❑ Heart: Normal S1, S2 with the PMI displaced laterally. Grade II/VI systolic ejection murmur heard at the apex without an S3, S4 or rub.
- ❑ Abdomen: Obese, with a scar in the right upper quadrant. Bowel sounds are normal and no pain to palpation is noted. An 8 cm tender pulsatile mass is palpated above the umbilicus.
- ❑ Perineum/GU: Normal.
- ❑ Rectal: Normal.
- ❑ Back: No CVA tenderness.
- ❑ Extremity: The right hip is flexed 45 degrees, but good range of motion is noted. Good capillary refill is present and all pulses are equal.
- ❑ Neuro: No focal deficits.

2.6 Laboratory:

- ❑ CBC: WBC 9.8, Hgb 12, Hct 32.5, Plt 200,000.
- ❑ Chemistry: Na 138, K 4.1, Cl 98, CO_2 20.
- ❑ BUN/Cr: 22/1.5.
- ❑ Glucose: 170.
- ❑ Ca/Mg: Normal.
- ❑ LFTs: Normal.
- ❑ Amylase/Lipase: Normal.
- ❑ PT and PTT: Normal.
- ❑ Cardiac enzymes: Normal.
- ❑ U/A: Trace blood and protein, otherwise no significant findings.

2.7 X-rays:

- ❑ Chest X-ray: Cardiomegaly.
- ❑ Pelvis X-ray: Normal.
- ❑ KUB: Calcified aortic aneurysm.

2.8 Special Tests:

- ❑ ECG: Left bundle branch block.

2.9 Critical Actions:

- ☑ Elicit a history of passing out and falling.
- ☑ Identify the presence of a pulsatile mass in the abdomen.
- ☑ Start a normal saline bolus.
- ☑ Start large bore IVs.
- ☑ Type and crossmatch for 8 units.* (8u?) would x for 2u
- ☑ Obtain early consultation with a vascular surgeon.

2.10 Pearls:

❑❑ **What is the primary cause of an abdominal aortic aneurysm?**

Atherosclerosis, which weakens the aortic wall. It is present in 96% of these cases. Other causes such as congenital abnormalities, infection, and trauma are relatively uncommon.

❑❑ **What is the mechanism by which the aneurysm produces pain?**

Pain may be caused by: 1) A rapid expansion of the aneurysm, 2) pressure of the aneurysm on surrounding structures such as nerves, and 3) the presence of free blood in the abdomen or retroperitoneum from a leaking or ruptured aneurysm.

CASE 3 (Shock in an Infant)

Examiner

This child has many problems but the most pressing is profound dehydration. However, she has not been vomiting but diarrhea has been present for three days. Her mother has been giving the child tap water for the past two days. In addition, her two older siblings have also had diarrhea for the past 2 days.

If the candidate does not aggressively fluid resuscitate, make the child's seizure intractable, possibly requiring intubation. A septic work-up is required even though the seizure is due to hyponatremia. Make it impossible for a peripheral line to be started in order that an intraosseous or central line must be started. Have the candidate describe the procedure in detail.

3.1 Introduction:

A 12 month old female presents with her mother with a three day history of diarrhea, vomiting and poor feeding.

Vital Signs are: BP 50, Doppler, P 190, R 56, T 100.2 °F, Wt 10 kg.

3.2 Primary Survey:

- ❑ General: 12 month old female lying quiet, toxic appearing.
- ❑ Airway: Intact.
- ❑ Breathing: Tachypneic without retractions.
- ❑ Circulation: Capillary refill > 4 seconds, distal pulses absent.
- ❑ Disability: Pupils normal, child moans to painful stimuli.
- ❑ Exposure: No gross abnormalities.

3.3 Management:

- ❑ Initiate IV rehydration with NS in 20 mL/kg boluses. It will take a total of three boluses to normalize the vital signs and stop the seizures.
- ❑ Order appropriate labs, X-rays, including blood, urine and stool cultures.
- ❑ Access intravenously by intraosseous or central route.

- ❑ Place on O_2, cardiac monitor, and pulse oximeter.

3.4 History:

- ❑ Allergies: None.
- ❑ Medications: None.
- ❑ PMH: Normal spontaneous vaginal delivery, full-term, uncomplicated pregnancy. No significant illnesses or injuries.
- ❑ Last meal: 24 hours ago.
- ❑ Family: No family history of seizures.
- ❑ Records: None.
- ❑ Immune: Up to date.
- ❑ Doctor: Family doctor is available to answer any questions.
- ❑ Social: Child lives with both parents and two siblings. Mother is unaware of the dangers of giving tap water. No indications of any social problems.

3.5 Secondary Survey:

- ❑ General: If given adequate fluid, the child will become more alert.
- ❑ Skin: Doughy, poor turgor, no lesions or petechiae.
- ❑ HEENT: Sclera nonicteric, PERRL, eyes sunken, oral mucosa dry, pharynx normal, TMs normal.
- ❑ Neck: Supple, no meningeal signs.
- ❑ Chest: Nontender to palpation.
- ❑ Lungs: Clear, no grunting, no retractions.
- ❑ Heart: Tachy rate, no murmur.
- ❑ Abdomen: Non-tender, no masses, no organomegaly.
- ❑ Perineum/GU: Normal.
- ❑ Rectal: Heme negative.
- ❑ Back: Normal.
- ❑ Extremities: Cool extremities with absence of distal pulses and delayed capillary refill.
- ❑ Neuro: No focal deficits, normal DTRs.

3.6 Laboratory:

- ❑ CBC: WBC 14, Hgb 14.1, Hct 43, Plt 225,000.
- ❑ Differential: Polys 75, Bands 3, Lymph 20, Eos 0, Mono 2.
- ❑ Chemistry: Na 115, K 3.5, Cl 80, CO_2 13.
- ❑ BUN/Cr: 56/0.9.
- ❑ Glucose: 130.
- ❑ Ca/Mg: Normal.
- ❑ LFTs: Normal.
- ❑ PT/PTT: Normal.
- ❑ ABG: pH 7.27, pO_2 98, pCO_2 30, HCO_3 14.
- ❑ Cultures: Blood/urine/stool all pending.
- ❑ U/A: RBC 0-2, WBC 0-2, Ketones 2+, Specific gravity 1.025.

3.7 X-rays:

- ❑ CXR: Normal.

3.8 Special Tests:

- ❑ CSF: RBC 0, WBC 0, Protein/glucose normal, no organisms present, bacterial antigens negative.

3.9 Critical Actions:

- ☑ Obtain vascular access via central line or interosseous.
- ☑ Start fluid bolus therapy with 0.9 NS or LR.
- ☑ Re-evaluation of VS following each bolus.
- ❑ Lumbar puncture.
- ☑ Monitor cardiac responses.
- ☑ Obtain labs.
- ☑ Obtain a history of tap water ingestion.

3.10 Pearls:

❑❑ What are the signs of shock in an infant?

Tachycardia, tachypnea, delayed capillary refill, altered mental status, and weak or absent pulses, dry mucous membranes, sunken eyes, and decreased skin turgor. Hypotension is a late sign implying at least 25% loss of intravascular volume.

❑❑ What are the indications for rapid correction of hyponatremia?

Patients with a serum sodium level of less than 110 and an acute alteration in mental status, seizures, or focal findings should have their levels raised about 4-6 mEq/dL over a few hours.

CASE 4 (Child Abuse)

Examiner

This child has been abused and the mother's story is inconsistent. She first said the child fell while at the baby-sitter's house, and then she said her child fell off the couch.

Have the mother become upset and try to take the child home. Security must detain the mother and child. A total body survey is mandatory. The child requires a social service consult and a referral to the Department of Children and Family Services.

4.1 Introduction:

A 4 year old female is brought to the ED by her mother with a complaint of left elbow pain.

Vital Signs are: BP 85/65, P 110, R 20, T 103 °F.

4.2 Primary Survey:

- ❑ General: 4 year old WN/WD female sitting quietly but not responding to questions. She appears in moderate discomfort.
- ❑ Airway: Intact.
- ❑ Breathing: Normal.
- ❑ Circulation: Normal.
- ❑ Disability: Normal.
- ❑ Exposure: Old bruises noted.

4.3 History:

- ❑ Allergies: None.
- ❑ Medication: None.
- ❑ PMH: Mother describes patient as "sickly," "she hasn't been well a day in her life." The patient was born 4 weeks premature and had a cleft palate.
- ❑ Last meal : 2 hours ago.
- ❑ Family: Noncontributory.
- ❑ Records: Old records indicate a sibling died 2 years ago secondary to an unexplained skull fracture. The patient has had many ED visits for multiple different problems.
- ❑ Immune: Up to date.
- ❑ Doctor: The mother says she fired her last pediatrician and is looking for another one.
- ❑ Social: The mother states she has no job, no money, and is late on her rent payment. The patient was born out of wedlock and she has no family support. The child has been crying excessively for two days prior to the accident.

4.4 Secondary Survey:

- ❑ General: Patient doesn't speak and sits close to mom.
- ❑ Skin: Bruise presents to left buttocks, approximately 1 to 2 weeks old.
- ❑ HEENT: The left TM is red and bulging. Remainder of the exam is normal.
- ❑ Neck: Normal.
- ❑ Chest: Normal.
- ❑ Lungs: Normal.
- ❑ Heart: Normal.
- ❑ Abdomen: Normal.
- ❑ Perineum/GU: Normal.
- ❑ Rectal: Normal.
- ❑ Back: Two small bruises to the right scapular area, 7 to 10 days old.
- ❑ Extremities: The left elbow is swollen and tender, including the distal half of the humerus. Pulse and sensation are normal but passive flexion and extension at the elbow is limited.
- ❑ Neuro: Normal.

4.5 Laboratory:

- ❑ CBC: WBC 8, Hgb 14, Hct 48, Plt 300,000.
- ❑ Chemistry: Na 140, K 4, Cl 101, CO_2 24.
- ❑ BUN/Cr: 12/1.0.

- ❑ Glucose: 95.
- ❑ Ca/Mg: Normal.
- ❑ LFTs: Normal.
- ❑ PT/PTT: Normal.
- ❑ U/A: Normal.

4.6 X-rays:

- ❑ Elbow: There is an oblique fracture through the supracondylar area 2 cm proximal to the epiphysis of the capitellum. The radial head is intact and a posterior fat pad is present.
- ❑ Baby gram: Total body radiographic survey reveals multiple old healed fractures of the ribs with the skull and other long bones being normal.

4.7 Critical Actions:

- ☑ Identify a fractured humerus.
- ☑ Obtain a social history to identify risk factors associated with child abuse.
- ☑ Obtain a complete radiographic evaluation (total body).
- ☑ Admit with consultation of a pediatrician and social worker.
- ☑ File a report with the Department of Children and Family Services.
- ❑ Obtain help from hospital security if the mother and child attempt to leave.

4.8 Pearls:

❑❑ What is the most common cause of death in children suffering child abuse?

Intracranial injuries. One sixth of survivors suffer significant neurologic sequelae.

❑❑ What is the significance of retinal hemorrhages in children under 2 years of age?

They are pathognomonic for a subdural hematoma secondary to severe shaking by the caretaker. These children are too small to participate in activities which could produce significant head trauma.

CASE 5 (Digoxin Toxicity)

Examiner

This patient has severe digoxin toxicity with stable bradycardia. The toxicity has occurred over a long period of time. The patient refuses to answer questions. However, her family states that the patient has been experiencing nausea, vomiting, blurred vision, loss of appetite, lethargy, increasing confusion, and mild respiratory difficulty.

The candidate should give Digibind and admit the patient to the ICU. The family doctor will try to persuade the candidate to admit to a general medical floor.

5.1 Introduction:

A 70 year old female presents with poor appetite, nausea, vomiting, and blurred vision. The patient is accompanied by her family.

Vital Signs are: BP 130/94, P 52 irregular, R 22, T 98.2 °F.

5.2 Primary Survey:

- ❑ General: Uncooperative 70 year old female is alert, slightly tachypneic and is in no obvious distress.
- ❑ Airway: Intact.
- ❑ Breathing: Bilateral crackles in both bases.
- ❑ Circulation: Pulses diminished, capillary refill normal.
- ❑ Disability: Pupils equal and reactive, disoriented.
- ❑ Finger: Rectal normal.

5.3 Management:

- ❑ Start IV, O_2, and place on cardiac monitor.

5.4 History:

- ❑ Allergies: None.
- ❑ Medication: Furosemide, 40 mg q A.M., Digoxin, 0.25 mg once a day, and an unknown blood pressure pill.
- ❑ PMH: Hypertension, acute myocardial infarction 3 years ago with angioplasty, status/post cholecystectomy 20 years ago.
- ❑ Last meal: 10 hours ago.
- ❑ Events: The patient refuses to answer questions. Family states patient has become more dependent and detached for the past 4 to 6 weeks. Over the past 4 days the patient has been experiencing nausea, vomiting, blurred vision, loss of appetite, lethargy, increasing confusion, and mild respiratory difficulty.
- ❑ Family: Non-contributory.
- ❑ Records: None.
- ❑ Immune: Up to date.
- ❑ Doctor: The family physician is available for admission and consultation.
- ❑ Social: The patient's husband died of colon cancer 1 year ago. She lives with her daughter.

5.5 Secondary Survey:

- ❑ General: Patient is resistant to questioning and is becoming more confused.
- ❑ Skin: Warm, dry, no rash.
- ❑ HEENT: PERRLA, fundi normal.
- ❑ Neck: No JVD, No bruits.
- ❑ Chest: Normal.
- ❑ Lungs: Crackles in both bases.
- ❑ Heart: RRR normal S1, S2, S3 present. Grade II-VI systolic murmur present.
- ❑ Abdomen: Old well healed scar, otherwise normal.
- ❑ Pelvic: Normal.

- ❑ Rectal: Normal.
- ❑ Back: Normal.
- ❑ Extremities: Normal and equal pulses.

5.6 Laboratory:

- ❑ CBC: WBC 9.6, Hgb 12.1, Hct 38, Plt 220,000.
- ❑ Chemistry: Na 140, K 2.3, Cl 110, CO_2 30.
- ❑ BUN/Cr: 40/2.6.
- ❑ Glucose: 105.
- ❑ Ca/Mg: 5.2/1.8.
- ❑ LFTs: Normal.
- ❑ Amylase/Lipase: Normal.
- ❑ PT/PTT: Normal.
- ❑ Cardiac enzymes: Normal
- ❑ ABG: pH 7.39, pO_2 69, pCO_2 33, HCO_3 28.
- ❑ U/A: Normal.
- ❑ Digoxin: 10.5 ng/mL; (normal = 0.8-2.0 ng/mL).

5.7 X-rays:

- ❑ CXR: Mild pulmonary vascular congestion with cardiomegaly.

5.8 Special Test:

- ❑ ECG: Sinus bradycardia without ectopy.

5.9 Critical Actions:

- ❑ Obtain history from family.
- ☑ Obtain a potassium level.
- ☑ Place on monitor.
- ❑ Obtain a digoxin level.
- ☑ Give Digibind.
- ☑ Admit to the ICU.
- ☑ Start IV or po KCl.

5.10 Pearls:

❑❑ What are the common cardiac rhythm disturbances seen in digoxin toxicity?

PVCs are the most common arrhythmia seen. Others include sinus bradycardia, AV blocks, PAT with block, junctional tachycardia, ventricular tachycardia, ventricular fibrillation, and atrial fibrillation. Atrial flutter is uncommon.

❑❑ What conditions contribute to digoxin toxicity?

Advanced age, hypoxia, myocardial ischemia, renal impairment, hypothyroidism, hypokalemia, hypomagnesemia, and hypercalcemia.

CASE 6 (Multiple Trauma)

Examiner

This patient has multiple problems that could result in death. According to the EMTs, the patient was found outside of the car, unrestrained, with the car embedded into a tree. No other information is available and no identification was found at the scene.

The candidate should identify these problems in a systematic fashion, and treat them. Aggressive fluid resuscitation is required, and O negative blood should be started. Allow the patient to go to CT with a nurse only if appropriate fluids have been given.

6.1 Introduction:

A 20 year old unresponsive male is brought in by paramedics secondary to an MVA. The patient was unrestrained and was found outside a vehicle. The vehicle was severely damaged as a result of crashing into a tree.

Vital Signs are: BP 80/40, P 120, R 6.

6.2 Primary Survey:

- ❑ General: WN/WD male, unresponsive, in respiratory distress, with a cervical collar and spine board applied.
- ❑ Airway : Airway is patent but trismus is present.
- ❑ Breathing: Agonal, no paradoxical movement of the chest wall.
- ❑ Circulation: Pulses diminished in all four extremities.
- ❑ Disability: No eye opening or verbal response. Patient responds to pain with decorticate (flexion) posturing.
- ❑ Exposure: No other obvious signs of trauma.
- ❑ Finger: Rectal normal, pelvis stable, and no mid-face fractures.

6.3 Management:

- ❑ Intubate and check for placement.
- ❑ Perform a rapid sequence intubation by using appropriate medications.
- ❑ Initiate two large bore IVs with rapid infusion of 2 L of NS or LR.
- → ❑ Start O negative blood. Type and cross for 4 units of PRBCs.
- ❑ Insert a Foley catheter and a OG tube after appropriate exam.
- ❑ Administer tetanus, 0.5 cc IM.
- ❑ Obtain an ABG and correct the high pCO_2 by hyperventilating the patient.
- ❑ Perform DPL for abdomen.
- ❑ If DPL is positive and volume resuscitation improves, obtain a CT. Ensure that a nurse accompanies the patient to CT exam.

6.4 History:

- ❑ Allergies: Unknown.
- ❑ Medications: Unknown.

- ❑ PMH: Unknown.
- ❑ Last meal: Unknown.
- ❑ Family: Unable to contact any family members and paramedics have to leave on another call.
- ❑ Records: None.
- ❑ Immune: Unknown.
- ❑ Narcotics: Unknown.
- ❑ Doctor: Unknown.
- ❑ Social history: Unknown.

6.5 Secondary Survey:

- ❑ General: Patient remains unresponsive, blood pressure increases if 2 L are given. Temperature is 95 °F rectal if the candidate requests it.
- ❑ Skin: Multiple bruises to the head, face, chest, and abdomen.
- ❑ HEENT: Large left parietal scalp hematoma. Left pupil is 8 mm with the right at 4 mm, both nonreactive. TMs clear and the nose and oropharynx are normal.
- ❑ Neck: Immobilized, trachea midline, no distended veins.
- ❑ Chest: No crepitance to palpation. No paradoxical movement.
- ❑ Lungs: Unequal breath sounds with bagging.
- ❑ Heart: Tachycardia without a murmur or rub.
- ❑ Abdomen: Decreased bowel sounds, firm, distended, with bruising in the right upper quadrant.
- ❑ Pelvis: Stable, no crepitance.
- ❑ Rectal: Normal prostate, no gross blood.
- ❑ Back: Normal.
- ❑ Extremities: No deformities and pulses are weak but equal.
- ❑ Neuro: GCS 3. Patient paralyzed for intubation, unable to perform a complete exam.

6.6 Laboratory:

- ❑ CBC: WBC 17, Hgb 9.0, Hct 25, Plt 250,000.
- ❑ Chemistry: Na 138, K 3.8, Cl 102, CO_2 22.
- ❑ BUN/Cr: 16/0.9.
- ❑ Glucose: 106.
- ❑ Ca/Mg: Normal.
- ❑ LFTs: Normal.
- ❑ Amylase/Lipase: Normal.
- ❑ PT/PTT: Normal.
- ❑ Cardiac enzymes: Normal.
- ❑ ETOH: 220.
- ❑ Toxicology: Negative.
- ❑ ABG #1: Post intubation pH 7.32, pO_2 300, pCO_2 42, HCO_3 18, FIO_2 100%.
- ❑ ABG #2: After increasing rate pH 7.39, $p0_2$ 350, pCO_2 28, HCO_3 17.
- ❑ U/A: Negative for blood.

6.7 X-rays:

- ❑ CXR: 50% right pneumothorax. Normal mediastinum.
- ❑ C-Spine: Normal.

- ❑ Pelvis: Normal.
- ❑ CT Head: Large epidural hematoma at the left parietal lobe with a moderate midline shift.
- ❑ CT Abd/Pelvis: Moderate sized liver laceration with free fluid present in the abdomen.

6.8 Special Tests:

- ❑ ECG: Sinus tachycardia, otherwise normal.

6.9 Management:

- ❑ Rapid insertion of a chest tube.
- ❑ Consult neurosurgery and a general or trauma surgeon.
- ❑ Continue to monitor vital signs.

6.10 Critical Actions:

- ❑ Intubate and hyperventilate.
- ❑ Administer 2 L fluid bolus with warm NS or LR.
- ❑ Identify pneumothorax and chest tube placement.
- ❑ Consult neurosurgery for drainage of the epidural hematoma.
- ❑ Consult general surgery for repair of the liver laceration.
- ❑ Ensure that a nurse accompanies the patient to CT scan.

6.11 Pearls:

❑❑ What are the causes of an epidural hematoma and what is the characteristic CT finding?

An epidural hematoma is usually due to a skull fracture over the temporal area causing a laceration to the middle meningeal artery. An epidural may be due to a dural sinus tear or bleeding through a fracture from the calvarial diploe. However, the latter case is rare. CT scan demonstrates a focal, smooth-margined, biconvex high-density accumulation adjacent to the inner table with the frequent occurrence of a mass effect.

❑❑ Describe the complications associated with insertion of a chest tube.

Damage to the intercostal nerve, artery, and vein. Laceration or puncture of intrathoracic and/or abdominal organs. Incorrect tube position, extra or intrathoracically. Damage to the internal mammary vessels resulting in a hemopneumothorax. Infection, hematoma, subcutaneous emphysema, and a persistent pneumothorax may be exhibited.

CASE 7 (Triple)

Patient #1 (Henoch-Schonlein's Purpura)

Examiner

The first patient finished breakfast and began experiencing abdominal pain. The pain is sharp, generalized, without radiation. She is nauseated with one episode of vomiting but it is not accompanied with diarrhea or constipation. Her last bowel movement occurred today and was "normal." She does not complain of fever, chills, dysuria, hematuria, or urinary frequency.

It is not mandatory to obtain the diagnosis of Henoch-Schonlein purpura (HSP). Children with mild symptoms can be safely managed as outpatients but this patient's pediatrician is out of town so admit for observation. The work-up of Patient #1 can be interrupted and the other two patients can be completely treated and dispositioned first.

7.1 Introduction: (Patient #1)

A 6 year old female presents to the ED with a complaint of abdominal pain. She is carried in by her father and her mother is present also.

Vital signs are: BP 97/62, P 110, R 22, T 101.8 °F, Wt 21 kg.

7.2 Primary Survey:

- ❑ General: WN/WD 6 year old female in no acute distress. She is smiling and joking with her parents.
- ❑ Airway: Intact.
- ❑ Breathing: Normal.
- ❑ Circulation: Normal.
- ❑ Disability: Normal.
- ❑ Finger : Deferred to secondary survey.

7.3 History:

- ❑ Allergies: None.
- ❑ Medication: None.
- ❑ PMH: No illnesses or surgeries.
- ❑ Last meal: Patient ate breakfast 5 hours ago but vomited. She has not eaten since.
- ❑ Family: Noncontributory.
- ❑ Records: None.
- ❑ Immune: Up to date.
- ❑ Doctor: The patient's pediatrician has called twice before she ever arrived to the ED. She is available for information but will be unable to admit due to being out of town.
- ❑ Social: No risk factors for child abuse. She lives with both natural parents and an 8 year old brother.

7.4 Management:

- ❑ Order appropriate labs and X-rays.
- ❑ Consider calling the pediatrician early in the work-up.

Before completing the exam, the nurse asks you to see another patient who is in severe pain.

Patient #2 (HF Acid Burn)

Examiner

This is a simple case of a hydrofluoric acid (HF) burn to the hand. He can be completely worked up and dispositioned without interruption. If the candidate takes too long, have the third patient arrive, who requires immediate attention. Regardless of the disposition, close follow-up (within 12 to 24 hours) by a plastic/hand surgeon is required.

7.1 Introduction: (Patient #2)

A 45 year old male presents with a complaint of pain to the digits of his left hand.

Vital Signs are: BP 122/75, P 112, R 16, T 98.8 °F.

7.2 Primary Survey:

- ❑ General: A 45 year old male is sitting upright on the cart. He is in moderate discomfort, cooperative, but is in no obvious distress.
- ❑ Airway: Intact.
- ❑ Breathing: Normal.
- ❑ Circulation: Normal.
- ❑ Disability: Normal.

7.3 History:

- ❑ Allergies: None.
- ❑ Medication: None.
- ❑ PMH: No significant illnesses or injuries. No past surgeries.
- ❑ Last meal: 2 hours ago.
- ❑ Events : Patient states that while at work his fingers started to burn. He denies trauma but says he works with many different chemicals of unknown composition.
- ❑ Family : The employer is available by phone and states the patient spilled hydrofluoric acid on his work bench approximately 4 hours ago. He reported the spill but denied cutaneous exposure at that time. The employer also states that the patient was reprimanded earlier for not wearing gloves when working with hazardous material.
- ❑ Records: None.
- ❑ Immune: Up to date.
- ❑ Narcotics: Denies illicit drug use.
- ❑ Doctor: Occupational physician is available for consultation or information.
- ❑ Social: No alcohol or tobacco use.

7.4 Secondary Survey:

- ❑ General: Unchanged.
- ❑ Skin: Erythema, swelling, and blistering present on the dorsal and volar aspects of the distal phalanges of the left hand.
- ❑ HEENT: Normal.
- ❑ Neck: Normal.
- ❑ Chest: Normal.
- ❑ Lungs: Normal.
- ❑ Heart: Normal.

- ❑ Abdomen: Normal.
- ❑ Perineum/GU: Normal.
- ❑ Rectal: Deferred.
- ❑ Back: Normal.
- ❑ Extremities: Pulses equal, capillary refill is normal, full range of motion with associated pain is present to all digits of the left hand.
- ❑ Neuro: Normal.

7.5 Laboratory:

- ❑ None required, but if ordered all will be normal.

7.6 X-rays:

- ❑ Left hand: Normal.

7.7 Management:

- ❑ Wash the hand with large volumes of water.
- ❑ Subcutaneously inject 10% calcium gluconate into the affected areas.
- ❑ Give IV or po pain medications.
- ❑ Call a plastic/hand surgeon and admit or arrange follow-up (within 12 to 24 hours).

The nurse informs you that a new patient is in room 3 with a complaint of chest pain.

Patient #3 (Inferior Myocardial Infarction)

Examiner

This patient is having an acute inferior myocardial infarction. The patient states that his chest pain started 4 hours ago while sitting in a chair. The pain is "pressure like" with radiation to the neck and left arm. He has vomited twice and feels "light-headed". The pain has not gone away since the onset of the episode.

The candidate should confirm there are no absolute contraindications for thrombolytic therapy and start the infusion. A cardiologist should be consulted, and a heparin and nitroglycerin drip started (there is no cardiac catheterization lab available).

7.1 Introduction: (Patient #3)

A 65 year old male presents via ambulance with a complaint of chest pain and nausea.

Vital Signs are: BP 150/70, P 62, R 20, T 98.6 °F.

7.2 Primary Survey:

- ❑ General: A 65 year old male is sitting on the cart. He is pale, diaphoretic and in acute distress.
- ❑ Airway: Intact.

- ❑ Breathing: Tachypneic and labored. Speaking in full sentences.
- ❑ Circulation: Normal.
- ❑ Disability : Normal.
- ❑ Exposure: Medic alert tag with “Diabetes” on it.
- ❑ Finger : Heme negative otherwise, normal.

7.3 Management:

- ❑ Initiate two IVs and O_2 at 4-6 L. Place on pulse oximeter and cardiac monitor.
- ❑ Pain relief with sublingual nitroglycerin or morphine sulfate.
- ❑ Order appropriate labs, X-rays, and an ECG.

7.4 History:

- ❑ Allergies: Sulfa.
- ❑ Medication: Glipizide, 10 mg po bid, and Procardia, XL 60 mg po q day.
- ❑ PMH: Diabetes and hypertension.
- ❑ Last meal: 10 hours ago.
- ❑ Family: Father died of a “heart attack” when he was 50 years old. His wife is in the waiting room.
- ❑ Records: None.
- ❑ Immune: Up to date.
- ❑ EMTs: No other information to add.
- ❑ Narcotics: No illicit drug use.
- ❑ Doctor : The patient’s family physician is available for consultation and information about the patient.
- ❑ Social history: Married with four children and 6 grandchildren. He has smoked one pack per day for 40 years. Denies alcohol use.

7.5 Secondary Survey:

- ❑ General: Patient feels better with O_2 and is breathing easier.
- ❑ Skin: Pale, cool, moist.
- ❑ HEENT: Normal.
- ❑ Neck: No JVD or bruits.
- ❑ Chest: Normal.
- ❑ Lungs: Normal.
- ❑ Heart: RRR without a murmur or S3, S4.
- ❑ Abdomen: Soft, non-tender, no pulsatile mass, no organomegaly.
- ❑ Perineum/GU: Normal.
- ❑ Rectal: Normal tone, hemoccult negative.
- ❑ Back: Normal.
- ❑ Extremities: No edema, pulses equal.
- ❑ Neuro: Normal.

7.6 Laboratory:

- ❑ CBC: WBC 12, Hgb 15.0, Hct 42.4, Plt 220,000.
- ❑ Differential: Normal.

- ❑ Chemistry: Na 134, K 4.1, Cl 101, CO_2 23.
- ❑ BUN/Cr: 12/1.0.
- ❑ Glucose: 450.
- ❑ Ca/Mg: Normal.
- ❑ LFTs: Normal.
- ❑ Amylase/Lipase: Normal.
- ❑ PT/PTT: Normal.
- ❑ Cardiac enzymes: CPK 212, LDH 160, MB pending.
- ❑ ABG: pH 7.40, pO_2 80, pCO_2 40, HCO_3 24 (room air).
- ❑ U/A: Normal.

7.7 X-rays:

- ❑ CXR: Normal.

7.8 Special Tests:

- ❑ Cardiac monitor: Normal sinus rhythm without ectopy.
- ❑ Pulse oximeter: 90% on room air; 97% on 4-6 L of O_2..
- ❑ ECG: Acute ST-segment elevation in leads II, III, and AVF with reciprocal changes.

7.9 Management:

- ❑ Confirm the absence of contraindications for lytic therapy.
- ❑ Start thrombolytics.
- ❑ Consult cardiology.
- ❑ Administer aspirin po.
- ❑ Administer heparin and nitroglycerin IV.

Patient #1 (HSP)

7.5 Secondary Survey:

- ❑ General: Unchanged.
- ❑ Skin: There is a symmetric rash on the buttocks, posterior thighs, and lower legs. The rash is a maculopapular, erythematous, urticarial and blanches upon application of pressure. Some areas have turned into palpable, purpuric lesions that do not blanch. The size varies from 3 mm to several centimeters in diameter.
- ❑ HEENT: Normal.
- ❑ Neck: Supple, no Kernig's or Brudzinski's sign. No nodes.
- ❑ Chest: Normal.
- ❑ Lungs: Normal.
- ❑ Heart: Normal.
- ❑ Abdomen: Soft with mild tenderness diffusely; Bowel sounds are present, no masses, no rebound or guarding, no organomegaly.
- ❑ Perineum/GU: Normal.
- ❑ Rectal: Hemoccult positive stool otherwise, normal.
- ❑ Back: Normal.

- ❑ Extremities: Both knees have small effusions without redness or warmth. The patient has full range of motion of all joints but cries and limps when she tries to walk.
- ❑ Neuro: Normal.

7.6 Laboratory:

- ❑ CBC: WBC 16, Hgb 14, Hct 42, Plt 400,000.
- ❑ Differential: Polys 65, Bands 10, Lymphs 20, Eos 10, Mono 3.
- ❑ Chemistry: Na 139, K 4.2, Cl 101, CO_2 25.
- ❑ BUN/Cr : 10/0.6.
- ❑ Glucose: 96.
- ❑ Ca/Mg: Normal.
- ❑ LFTs: Normal.
- ❑ Amylase/Lipase: Normal.
- ❑ PT / PTT: Normal.
- ❑ Sed rate: 30.
- ❑ Blood cultures: Pending.
- ❑ U/A: Blood 3+, protein 2+, RBC 50/hpf, WBC 0, specific gravity 1.021.

7.7 X-rays:

- ❑ CXR: Normal.
- ❑ Abd series: Normal.
- ❑ Both knees: Normal.

7.8 Management:

If the diagnosis of Henoch-Schonlein purpura (HSP) is in doubt, admit for observation and further work-up. Children with mild symptoms can safely be observed as outpatients as long as an experienced primary care provider is available. However, this patient should be admitted for observation because her physician is out of town. The arthritis is easily treated with aspirin. Corticosteroids are of no benefit for skin and kidney complications of this disorder.

7.9 Critical Actions:

- ❑ Admit this patient for observation because her physician is not immediately available.
- ❑ Complete history and physical exam.
- ❑ Check platelets.
- ❑ Obtain kidney function tests.
- ❑ Obtain urine for analysis.
- ❑ Recognize the multisystem nature of the patient's problem.

7.10 Pearls: (Patient #1)

❑❑ What is the cause of Henoch-Schonlein's purpura?

The cause is unknown. It is believed that "something" elicits an allergic reaction which results in deposition of antibody-antigen complexes in the small vessels of the skin, synovium, kidney, and bowel leading to a vasculitis.

❑❑ What are the potential complications of HSP?

Chronic renal failure is the most common and serious complication with gastrointestinal hemorrhage and intussusception occurring less frequently.

Patient #2 (HF Acid Burn)

7.8 <u>Critical Actions</u>:

❑ Obtain a history of HF acid exposure.
❑ Treat with calcium gluconate.
❑ Call a plastic or hand surgeon and arrange a follow up in 12 to 24 hours.

7.9 <u>Pearls</u>: (Patient #2)

❑❑ Can calcium chloride be used for local infiltration?

No. Calcium chloride produces direct injury when injected into tissues.

❑❑ What metabolic abnormalities occurs with systemic HF poisoning?

Metabolic acidosis, severe hypocalcemia (due to the complexing of calcium by fluoride ions), hypomagnesemia, and hyperkalemia.

Patient #3 (Inferior Myocardial Infarction)

7.10 <u>Critical Actions</u>:

❑ Initial treatment with O_2, monitor, NTG, or morphine for pain.
❑ Start nitroglycerin drip.
❑ Administer heparin bolus and hourly infusion.
❑ Talk with a cardiologist.
❑ Evaluate for absolute contraindications to thrombolytic therapy.
❑ Start thrombolytic therapy.
❑ Admit to the CCU.

7.11 <u>Pearls</u>: (Patient #3)

❑❑ What is the clinical presentation in a patient with a right ventricular (RV) infarction?

Hypotension, jugular venous distention, clear lungs and Kussmaul's sign are seen. RV infarcts are due to a total occlusion of the right coronary artery and are present in 20 to 40% of patients with an inferior myocardial infarction.

❑❑ What are the ECG criteria for thrombolytic therapy?

One or more of the following: 1) $\geq$ 1 mm ST-segment elevation in $\geq$ 2 contiguous limb leads, 2) $\geq$ 2 mm ST-segment elevation in $\geq$ 2 contiguous precordial leads, 3) New left bundle branch block in context of symptoms consistent with infarction.

CASE 8 (Cardiac Arrest)

Examiner

This patient is in full cardiopulmonary arrest. His wife states that her husband was doing well, ate lunch, and walked upstairs to bed. She discovered him there, not breathing.

The candidate should give appropriate telemetry orders and follow ACLS guidelines when the patient arrives. Once asystole has occurred the candidate should verify this, terminate the code, and inform the family.

8.1 Introduction:

A telemetry calls from the paramedics: "We have a 60 year old male unresponsive for 5 minutes prior to our arrival. At this time he is in full cardiopulmonary arrest and we are unable to intubate or start an IV. Our estimated time of arrival is 5 minutes."

8.2 Management:

- ❑ Instruct the paramedics to initiate CPR.
- ❑ Deliver O_2 at 100% by a bag-valve-mask system.
- ❑ Order a rhythm strip sent, interpret this as ventricular fibrillation and order immediate defibrillation at 200 joules.

The patient arrives to the department with his wife and paramedics. They inform you they defibrillated at 200, 300, and 360 joules.

Vital Signs are: BP 0, P 0, R 0, T 97.0 °F.

8.3 Primary Survey:

- ❑ General: This patient is an obese 60 year old male, cyanotic and he is in cardiopulmonary arrest.
- ❑ Airway: Airway is clear.
- ❑ Breathing: No spontaneous respirations.
- ❑ Circulation: No pulses, no dependent lividity.
- ❑ Disability : Pupils fixed and dilated, GCS 3.
- ❑ Exposure: No medic alert tags; Atraumatic skin.
- ❑ Finger: Rectal heme negative, normal prostate.

8.4 Management:

- ❑ Quick look with the defib paddles.
- ❑ Recognize V-fib and immediately defibrillate with 360 joules.
- ❑ Intubate.
- ❑ Start two IVs.
- ❑ Continue CPR and follow ACLS protocol.
- ❑ Place the patient on a cardiac monitor and pulse oximeter.

8.5 History:

- ❑ Allergies: Sulfa.
- ❑ Medication: Capoten, 25 mg po tid, Propranolol, 40 mg po tid, nitroglycerin, SL prn chest pain.
- ❑ PMH: Hypertension, angina, gout. No surgeries or hospitalizations.
- ❑ Family: A younger brother died last year from an acute myocardial infarction.
- ❑ Records: None.
- ❑ Immune: Up to date.
- ❑ Narcotics: No history of illicit drug use.
- ❑ Doctor: His family physician is available for consultation.
- ❑ Social history: Patient is a local police officer. He is married with four children and three grand children. He smokes two packs of cigarettes per day for 45 years but he does not consume alcohol.

8.6 Secondary Survey:

- ❑ General: No change in the patient's status.
- ❑ Skin: Cyanosis present; No bruises, abrasions or lacerations.
- ❑ HEENT: Normocephalic and atraumatic head. ET tube in place. Pupils remained fixed and dilated.
- ❑ Chest: Rises and falls equally when bagged.
- ❑ Lungs: Breath sounds equal but not spontaneous.
- ❑ Heart: No heart sounds. Unable to palpate a PMI.
- ❑ Abdomen: Obese, distended, no bowel sounds.
- ❑ Perineum/GU: Normal.
- ❑ Rectal: No sphincter tone, heme negative.
- ❑ Back: Normal.
- ❑ Extremities: No pulses, 3+ pitting edema to the lower legs.
- ❑ Neuro: GCS 3, toes equivocal. No DTRs.

8.7 Management:

- ❑ The rhythm decompensates to asystole.
- ❑ Check for proper lead placement and confirm asystole in two contiguous leads.
- ❑ Confirm the absence of vital signs and terminate the code.
- ❑ Inform the family.

8.8 Critical Actions:

- ☑ Recognize V-fib in the field and defibrillate.
- ☑ Use appropriate ACLS protocol for V-fib.
- ☑ Establish an airway.
- ☑ Verify asystole and terminate code.
- ☑ Talk with family and offer further assistance.

8.9 Pearls:

❑❑ What is the mechanism of action of nitroglycerin?

Nitroglycerin is a smooth muscle dilator resulting in dilatation of large coronary arteries and veins.

This results in an increased oxygen delivery to the heart and peripheral pooling of blood, thereby decreasing venous return, ventricular filling pressure and left ventricular work.

❑❑ **How does defibrillation of a fibrillating heart work?**

Passing a current through a fibrillating heart depolarizes the cells and allows them to repolarize uniformly, thus restoring organized, coordinated contractions.

CASE 9 (Testicular Torsion)

Examiner

This patient has an acute testicular torsion which requires immediate intervention. His lower abdominal pain started abruptly, 1 hour ago while running in gym class. The pain is constant, severe, and starts in the right lower quadrant radiating to the right testicle. Associated nausea, vomiting, anorexia, and normal bowel pattern are also evident. A similar episode occurred two days ago but was not as intense, and resolved spontaneously.

His parents are not present but care should still be given. The urologist is unavailable for 30 to 45 minutes so obtain a scan to secure the diagnosis after talking with him. When results are obtained, immediately call the urologist back and he will allow the patient to be sent to the OR. The parents arrive before the patient goes to the OR and sign the consent form.

9.1 Introduction:

A 15 year old male patient presents with acute abdominal pain. He is accompanied by his high school coach and you are unable to locate his parents.

Vital Signs are: BP 130/92, P 116, R 30, T 99.6 °F, Wt 145 lbs.

9.2 Primary Survey:

- ❑ General: The patient is a WN/WD male, pale, diaphoretic, in severe discomfort.
- ❑ Airway: Intact.
- ❑ Breathing: Normal.
- ❑ Circulation: Normal.
- ❑ Disability: Normal.
- ❑ Exposure: No medic alert tags.
- ❑ Finger: Normal rectal exam.

9.3 History:

- ❑ Allergies: None.
- ❑ Medications: None.
- ❑ PMH: No hospitalizations or surgeries.
- ❑ Last meal: 4 hours ago.
- ❑ Family: Noncontributory.

- ❑ Records: None.
- ❑ Immune: Up to date.
- ❑ Narcotics: No illicit drug use.
- ❑ Doctor: None.
- ❑ Social: Patient is not sexually active. No alcohol or tobacco use.

9.4 <u>Secondary Survey</u>:

- ❑ General: If medicated, patient is more comfortable but still in pain.
- ❑ Skin: Normal.
- ❑ HEENT: Normal.
- ❑ Neck: Supple, no nodes.
- ❑ Chest: Normal.
- ❑ Lungs: Normal.
- ❑ Heart: Normal.
- ❑ Abdomen: Unable to fully evaluate due to diffuse guarding. Bowel sounds are present, no point tenderness, no organomegaly.
- ❑ Perineum/GU: The scrotum appears tense and slightly edematous. The right testicle is very tender and difficult to examine. The epididymis and cord cannot be localized as the source of pain. The cremasteric reflex is absent, the testicle is elevated and is in a horizontal position.
- ❑ Rectal: Normal.
- ❑ Back: No CVA tenderness.
- ❑ Extremities: No edema.
- ❑ Neuro: Normal.

9.5 <u>Management</u>:

- ❑ Immediately consult a urologist (who states he will be in the OR another 30 to 45 minutes).
- ❑ Obtain a duplex color Doppler ultrasound.
- ❑ Keep the patient NPO.
- ❑ Obtain appropriate labs.
- ❑ Try to contact his parents.
- ❑ Start IV.
- ❑ Give pain medication.

9.6 <u>Laboratory</u>:

- ❑ CBC: WBC 15,000, Hgb 14.5, Hct 44, Plt 250,000.
- ❑ Chemistry: Normal.
- ❑ BUN/Cr: 13/0.9.
- ❑ Glucose: 98.
- ❑ Ca/Mg: Normal.
- ❑ LFTs: Normal.
- ❑ Amylase/Lipase: Normal.
- ❑ PT/PTT: Normal.
- ❑ U/A: Normal.

9.7 Special Tests:

❑ Testicular scan: Normal arterial flow to the left testicle with markedly diminished flow to the right testicle noted.

9.8 Critical Actions:

❑ Attempt to contact parents but do not delay care while seeking consent.
❑ Recognize right testicular tenderness.
❑ Suspect testicular torsion and consult urology before obtaining a testicular scan.
❑ Obtain a U/A.
❑ Prepare the patient for surgery.
❑ Attempt manual detorsion.
❑ Provide pain relief.

9.9 Pearls:

❑❑ What is the utility of the radionuclide scan and Doppler ultrasound in the diagnosis of testicular torsion?

The radionuclide scan involves the injection of a radioactive substance and documentation of this substance in the testis, thus demonstrating arterial flow. It has a 90% to 100% accuracy rate in determining testicular blood flow. This exam is invasive, time-consuming, and reader dependent while providing little anatomic information. Duplex color Doppler ultrasonography is the diagnostic test of choice with a sensitivity approaching 100%. It provides information on both anatomy and arterial perfusion, is noninvasive, and quicker to obtain. These studies are truly adjunctive and in no way should preclude or delay surgical exploration once the diagnosis of testicular torsion is suspected.

❑❑ What are the limits of viability for a torsed testicle?

A 100% salvage rate is seen with detorsion within 6 hours after onset of pain. Beyond 12 hours, the rate drops to 20%. After 24 hours, the salvage rate approaches zero.

CASE 10 (Carbon Monoxide Poisoning)

Examiner

The EMTs are the key to an early diagnosis. If the candidate interviews them, he/she will find out the patient lives in an old house and all the other family members have been sick with "the flu". The patient states that he developed sub-sternal chest pain while walking upstairs from the basement to his bedroom. The pain is "pressure-like" without radiation, but with associated dyspnea, nausea, and diaphoresis. He took one nitroglycerin pill after which he felt faint and passed out. He presently has some chest pain, mild dyspnea, nausea, and a severe headache.

The patient should be treated with 100% O_2 and arrangement should be made to transfer the patient to a hyperbaric chamber. The family should be instructed to present to the ED for evaluation.

10.1 Introduction:

A 60 year old male presents, via ambulance, with a complaint of chest pain, dyspnea, and fainting.

Vital Signs are: BP 160/90, P 110, R 26, T 99.2 °F.

10.2 Primary Survey:

- ❑ General: The patient is a pale, cachectic 60 year old male, diaphoretic and hyperventilating.
- ❑ Airway: Intact.
- ❑ Breathing: Tachypneic; Breath sounds distant.
- ❑ Circulation: Pulses equal and strong.
- ❑ Disability: Pupils equal and reactive, GCS 15.
- ❑ Exposure: Medic alert tag stating "Heart disease".
- ❑ Finger: Rectal normal, heme negative.

10.3 Management:

- ❑ Initiate O_2 100% nonrebreather.
- ❑ Place on cardiac monitor and pulse oximeter.
- ❑ Order appropriate labs, ECG, and CXR.
- ❑ Start IV.

10.4 History:

- ❑ Allergies: None.
- ❑ Medication: NTG prn and various inhalers.
- ❑ PMH: COPD and angina. No previous surgery.
- ❑ Last meal: 4 hours ago.
- ❑ Family: Mother and father died from a "heart attack" in their 50's.
- ❑ Records: Available along with an old ECG.
- ❑ Immune: Unknown.
- ❑ EMTs: EMTs state that according to the family everyone has been sick with "the flu".
- ❑ Narcotics: No illicit drug use.
- ❑ Doctor: The patient has a specialist in pulmonary who is available for consultation.
- ❑ Social: Patient smokes 1 pack per day and his smoking has been confined to the basement by his pregnant daughter.

10.5 Secondary Survey:

- ❑ General: Anxiety has decreased since he was placed on O_2.
- ❑ Skin: Pale, diaphoretic.
- ❑ HEENT: Normal.
- ❑ Neck: Supple without lymphadenopathy.
- ❑ Chest: Normal.
- ❑ Lungs: Decreased breath sounds bilaterally with few basilar crackles present. Slight wheezing with a prolonged expiratory phase is also noted.
- ❑ Heart: Tachycardia without an S3, S4 or murmur.

- ❑ Abdomen: Normal.
- ❑ Perineum/GU: Normal.
- ❑ Rectal: Normal.
- ❑ Back: Normal.
- ❑ Extremities: Normal.
- ❑ Neuro: Cranial nerves, motor/sensory exam, coordination, and cerebellar signs are all normal. He is oriented to person and place but thinks it is 1958. He also has lapses in short term memory.

10.6 Laboratory:

- ❑ CBC: WBC 12, Hgb 14.4, Hct 45.4, Plt 260,000.
- ❑ Chemistry: Na 138, K 4.2, Cl 101, CO_2 20.
- ❑ BUN/Cr: 18/1.4.
- ❑ Glucose: 110.
- ❑ Ca/Mg: Normal.
- ❑ LFTs: Normal.
- ❑ Amylase/Lipase: Normal.
- ❑ PT/PTT: Normal.
- ❑ Cardiac enzymes: CPK 200, LDH 230, SGOT 26, CKMB 1%.
- ❑ ABG: pH 7.39, pO_2 70, pCO_2 30, HCO_3 21, Saturation 95%.
- ❑ CO Hgb: 35%.
- ❑ U/A: Normal.

10.7 X-rays:

- ❑ CXR: Changes consistent with COPD, no acute infiltrate.

10.8 Special Tests:

- ❑ ECG: Sinus tachycardia without ectopy. No changes as compared to old ECGs.
- ❑ Cardiac monitor: Sinus tachycardia.
- ❑ Pulse oximeter: 96% on room air.

10.9 Management:

- ❑ Once the CO results are known, call the family and have them come to the ED for evaluation.
- ❑ Arrange for transfer to a hyperbaric chamber.
- ❑ Continue treating with 100% O_2 and consider administering a treatment of nebulized albuterol.

10.10 Critical Actions:

- ☑ Assess ABCs. Place on O_2, IV, and cardiac monitor.
- ☑ Interview the EMTs to determine why the whole family has the "flu".
- ☑ Obtain an ECG, ABG, and CO Hgb level.
- ☑ Recognize CO poisoning.
- ☑ Treat with 100% O_2.
- ☑ Contact family members and arrange for evaluation and testing.
- ☑ Transfer the patient to a hyperbaric chamber.

10.11 Pearls:

❑❑ **What are the indications for hyperbaric oxygen therapy in CO poisoning?**

All patients with coma or loss of consciousness, neurologic findings, ischemic chest pain (ECG changes or arrhythmias), CO Hgb level greater than 30%, and mental status changes that do not resolve after 3 hours of 100% oxygen therapy. Also consider its use for pregnant women, patients with a history of coronary artery disease, and a CO Hgb level greater than 25-30%.

❑❑ **What is the effect of 100% oxygen therapy in the treatment of CO poisoning?**

The half-life of CO is decreased to 40 to 80 minutes from about 6 hours on room air. Hyperbaric oxygen therapy decreases the elimination half-life to $\geq$ 20 minutes.

CASE 11 (Meningitis)

Examiner

This is a case of meningitis in a young female with focal neurologic deficits. Several days before admission, patient states she was suffering from a severe sore throat. This resolved but last night she started having a headache and a fever that did not subside with Tylenol.

You must order a temperature early and obtain a CT scan of the head before an LP because she has neuro deficits. The physician should start antibiotics before allowing the patient to go to the radiology department for her scan. You may use any of the appropriate approved antibiotic regimes as long as it covers the potential organisms involved. Consult a neurologist or internist and admit the patient to the intensive care unit.

11.1 Introduction:

The paramedics present with a 21 year old female with a complaint of headache and weakness.

Vital Signs are: BP 128/70, P 80, R 16.

11.2 Primary Survey:

- ❑ General: This is a WN/WD 21 year old female, appearing lethargic. However, she is arousable and is able to follow commands.
- ❑ Airway: Intact.
- ❑ Breathing: Normal.
- ❑ Circulation: Rapid full pulses. Normal capillary refill.
- ❑ Disability: Pupils equal and reactive, GCS 15.
- ❑ Exposure: Normal.
- ❑ Finger: Normal.

11.3 History:

- ❑ Allergies: None.
- ❑ Medications: None.

- ❑ PMH: No significant illnesses or surgeries. Last menstrual period 3 weeks ago.
- ❑ Last meal: 6 hours ago.
- ❑ Family: Noncontributory.
- ❑ Records: None.
- ❑ Immune: Up to date.
- ❑ Narcotics: No illicit drug use.
- ❑ Social history: No alcohol or tobacco use. She lives with her parents and attends college.

11.4 Secondary Survey:

- ❑ Temperature: 103.7 °F.
- ❑ General: Unchanged.
- ❑ Skin: Warm, dry intact, no petechiae.
- ❑ HEENT: She does not look past the midline when asked to look right. The right pupil is 2 mm larger than the left and discs are flat. Oropharynx is red without exudates.
- ❑ Neck: Rigid, no adenopathy. Positive Kernig's and Brudzinski's signs.
- ❑ Chest: Normal.
- ❑ Lungs: Clear to auscultation.
- ❑ Heart: RRR, normal S1, S2, no S3, S4.
- ❑ Abdomen: Normal.
- ❑ Perineum/GU: Normal.
- ❑ Rectal: Normal.
- ❑ Back: Normal.
- ❑ Extremities: Normal.
- ❑ Neuro: Cranial nerves - Right homonymous hemianopsia with a right facial droop, right upper extremity weakness and decreased sharp/dull discrimination to that extremity. DTRs are normal. No Babinski reflex. Unable to fully cooperate for an adequate cerebellar exam. She is oriented only to person and birthday, no dysarthria.

11.5 Laboratory:

- ❑ CBC: WBC 16.8, Hgb 12.7, Hct 36.4, Plt 250,000.
- ❑ Differential: Polys 80, Bands 46, Lymphs 15, Eos 1, Mono 4.
- ❑ Chemistry: Na 142, K 3.7, Cl 101, CO_2 24.
- ❑ BUN/Cr: 12/0.7.
- ❑ Glucose: 194.
- ❑ Ca/Mg: Normal.
- ❑ Liver Function: SGOT 21, SGPT 24, Alk Phos 60, GGTP 10, Bili 0.8.
- ❑ Amylase/Lipase: Normal.
- ❑ PT/PTT: Normal.
- ❑ ABG: pH 7.42, pCO_2 32, pO_2 97, HCO_3 23.
- ❑ U/A: Normal.

11.6 X-rays:

- ❑ CXR: Normal.
- ❑ CT head: Normal.

11.7 Special Tests:

- ❑ ECG: Normal.
- ❑ Spinal tap: Opening pressure 500, Protein 480, Glu 8, WBC 17,000, Segs 93%, Lymphs 3%, Monos 4%, RBCs 660. Gram's Stain positive for gram positive cocci with many PMNs. Latex pending.

11.8 Management:

- ❑ Start IV.
- ❑ Place on cardiac monitor and pulse oximeter.
- ❑ Administer antibiotics before CT scan.
- ❑ Perform LP.
- ❑ Admit to the ICU.
- ❑ Consult a neurologist or internist.

11.9 Critical Actions:

- ☑ Examine the neck.
- ☑ Determine temperature.
- ☑ Perform a thorough neurologic exam.
- ☑ Perform a CT before LP.
- ☑ Perform an LP.
- ☑ Administer antibiotics (given before allowing patient to go for CT scan).
- ☑ Admit to the ICU.
- ☑ Consult a neurologist or internist.

11.10 Pearls:

❑❑ What are the common bacterial pathogens that cause meningitis in this age group?

Streptococcus pneumoniae is the most common followed by *Neisseria meningitidis* and *Haemophilus influenzae.*

❑❑ Which patients are at risk for meningitis?

It most often occurs in the very young or the very old. Other individuals at risk include immunocompromised patients (HIV infected or splenectomized patients), immunosuppressed patients, alcoholics, patients with recent neurosurgical procedures, and patients with underlying infections such as pneumonia, sinusitis, mastoiditis, or otitis media.

CASE 12 (Burn)

Examiner

A man is brought in by his wife who states that the patient was burning a pile of wood approximately 10 minutes ago. A flash occurred and a gas can exploded while in his hands. He was thrown 10 feet but he is still conscious.

Immediate rapid sequence intubation is required and should be performed using in-line c-spine immobilization and appropriate medications. The candidate should administer fluids per the Parkland formula and may use the Lund and Browder chart to accurately calculate the percent of body involvement. This patient requires transfer to a burn unit.

12.1 Introduction:

A 45 year old male presents with his wife complaining of burns to the face.

Vital Signs are: BP 100/60, P 120, R 24, T 98.2 °F, Wt 80 kg.

12.2 Primary Survey:

- ❑ General: Patient is sitting upright, anxious, alert, tachypneic and is in obvious discomfort.
- ❑ Airway: Redness and swelling to the oropharynx with soot present in the nose and mouth.
- ❑ Breathing: Tachypnea with a cough present.
- ❑ Circulation: Capillary refill is delayed, all pulses are equal.
- ❑ Disability: He is alert and oriented to person, place, and time, GCS 15.
- ❑ Exposure: Second degree burns are present on the face, neck, chest, and both upper extremities.
- ❑ Finger: Rectal normal.

12.3 Management:

- ❑ Perform immediate rapid sequence intubation.
- ❑ Protect c-spine.
- ❑ Place on cardiac monitor and pulse oximeter. Start two large bore IVs.
- ❑ Use the Parkland formula to calculate fluid requirements.
- ❑ Administer tetanus prophylaxis.
- ❑ Administer pain medication and an H_2 blocker.
- ❑ Order appropriate labs and X-rays.

12.4 History:

- ❑ Allergies: None.
- ❑ Medications: None.
- ❑ PMH: No previous illnesses or injuries.
- ❑ Last meal: 1 hour ago.
- ❑ Family: Noncontributory.
- ❑ Records: None.
- ❑ Immune: 15 years ago.
- ❑ EMTs: They have no new information to add.
- ❑ Narcotics: No history of illicit drug use.
- ❑ Doctor: None.
- ❑ Social: Married with two children. No alcohol or tobacco use.

12.5 Secondary Survey:

- ❑ General: Patient paralyzed, sedated, and intubated.

- ❑ Skin: The total surface involved is approximately 20%, all of which are second-degree (deep partial-thickness) in nature. The areas include the volar aspect of each arm (hands are spared), the anterior neck, the entire face, and chest.
- ❑ HEENT: The entire face is burned. PERRLA, EOM-I, Fundi normal, conjunctiva injected. ET tube in place.
- ❑ Neck: Redness and swelling present.
- ❑ Chest: No burns present. The chest rises and falls without difficulty.
- ❑ Lungs: Coarse breath sounds bilateral.
- ❑ Heart: Tachycardia present with a regular rate and rhythm, normal S1 and S2, without a murmur.
- ❑ Abdomen: Normal.
- ❑ Back: Normal.
- ❑ Extremities: Normal.
- ❑ Neuro: Patient intubated, paralyzed, and sedated. Before intubation no focal deficits were noted.

12.6 Laboratory:

- ❑ CBC: WBC 17, Hgb 13.2, Hct 44, Plt 240,000.
- ❑ Chemistry: Na 135, K 4.5, Cl 108, CO_2 24.
- ❑ BUN/Cr: 6/1.0.
- ❑ Glucose: 150.
- ❑ Ca/Mg: Normal.
- ❑ LFTs: Normal.
- ❑ Amylase/Lipase: Normal.
- ❑ PT/PTT: Normal.
- ❑ Cardiac enzymes: Normal.
- ❑ ABG: pH 7.42, pO_2 75, pCO_2 28, HCO_3 22, (pre-intubation).
- ❑ CO Hgb: 1%, if checked.
- ❑ U/A: No myoglobin or blood.

12.7 X-rays:

- ❑ CXR: Diffuse infiltrates bilateral. Normal heart size and mediastinum.
- ❑ C-Spine: Normal.
- ❑ CT head: Normal.

12.8 Special Tests:

- ❑ ECG: Sinus tachycardia without ectopy.

12.9 Management:

- ❑ Cleanse all wounds
- ❑ Dress the burns with sterile gauze or sheets.
- ❑ Examine the cornea for burns.
- ❑ Do not apply antibiotic ointment to the burns or start parenteral antibiotics.
- ❑ You may debride blisters to prevent further damage to burned tissue.
- ❑ Hydrate via IV.
- ❑ Provide pain management.

12.10 Critical Actions:

- ☑ Perform a rapid sequence intubation.
- ☑ Correctly calculate the fluid requirements.
- ☑ Administer tetanus prophylaxis.
- ☑ Acquire pertinent history.
- ☑ Evaluate c-spine.
- ☑ Consult with and transfer to a burn unit.
- ☑ Relieve patient's pain.
- ☑ Do not expose the burns to any type of antibiotic ointment.
- ❑ Apply dry sterile dressings to burns.

12.11 Pearls:

❑❑ What conditions mandate transfer to a burn unit?

1) Major partial-thickness burns of > 25% in the 10 to 50 year old age group.
2) Major partial-thickness burns of > 20% in children younger than 10 years or in adults older than 50 years.
3) Any full-thickness burn greater than 10% of total body surface area.
4) Any burn involving the hands, face, feet, perineum, joints, circumferential in nature, associated inhalation injury or complicated by fractures or trauma.
5) Electrical burns and burns in patients who are at risk due to underlying conditions should also be considered for transfer.

❑❑ What is the role of prophylactic parenteral antibiotics?

They are not to be started in the ED.

CASE 13 (Triple)

Patient #1 (Tetanus)

Examiner

The patient states he awoke from sleep with pain, stiffness, and a muscle spasm in his neck, jaw, and shoulders. He is unable to fully open his mouth and he complains of odynophagia and dysphagia if asked. He remembers falling to the ground in the railyard about 4 days ago while on a drinking binge. As a result, he hit his left lower leg but he did not loose consciousness.

This patient is stable but the candidate should perform a complete body search for injuries. An immunization history is important. If the candidate focuses completely on a c-spine injury, have the patient complain of trismus, increasing pain, and dysphagia. Make the candidate work to get the patient into the ICU by having the consulting internist be resistant to this idea.

13.1 Introduction: (Patient #1)

A 68 year old male presents with a complaint of stiffness to the neck and jaw for 4 hours.

Vital Signs are: BP 140/82, P 110, R 30, T 98.9 °F, Wt 80 kg.

13.2 Primary Survey:

- ❑ General: Poorly nourished male presents in moderate discomfort. He moves his head, neck, and upper torso as a unit. He is not in respiratory distress.
- ❑ Airway : The airway is intact but there is midline c-spine pain to palpation.
- ❑ Breathing: Intact.
- ❑ Circulation: Intact.
- ❑ Disability: GCS 15, PERRLA.
- ❑ Exposure: No medic alert tags. If the candidate asks for skin lesions, contusions, or lacerations, make them specifically ask about the left lower leg.
- ❑ Finger: May be deferred to secondary survey.

13.3 Management:

- ❑ Initiate c-spine immobilization.
- ❑ You may order appropriate diagnostic studies now or after the history and secondary survey.
- ❑ Start IV and place the patient on a pulse oximeter and monitor.

13.4 History:

- ❑ Allergies: None.
- ❑ Medications: Procardia once a day.
- ❑ PMH: Hypertension. Hernia repair in 1980.
- ❑ Last meal: 24 hours ago.
- ❑ Family: Non-contributory, no family or friends present for information.
- ❑ Records: None.
- ❑ Immune: "Many years" since his last Td immunization.
- ❑ EMTs: N/A.
- ❑ Narcotics: No illicit drug use.
- ❑ Doctor: None.
- ❑ Social: Drinks one case of beer a day and smokes two packs of cigarettes per day.

13.5 Secondary Survey:

- ❑ General: Poorly nourished, poorly kept male who is alert but uncomfortable. He is not in respiratory distress.
- ❑ Skin: Well hydrated, 5 cm full-thickness laceration to the left lower leg at the calf. The wound edges are necrotic and red streaks are present. It is very painful to the touch.
- ❑ HEENT: Cataract in the left eye, otherwise, normal exam.
- ❑ Jaw : The patient is unable to open his mouth more than 3 cm. No palpable tenderness, TMJ crepitation, or deformity noted. There is tightness noted to the masseter and temporalis muscles.
- ❑ Neck: Paraspinal and midline tenderness is present. Negative Brudzinski's and Kernig's. Greatly diminished range of motion.
- ❑ Chest : Normal.
- ❑ Lungs: Normal.
- ❑ Heart: Normal.

- ❑ Abdomen: Normal.
- ❑ Perineum/GU: Normal.
- ❑ Rectal: Normal.
- ❑ Back: Normal.
- ❑ Extremities: Large laceration to the left lower leg at the calf. Pulses are present and equal, no edema. No crepitance. Inspection of the wound reveals an embedded sliver of wood.
- ❑ Neuro: A/O X 3, GCS 15. Cranial nerves intact. Motor and sensory exam are normal and symmetric. DTRs are brisk without clonus. Negative Trousseau's and Chvostek's signs. Toes down-going. Normal cerebellar exam.

13.6 Management:

- ☑ Don't suture the wound.
- ☑ Administer tetanus immune globulin (TIG or Hyper-TET), 500-5000 units IM.
- ☑ Administer 0.5 mL of tetanus toxoid IM.
- ☑ Treat the pain and spasm.
- ☑ Continue c-spine care until X-rays are back.
- ☑ Obtain blood and wound cultures and start antibiotics. You may use metronidazole, tetracycline, erythromycin, penicillin, or a cephalosporin.
- ❑ Administer thiamine and folic acid IV.
- ❑ Consider magnesium sulfate due to his poor nutrition and chronic alcohol abuse.

The nurse informs you that another patient is in room 2. He is upset and wants to sign out against medical advise.

Patient #2 (Exudative Pharyngitis)

Examiner

This patient has a sore throat that has been hurting for two days with the fever starting today. He also complains of headache, dysphagia, and neck pain. In addition, he is very upset because of his discomfort and his perceived long wait.

It is important that the candidate calms the patient and helps ease his discomfort. This patient may be discharged but a follow-up should be arranged.

13.1 Introduction: (Patient #2)

A 22 year old male presents with a complaint of a sore throat.

Vital Signs are: BP 120/60, P 110, R 18, T 102.3 °F.

13.2 Primary Survey:

- ❑ General: WN/WD male appearing ill and upset about waiting to be seen.
- ❑ Airway: Intact.
- ❑ Breathing: Normal.

- ❑ Circulation: Normal.
- ❑ Disability: GCS 15, PERRLA.
- ❑ Exposure: Patient refuses to disrobe.
- ❑ Finger: Deferred at this time.

13.3 Management:

- ❑ The patient is stable, labs and treatment may be deferred until completion of the history and secondary survey.

13.4 History:

- ❑ Allergies: None.
- ❑ Medications: None.
- ❑ PMH: No illnesses or injuries. No past surgeries.
- ❑ Last meal: 2 hours ago.
- ❑ Family: His wife was diagnosed with "strep" throat last week.
- ❑ Records: None.
- ❑ Immune: Up to date.
- ❑ EMTs: Not applicable.
- ❑ Narcotics: No illicit drug use.
- ❑ Doctor: None.
- ❑ Social: No alcohol or tobacco use.

13.5 Secondary Survey:

- ❑ General: The patient appears uncomfortable but more relaxed if the candidate's interaction is appropriate.
- ❑ Skin: No rash or petechiae.
- ❑ HEENT: The oropharynx is injected with enlarged palatine tonsils and exudates present. The uvula is midline with no asymmetric enlargement of the tonsils or swelling of the pharynx. PERRLA, EOM-I, TMs normal. No retropharyngeal swelling on fluctuance.
- ❑ Neck: No meningeal signs, many anterior cervical lymph nodes.
- ❑ Chest: Normal.
- ❑ Lungs: Clear.
- ❑ Heart: Tachycardia, regular rhythm, no murmur.
- ❑ Abdomen: No organomegaly.
- ❑ Perineum/GU: Appropriate to defer
- ❑ Rectal: Appropriate to defer.
- ❑ Back: Normal.
- ❑ Neuro: Intact.

13.6 Laboratory:

- ❑ CBC: WBC 17,000, Hgb 15, Hct 45, Plt 250,000.
- ❑ Chemistry: Normal.
- ❑ BUN/Cr: Normal.
- ❑ Glucose: Normal.

- ❑ LFTs: Normal.
- ❑ Monospot: Negative.
- ❑ Rapid Strep: Positive.

13.7 X-rays:

- ❑ CXR: Normal
- ❑ Lateral Neck: Normal.

13.8 Management:

- ☑ Establish good relations and convince the patient to stay.
- ☑ Treat the patient's fever with acetaminophen or ibuprofen.
- ☑ Treat with penicillin, IM or po.
- ☑ Arrange follow-up with an internist by phone or instruct to return to the ED in 1 to 2 days.

The charge nurse informs you that a "bad" trauma is in room 3.

Patient #3 (Multiple Trauma)

Examiner

This patient is unable to communicate and has sustained a bladder rupture, tibial fracture, c-spine injury, and a pelvic fracture. The patient appears pale, with shallow and sonorous respirations. He also smells of alcohol.

Rapid intubation while maintaining c-spine precaution is required. If rapid fluid resuscitation is not performed, have a nurse continually announce a BP of 80/P. Insertion of a Foley catheter before a urethrogram is a dangerous act. Have the candidate describe how to perform a urethrogram.

13.1 Introduction: (Patient #3)

The EMTs present with a 50 year old male who was struck by a car and thrown 20 feet.

Vital Signs are: BP 88/45, P 118, R 22.

13.2 Primary Survey:

- ❑ General: The patient appears pale, with shallow and sonorous respirations, smelling of alcohol.
- ❑ Airway: Responds to pain by incomprehensible "gurgling" sounds.
- ❑ Breathing: Shallow sonorous respirations, lungs clear to auscultation.
- ❑ Circulation: Pale skin, rapid and thready pulse, and delayed capillary refill.
- ❑ Disability: GCS 8. Pupils equal and reactive.
- ❑ Exposure: No medic alert tags, bruising and swelling to the left leg.
- ❑ Finger: High riding prostate, no blood per rectum. Blood at the meatus. No scrotal swelling or hematoma. Pelvis stable.

13.3 Management:

- ❑ Recognize the airway problem and perform a jaw thrust or chin lift maneuver to relieve the obstruction. Perform a rapid sequence intubation with head injury and c-spine precautions.
- ❑ Evaluate for proper placement of the ETT.
- ❑ Recognize shock and treat with 2 large bore IVs, infusing 2 L of LR or NS.
- ❑ Order appropriate labs, and X-rays.
- ❑ Place the patient on a cardiac monitor and pulse oximeter.
- ❑ Insert a NG tube after checking for midface fractures or a basilar skull fracture.
- ❑ DO NOT insert a Foley catheter.
- ❑ Check vital signs frequently.

13.4 History:

- ❑ Allergies: Unknown.
- ❑ Medications: Unknown.
- ❑ PMH: Unknown.
- ❑ Last Meal: Unknown.
- ❑ EMTs: The patient was hit by a car and thrown a long distance. No witnesses are available. No identification was found on the patient.

13.5 Secondary Survey:

- ❑ Vital signs: BP 120/80, P 100, R 18 (bagged), T 99.0 °F.
- ❑ General: Patient is intubated, respirations per bag-valve-mask without difficulty.
- ❑ Skin: Bruising to the left knee.
- ❑ HEENT: There is soft tissue swelling and an abrasion to the forehead but no palpable fracture. Eyes open to painful stimuli, PERRLA, EOM-I. Fundi normal.
- ❑ Neck: Immobilized with a collar. There is no crepitance or palpable defect.
- ❑ Chest: No obvious injury, no crepitus.
- ❑ Lungs: Clear to auscultation
- ❑ Heart: Tachycardia without murmur.
- ❑ Abdomen: Distended and firm to palpation. Bowel sounds are absent.
- ❑ Perineum/GU: Blood at meatus, perineal hematoma present.
- ❑ Pelvis: Pain and crepitus on compression of the symphysis pubis.
- ❑ Back: Normal
- ❑ Extremities: Bruising and swelling of the left knee, with ligaments intact and a tense effusion are present. All pulses are present and equal. No other deformities noted.
- ❑ Neuro: No focal findings, DTRs are equal, GCS 8 prior to intubation.

13.6 Laboratory:

- ❑ CBC: WBC 14, Hgb 15.2, Hct 45.5, Plt 295.
- ❑ Chemistry: Na 140, K 4.2, Cl 101, CO_2 23.
- ❑ BUN/Cr: 14/1.0.
- ❑ Glucose: 125.
- ❑ Ca/Mg: Normal.
- ❑ LFTs: Normal.

- ❑ ABG: pH 7.39, pO_2 65, pCO_2 3, HCO_3 22, (room air).
- ❑ ETOH: 350.
- ❑ U/A: Gross blood.

13.7 X-rays:

- ❑ CXR: Normal.
- ❑ C-spine: C6-C7 subluxation.
- ❑ Pelvis: Fractured symphysis pubis and left pubic rami.
- ❑ Left knee: Non-displaced tibial plateau fracture.
- ❑ Retrograde Urethrogram: Urethra intact. Extra-peritoneal bladder rupture with extravasation of dye present.
- ❑ Cystogram: Extravasation of dye.
- ❑ CT head: Normal.
- ❑ CT abdomen: Liver laceration.

13.8 Special Tests:

- ❑ ECG: Sinus tachycardia.

13.9 Critical Actions:

□ tetanus booster

- ☑ Consult neurosurgery for the c-spine fracture.
- ☑ Maintain of c-spine precautions.
- ☑ Consult urology for bladder repair.
- ☑ Splint the right leg and consult orthopedics.
- ☑ Consult a trauma or general surgeon.
- ❑ Send the patient to the OR for c-spine stabilization, bladder repair, and exploratory laparotomy.
- ☑ Recognize hypotension and treat with fluids.
- ☑ Intubate early.
- ☑ Do not insert a Foley catheter until urethrogram is completed and it shows an intact urethra.

Patient #1 (Tetanus)

The nurse has irrigated the patient's leg wound and asks which suture you would like.

13.7 Laboratory:

- ❑ CBC: WBC 11, Hgb 15, Hct 45, Plt 300,000.
- ❑ Chemistry: Normal.
- ❑ BUN/Cr: Normal.
- ❑ Glucose: 110.
- ❑ Ca/Mg: Normal.
- ❑ LFTs: Normal.
- ❑ Amylase/Lipase: Normal.
- ❑ PT/PTT: Normal.
- ❑ Blood cultures: Pending.
- ❑ Gram's stain: Gram positive club-shaped rods.

- ❑ U/A: Normal.

13.8 X-rays:

- ❑ C-spine: Normal.

13.9 Special Tests:

- ❑ ECG: Sinus tachycardia, no other abnormality noted.
- ❑ Pulse oximeter: 100% on room air.
- ❑ Cardiac monitor: Sinus tachycardia.

13.10 Critical Actions:

- ❑ Obtain a history of the fall with a leg laceration.
- ❑ Obtain immunization history.
- ❑ Don't suture the wound.
- ❑ Administer tetanus toxoid.
- ❑ Treat the spasm and pain.
- ❑ Admit to the ICU.
- ❑ Consult a surgeon to explore, debride, and remove the foreign body.

13.11 Pearls: (Patient #1)

❑❑ What is the differential diagnosis of tetanus?

Strychnine poisoning, dystonic reaction, hypocalcemia tetany, peritonsillar abscess, parotiditis, meningitis, subarachnoid hemorrhage, rabies, temporomandibular joint disease.

❑❑ What is the role of TIG in the treatment of tetanus?

TIG neutralizes circulating tetanospasmin and toxin in the wound but not the toxin that is already present in the nervous tissue. The administration of TIG decreases mortality.

Patient #2 (Exudative Pharyngitis)

13.9 Critical Actions:

- ❑ Establish good rapport with the patient and convince him to stay.
- ❑ Diagnose Streptococcal pharyngitis.
- ❑ Treat with the appropriate antibiotics.
- ❑ Arrange follow up.
- ❑ Treat the fever.

13.10 Pearls: (Patient #2)

❑❑ **What are the objectives in treating Streptococcal pharyngitis?**

Prevent rheumatic fever, peritonsillar abscess and cellulitis, suppurative cervical lymphadenitis, and retropharyngeal abscess. Treatment also hastens clinical recovery.

❑❑ **What is the antibiotic of choice for the treatment of Group A β-hemolytic Streptococcal pharyngitis?**

A single dose of penicillin, 1.2 million units IM, or oral penicillin, 250 mg po tid for 10 days, effectively eradicates the infection and prevents rheumatic fever. Alternatives to penicillin include erythromycin, Cephalosporins, clindamycin, and azithromycin.

Pearls: (Patient #3)

❑❑ **In evaluating genitourinary trauma, what is the proper sequence of studies to evaluate the kidneys, bladder, and urethra?**

Perform a retrograde urethrogram first if blood is present at the urethral meatus. If a bladder injury is suspected, an IVP is performed, after a urethrogram, to avoid residual contrast from obscuring the lower ureter.

❑❑ **What are the contraindications to insertion of a Foley catheter?**

Blood at the urethral meatus, "floating" or "high-riding" prostate, perineal hematoma, and a midline pelvic fracture or dislocation. A urethrogram should be performed first when any of these findings are present.

CASE 14 (Ventricular Tachycardia)

Examiner

This previously healthy patient was sitting at his desk at work when he started feeling "funny". He denies chest pain or pressure, but some nausea and diaphoresis are noted. He has no history of similar complaints and the event started one hour before arrival to the ED. He drove himself to the ED.

This patient has unstable V-tach requiring cardioversion. The candidate may try adenosine first, but this will not work. If the candidate does not identify V-tach and treat appropriately, the patient will decompensate. Consult cardiology and admit to the ICU.

14.1 Introduction:

A 52 year old male presents, via a private automobile, with a complaint of not "feeling well".

Vital Signs are: BP 80/P, P 120, R 24, T 98.3 °F.

14.2 Primary Survey:

- ❑ General: WN/WD male appears anxious, uncomfortable, in mild respiratory distress.
- ❑ Airway: Intact.

- ❑ Breathing: Tachypneic but not labored.
- ❑ Circulation: Pulses are equal and thready.
- ❑ Disability: Normal.
- ❑ Exposure: No medic alert tags.
- ❑ Finger: Normal rectal. Heme negative.

14.3 Management:

- ❑ Start IV and O_2. Place on pulse oximeter and cardiac monitor.
- ❑ Order appropriate labs, X-rays, and an ECG.
- ❑ Perform synchronized cardioversion with sedation. You may use adenosine first.

14.4 History:

- ❑ Allergies: None.
- ❑ Medications: None.
- ❑ PMH: No significant injuries or illnesses. No past surgeries.
- ❑ Last meal: 2 hours ago.
- ❑ Family: No family history of heart disease.
- ❑ Records: None.
- ❑ Immune: Up to date.
- ❑ Narcotics: Denies use of illicit drugs.
- ❑ Doctor: No family physician.
- ❑ Social: Denies alcohol use but smokes one pack of cigarettes per day and has done so for 32 years. He is married with two children.

14.5 Secondary Survey:

- ❑ Vital signs: BP 120/80, P 80, R 16.
- ❑ General: After treatment he feels and looks better.
- ❑ Skin: Initially it was pale, cool, and moist but after treatment it is warm and dry with good color.
- ❑ HEENT: Normal.
- ❑ Neck: Normal.
- ❑ Chest: Normal.
- ❑ Lungs: Normal.
- ❑ Heart: RRR with a normal S1, S2 no S3 or S4 and no murmur; Normal PMI.
- ❑ Abdomen: Normal.
- ❑ Perineum/GU: Normal.
- ❑ Rectal: Normal.
- ❑ Extremities: Normal.
- ❑ Neuro: Normal.

14.6 Laboratory:

- ❑ CBC: WBC 9, Hgb 14, Hct 45, Plt 250,000.
- ❑ Chemistry: Na 135, K 4.0, Cl 102, CO_2 24.
- ❑ BUN/Cr: 10/1.0.
- ❑ Glucose: 102.
- ❑ Ca/Mg: Normal.

- ❑ LFTs: Normal.
- ❑ Amylase/Lipase: Normal.
- ❑ PT/PTT: Normal.
- ❑ Cardiac enzymes: CPK 220, LDH 300, SGOT 32, CKMB 2%.
- ❑ ABG: pH 7.45, pO_2 95, pCO_2 30, HCO_3 24, Saturation 100%.
- ❑ U/A: Normal.

14.7 X-rays:

- ❑ CXR: Normal.

14.8 Special Tests:

- ❑ ECG: Ventricular tachycardia at a rate of 140. The post-treatment ECG reveals normal sinus rhythm.

14.9 Critical Actions:

- ☑ Recognize V-tach on the ECG.
- ☑ Cardiovert.
- ☑ Admit to the ICU.
- ☑ Obtain cardiology consult.

14.10 Pearls:

❑❑ What ECG findings are suggestive of ventricular tachycardia?

Wide QRS complex, rate greater than 100, regular rhythm, QRS axis is usually constant, extreme right axis deviation, and concordance in all leads.

❑❑ What are the causes of ventricular tachycardia?

The most common causes are ischemic heart disease and acute myocardial infarction. Other less common causes include hypertrophic cardiomyopathy, mitral valve prolapse, and toxicity from drugs (digoxin, quinidine, procainamide, sympathomimetics).

CASE 15 (Organophosphate Poisoning)

Examiner

According to this patient's brother, who arrives later than the patient, the victim just started a new job with an exterminating company. He was previously healthy and had no complaints before leaving for work today.

This patient requires immediate intubation with c-spine immobilization, IV rehydration, nasogastric suctioning, and Foley catheterization. A coma protocol should be instituted but the patient will not respond. During the initial stabilization one of the treating EMTs complains of nausea. Candidate should recognize a potential toxic exposure and take protective measures, such as bag patient's clothing, wear protective mask and gloves, decontaminate the patient's skin by washing with soap and water, and decontaminate the GI tract with activated charcoal.

15.1 Introduction:

A 17 year old male in acute respiratory distress arrives by a basic EMT ambulance. No treatment has been given and his brother is on the way by a private auto.

The EMTs complain of nausea.

Vitals Signs are: BP 80/40, P 48, R 45, T 100.5 °F.

15.2 Primary Survey:

- ❑ General: A WN/WD 17 year old male presents unconscious with vomitus on clothing.
- ❑ Airway: Excessive oral secretions are present and the gag reflex is absent.
- ❑ Breathing: Rapid shallow respirations are present.
- ❑ Circulation: Capillary refill is delayed, peripheral pulses are weak.
- ❑ Disability: Eyes do not open to painful stimuli, verbal response is absent, and decerebrate posturing is present. Pupils are pinpoint.
- ❑ Exposure: No medic-alert tags; no lesions, abrasions, burns, or lacerations.
- ❑ Finger: Rectal normal. Patient is incontinent of urine and stool.

15.3 Management:

- ❑ Intubate with c-spine immobilization.
- ❑ Start IV with aggressive fluid resuscitation.
- ❑ Insert NG tube and a Foley catheter. Place on cardiac monitor and pulse oximeter.
- ❑ Decontaminate the patient.
- ❑ Give activated charcoal to decontaminate the GI tract.

The nurse tells you the patient's brother has arrived and is in the waiting room.

15.4 History:

- ❑ Allergies: None.
- ❑ Medications: None.
- ❑ PMH: No significant past illnesses or injuries. No past surgeries.
- ❑ Last meal: Unknown.
- ❑ Family: Noncontributory.
- ❑ Records: None.
- ❑ Immune: Unknown.
- ❑ EMTs: They were called to the scene by a bystander which noticed the patient unconscious in an unmarked private van. The EMTs noted no signs of trauma, no unusual smells, no drug paraphernalia, no alcohol bottles or cans and no pill bottles.
- ❑ Narcotics: No history of drug or alcohol abuse according to the brother.
- ❑ Doctor: No family physician.
- ❑ Social: No tobacco or alcohol use. He lives with his brother and is a freshman in college.

15.5 Secondary Survey:

- ❑ Skin: Normal color but diaphoretic.

- ❑ HEENT: Pupils are pinpoint, profuse tearing is present, oropharynx is full of secretions.
- ❑ Neck: Normal.
- ❑ Chest: Normal.
- ❑ Lungs: Shallow respirations, expiratory wheezes are present with few bibasilar crackles.
- ❑ Heart: Bradycardia with normal heart tones and no murmur present.
- ❑ Abdomen: Bowel sounds are hyperactive.
- ❑ Perineum/GU: Normal.
- ❑ Rectal: Normal sphincter tone. Heme negative. Brown colored, liquid stool.
- ❑ Back: Normal.
- ❑ Extremities: Muscle fasciculations are diffusely present.
- ❑ Neuro: Minimal flexion response to pain. DTRs are hyperactive and symmetric and toes are downgoing.

15.6 Laboratory:

- ❑ CBC: WBC 15, Hgb 13.5, Hct 39.5, Plt 300,000.
- ❑ Chemistry: Na 138, K 3.0, Cl 108, CO_2 14.
- ❑ BUN/Cr: 18/1.1.
- ❑ Glucose: 120.
- ❑ Ca/Mg: Normal.
- ❑ LFTs: Normal.
- ❑ Amylase/Lipase: Normal.
- ❑ PT/PTT: Normal.
- ❑ Cardiac enzymes: Normal.
- ❑ ABG: pH 7.12, pO_2 45, pCO_2 52, (on arrival).
- ❑ ABG: pH 7.34, pO_2 70, pCO_2 30, (after intubation).
- ❑ Lactate: 5.0 mEq/L.
- ❑ Serum Osm: 298 mOsm/kg.
- ❑ U/A: Protein 3+, Glucose 2+, Specific gravity 1.020.

15.7 X-rays:

- ❑ CXR: Mild pulmonary vascular congestion.
- ❑ C-spine series: Normal.

15.8 Special Tests:

- ❑ ECG: Sinus bradycardia.
- ❑ Serum cholinesterase and RBC cholinesterase: Pending.

15.9 Management:

- ❑ Contact the patient's employer to determine which insecticide was used (organophosphate called Parathion).
- ❑ Contact Poison Control.
- ❑ Order atropine, 0.05 mg/kg/dose IV q 5-15 minutes and 2-PAM (pralidoxime) 25-50 mg/kg/dose IV.
- ❑ Consult an internist and admit to the ICU.

15.10 Critical Actions:

- ❑ Intubate with c-spine immobilization.
- ❑ Start IV rehydration.
- ❑ Recognize the toxidrome and decontaminate.
- ❑ Initiate coma protocol.
- ❑ Consult Poison Control and an internist.
- ❑ Contact the employer to determine which insecticide was used.

15.11 Pearls:

❑❑ What is the most frequent cause of treatment failure in organophosphate poisoning?

Inadequate atropinization. Large doses of atropine, 20-40 mg/day, may be required.

❑❑ What is the difference between organophosphate and carbamate poisoning?

Carbamates are less toxic and have a shorter duration of action. Signs and symptoms usually disappear within 8 hours after exposure. Carbamates are more rapidly absorbed through the skin than organophosphates but CNS effects are less, due to poor penetration of the blood-brain barrier.

CASE 16 (Febrile Seizure)

Examiner

Earlier today this patient seemed irritable, warm to the touch, and consumed less formula, according to his mother. He was sitting on his mother's lap when he stiffened, rolled his eyes back, and began having clonic-tonic movements of all the extremities for approximately 2 minutes. In addition, the patient received a DPT injection yesterday.

This patient has experienced a simple febrile seizure secondary to the DPT shot. The candidate may either admit the patient or discharge with follow up in 24 hours. If a CT scan is ordered, antibiotics should be started before the patient leaves the department.

16.1 Introduction:

A 4 month old male who is actively seizing presents in the arms of his mother.

Vital Signs are: BP 70, P 140, R 32, Wt 11 lbs (5 kg).

16.2 Primary Survey:

- ❑ Airway: Airway patent, no pooling of secretions, gag reflex intact.
- ❑ Breathing: Stridorous and irregular respirations.
- ❑ Circulation: Decreased capillary refill, normal pulses.
- ❑ Disability: Pupils equal and reactive. Spontaneous eye opening, localizes to pain, grunting verbal response.

- ❑ Exposure: No rash, petechiae, or signs of trauma.
- ❑ Finger: Normal.

16.3 Management:

- ❑ Stabilize the airway and start O_2.
- ❑ Place the patient on a cardiac monitor and pulse oximeter.
- ❑ Obtain a bedside blood glucose.
- ❑ Obtain a rectal temperature.
- ❑ After determining the patient to be febrile (103.5 °F), administer acetaminophen 15 mg/kg po or pr, or ibuprofen, 10 mg/kg po.
- ❑ Start IV with a 20 mL/kg bolus of normal saline.
- ❑ Obtain appropriate labs and X-rays.
- ❑ Give an appropriate benzodiazepine IV or PR, if the seizure lasts longer than 10 minutes.
- ❑ If a head CT is ordered, give antibiotics before the patient leaves the department.

16.4 History:

- ❑ Allergies: None.
- ❑ Medications: None.
- ❑ PMH: No significant illnesses, normal spontaneous vaginal delivery at 41 weeks of gestation. Birth weight 7 lbs, 8 oz. No past surgeries.
- ❑ Last meal: Drank 2 ounces of formula 3 hours ago.
- ❑ Family: Negative.
- ❑ Records: None.
- ❑ Doctor: Dr. Pediatrician.
- ❑ Social history: Patient lives with natural parents and one sibling. No risk factors for abuse.

16.5 Secondary Survey:

- ❑ General: WN/WD, unresponsive, no respiratory distress.
- ❑ Skin: Warm, moist, no rash.
- ❑ HEENT: Head normocephalic/atraumatic, fontanels open and flat. PERRL, TMs normal, nose and throat are clear.
- ❑ Neck: Supple, no nodes, no meningeal signs.
- ❑ Chest: Normal.
- ❑ Lungs: Tachypnea, no wheezing.
- ❑ Heart: Tachycardic rate, regular rhythm, no murmur.
- ❑ Abdomen: Soft, BS present, no mass, no organomegaly.
- ❑ Perineum/GU: Normal.
- ❑ Rectal: Normal sphincter tone, heme negative.
- ❑ Back: Normal.
- ❑ Extremities: Normal.
- ❑ Neuro: Postictal. Cranial nerves intact as best as can be determined. DTRs normal.

16.6 Laboratory:

- ❑ CBC: WBC 14, Hgb 11.5, Hct 35.6, Plt 350,000.

- ☐ Differential : Normal.
- ☐ Chemistry: Na 140, K 3.8, Cl 101, CO_2 24.
- ☐ BUN/Cr: 17/0.7.
- ☐ Glucose: 102.
- ☐ Ca/Mg: 9.0/2.0.
- ☐ LFTs: Normal.
- ☐ Blood Cultures: Pending.
- ☐ U/A: Normal.
- ☐ Urine Culture: Pending.

16.7 X-ray:

- ☐ CXR: Right lower lobe infiltrate.
- ☐ CT head: Normal.

16.8 Special Tests:

- ☐ CSF: Appearance, Clear.
- ☐ Cell count: WBC 2, RBC 0.
- ☐ Glucose: 65.
- ☐ Protein: 30.
- ☐ Gram stain: No organisms.
- ☐ CIE/Latex: Negative.
- ☐ Culture: Pending.

16.9 Critical Actions:

- ☒ Protect the airway.
- ☒ Stat serum glucose.
- ☒ Obtain a rectal temperature.
- ☒ Lower the temperature with antipyretics.
- ☐ Administer antibiotics before obtaining the head CT scan and before admission.
- ☒ Instruct follow-up with a pediatrician in 24 hours if candidate does not admit.

16.10 Pearls:

☐☐ What are the usual characteristics of a simple febrile seizure?

1) Temperature greater than 100 °F with a rapid rise.
2) Age between 3 months and 5 years.
3) Generalized tonic-clonic, nonfocal.
4) Short postictal period.
5) Seizure lasts less than 15 minutes.

☐☐ What are the risk factors for recurrent febrile seizures?

1) First degree relative with epilepsy.
2) First degree relative with febrile seizures.
3) Complex first febrile seizure.

4) Age younger than 12 months at the time of the initial febrile seizure.
5) Increased infectious exposure due to day care attendance.

❑❑ **What is the incidence of developing epilepsy in the future?**

Febrile seizures do not cause epilepsy but there is a 1% chance of developing this by age 7 years. The incidence of epilepsy in children without a history of febrile seizures is 0.4%.

CASE 17 (Ectopic Pregnancy)

Examiner

A pregnant women presents to the ED with abdominal pain that started one week ago and it has progressively worsened. She describes the pain as diffuse, sharp, constant, and nonradiating. She also is experiencing nausea. The patient denies vaginal discharge but complains of dysuria without hematuria. No history of similar complaints. Her last menstrual period was approximately 7 weeks ago and she had some vaginal bleeding 3 days ago.

This patient has an acutely ruptured ectopic pregnancy. If IV fluids are started, the patient will respond by "feeling better," and her BP will increase to 100/P. You may have the candidate perform a culdocentesis by making the ultrasound difficult to obtain. Immediately upon finishing the culdocentesis, have the gynecologist with the ultrasound machine arrive in the ED.

17.1 Introduction:

A 28 year old female presents with a complaint of lower abdominal pain.

Vital Signs: BP 100/70, P 108, R 22, T 98.9 °F.

17.2 Primary Survey:

❑ General: WN/WD female sitting up, appears uncomfortable and pale but is in no immediate distress.
❑ Airway: Normal.
❑ Breathing: Tachypnea but no distress.
❑ Circulation: Strong, rapid, and equal pulses. Normal capillary refill.
❑ Disability: Normal.
❑ Exposure: No medic alert tags.

17.3 Management:

❑ Because the patient is stable, the candidate may not initiate treatment until a full history is completed.

17.4 History:

❑ Allergies: None.
❑ Medications: Sulfa.

- ❑ PMH: Ectopic pregnancy 5 years ago treated with methotrexate. No past surgeries.
- ❑ Last meal: 6 hours ago.
- ❑ Family: Non-contributory.
- ❑ Records: None.
- ❑ Immunizations: Up to date.
- ❑ Narcotics: No illicit drug use.
- ❑ Doctor: Patient has a gynecologist.
- ❑ Social history: The patient is married, has no children and works as a lawyer for a personal injury firm. She denies alcohol and tobacco use.

During the history the patient becomes dizzy, nauseated, and complains of increasing abdominal pain. If asked, the new vital signs are BP 80/P, P 120, R 22.

17.5 <u>Management</u>:

- ❑ Administer 1 L bolus of LR or 0.9 NS.
- ❑ Place the patient on a pulse oximeter and cardiac monitor.
- ❑ Start O_2.
- ❑ Consult Ob/Gyn.
- ❑ Obtain appropriate labs.
- ❑ Order a stat pelvic ultrasound.
- ❑ Type and cross for 2 units of packed RBCs.

17.6 <u>Laboratory</u>:

- ❑ CBC: WBC 13.2, Hgb 7.1, Hct 21.2, Plt 220,000
- ❑ Differential: Normal.
- ❑ Chemistry: Na 141, K 4.1, Cl 110, CO_2 24.
- ❑ BUN/Cr: 14/0.7.
- ❑ Glucose: 105.
- ❑ LFTs: Normal.
- ❑ Amylase/Lipase: Normal.
- ❑ B-HCG: 2200.
- ❑ Type and Rh: B+.
- ❑ U/A: Normal.
- ❑ Urine pregnency test: Positive.

17.7 <u>Special Tests</u>:

- ❑ Ultrasound: No intrauterine pregnancy, free fluid in the culdosac. However, there is a possibility of an ectopic pregnancy.

17.8 <u>Secondary Survey</u>:

- ❑ General: After a fluid bolus, the nausea and dizziness is gone but the abdominal pain is worse.
- ❑ Skin: Pale, cool, dry.
- ❑ HEENT: Normal.
- ❑ Neck: Normal.

- ❑ Chest: Normal.
- ❑ Lungs: Normal.
- ❑ Heart: Tachycardia without a murmur.
- ❑ Abdomen: Mild distention, bowel sounds are diminished, pain to palpation in the suprapubic region. Rebound and guarding present.
- ❑ Pelvic: The uterus is 6 to 7 weeks in size with tenderness to palpation of both adnexa. No adnexal mass palpable. The cervical os is closed and no blood is present in the vaginal vault. Positive Hagar and Chadwick's sign.
- ❑ Rectal: Normal.
- ❑ Extremities: No edema.
- ❑ Neuro: Normal.

17.9 Management:

- ❑ After the ultrasound is completed, the gynecologist will take the patient to the OR.

17.10 Critical Actions:

- ❑ Obtain a menstrual history.
- ❑ Start IV rehydration.
- ❑ Order a pelvic ultrasound.
- ❑ Consult Ob/Gyn.
- ❑ Type and cross for 2 to 4 units of packed RBCs.

17.11 Pearls:

❑❑ What is the classic triad of symptoms in ectopic pregnancy?

Abdominal pain, amenorrhea, and vaginal bleeding. This is seen 15% of ectopic pregnancies.

❑❑ What is the most common sign?

Tenderness on pelvic exam is the most common sign and is present in 85% to 97% of cases.

❑❑ When can a gestational sac be detected in the uterus by transvaginal ultrasound?

Five to six weeks of gestation corresponding to a quantitative β-HCG >2000 mIU/mL.

CASE 18 (Toxic Epidermal Necrolysis)

Examiner

The patient complained of dysuria 5 days ago so a friend gave her an unknown "bladder" antibiotic. After taking the pills for one day, she noted large, red, painful lesions on her chest, legs, and arms. Within 24 hours, blisters formed and denuded skin developed. She also complained of anorexia, fever, joint aches, and malaise. She stopped taking the medication and disposed of them after the rash appeared.

The candidate should recognize a life-threatening dermatosis and use appropriate burn care (including the Parkland formula). This patient should be transferred to a burn center.

18.1 Introduction:

A 26 year old female arrives by ambulance with a complaint of worsening rash over the past 5 days.

Vital Signs: BP 110/60, P 112, R 22, T 100.6 °F.

18.2 Primary Survey:

- ❑ General: WN/WD female, awake and oriented but lethargic. She is in no distress but appears uncomfortable.
- ❑ Airway: Intact.
- ❑ Breathing: Normal.
- ❑ Circulation: Capillary refill delayed, rapid pulse rate.
- ❑ Disability: Normal.
- ❑ Exposure: No medic alert tags. Large areas of denuded skin and blisters are present.
- ❑ Finger: Normal.

18.3 Management:

- ❑ Recognize the life-threatening dermatoses.
- ❑ Start 2 large bore IVs.
- ❑ Use the Parkland burn formula to calculate fluid needs.
- ❑ Place the patient on a cardiac monitor and pulse oximeter.
- ❑ Order appropriate diagnostic tests.
- ❑ Use burn technique to handle the patient.
- ❑ Consult a burn specialist and arrange for transfer to a burn unit.

18.4 History:

- ❑ Allergies: None.
- ❑ Medications: An unknown, large, white pill given to her by a friend.
- ❑ PMH: 2 pregnancies, both normal spontaneous vaginal deliveries. No other significant illnesses or injuries. No past surgeries.
- ❑ Last meal: 3 hours ago.
- ❑ Family: Contact her friend and find out whether the medication she gave the patient was a sulfonamide.
- ❑ Records: None.
- ❑ Immune: Up to date.
- ❑ EMTs: In the ED break room.
- ❑ Narcotics: Denies illicit drug use.
- ❑ Doctor: None.
- ❑ Social history: Married, 2 children. No alcohol or tobacco use.

18.5 Secondary Survey:

- ❑ General: No change since arrival to the ED.
- ❑ Skin: Blistering with denuded areas present, positive Nikolsky's sign. Sixty percent of the body surface is involved.
- ❑ HEENT: No oral lesions, conjunctiva clear.

- ❑ Neck: Normal.
- ❑ Chest: Lesions present.
- ❑ Lungs: Tachypnea but no respiratory distress. Lungs clear to auscultation.
- ❑ Heart: Tachycardia without a murmur.
- ❑ Abdomen: Lesions present otherwise, normal.
- ❑ Pelvic: No rash, no vaginal discharge, normal bimanual exam.
- ❑ Rectal: No lesions, normal tone, heme negative.
- ❑ Back: Lesions present.
- ❑ Extremities: Normal except for lesions that include the dorsum of the hands. The feet are spared.
- ❑ Neuro: Normal.

18.6 Laboratory:

- ❑ CBC: WBC 19, Hgb 12, Hct 36, Plt 275,000.
- ❑ Differential: Poly 45, Bands 25, Lymph 25, Eos 2, Mono 1.
- ❑ Chemistry: Na 140, K 4.5, Cl 98, CO_2 14.
- ❑ BUN/Cr: 20/2.0.
- ❑ Glucose: 90.
- ❑ Ca/Mg: Normal.
- ❑ LFTs: Elevated.
- ❑ Amylase/Lipase: Normal.
- ❑ PT/PTT: Normal.
- ❑ ABG: pH 7.30, pO_2 95, pCO_2 36, HCO_3 15.
- ❑ B-HCG: Negative.
- ❑ Blood cultures: Pending.
- ❑ U/A: Specific gravity 1.025, WBC 100, RBC 10, Bacteria Large amount, Protein 3+ Ketones 3+.
- ❑ Urine culture: Pending.

18.7 Critical Actions:

- ❑ Obtain the diagnosis and cause of toxic epidermal necrolysis.
- ❑ Use the Parkland formula to determine fluid requirements.
- ❑ Use burn technique to handle the patient.
- ❑ Admit to a burn unit.
- ❑ Consult a burn specialist.

18.8 Pearls:

❑❑ What is the etiology of toxic epidermal necrolysis?

TEN is precipitated by drugs like sulfonamides, barbiturates, phenytoin, phenylbutazone, or penicillin. Rare causes include a graft-versus-host reaction (after a bone marrow transplant) or administration of blood products.

❑❑ What differentiates Staphylococcal Scalded Skin Syndrome from TEN?

SSSS contracted by children less than 5 years old is due to a *Staph* toxin that spares the mucous membranes. Cleavage occurs within the epidermis, and has a mortality rate of less than 5%. TEN occurring primarily in

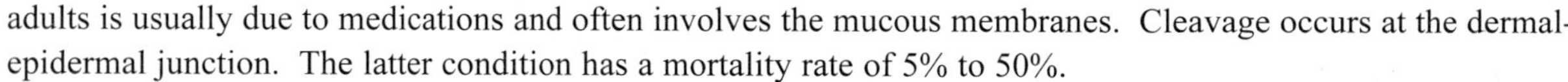

adults is usually due to medications and often involves the mucous membranes. Cleavage occurs at the dermal-epidermal junction. The latter condition has a mortality rate of 5% to 50%.

❑❑ **What are the complications of TEN?**

Sepsis, hypovolemia, pulmonary edema, electrolyte disturbances, renal failure, and death.

CASE 19 (Boerhaave's Syndrome)

Examiner

According to his wife, this patient has been feeling "sick to his stomach" over the past 2 days. After eating breakfast this morning, he began vomiting. He drank some Pepto-Bismol and began complaining of severe left sided chest pain. About 2 hours ago, he became feverish, short of breath, and the pain worsened. He was previously healthy with no recent trauma noted.

The patient requires immediate intubation and fluid resuscitation. It is appropriate to do a "cardiac" work-up, which will be negative. Once the diagnosis is made, appropriate antibiotics must be started in the ED.

19.1 Introduction:

A 62 year old male is brought in by his wife with a complaint of severe chest pain.

Vital Signs are: BP 92/50, P 122, R 26, T 102.5 °F.

19.2 Primary Survey:

- ❑ General: This is a WN/WD diaphoretic, anxious male.
- ❑ Airway: Airway is patent, gag reflex intact.
- ❑ Breathing: Breath sounds are diminished on the left side, he is tachypneic, neck veins are flat, and the trachea is midline.
- ❑ Circulation: Skin is pale, capillary refill is delayed, and patient is tachycardic.
- ❑ Disability: GCS 15, PERRLA.
- ❑ Exposure: No medic alert tags.
- ❑ Finger: Rectal normal.

19.3 Management:

- ❑ Start 2 large bore IVs of LR or 0.9 NS.
- ❑ Administer multiple 250 cc fluid boluses until the pressure increases.
- ❑ Place on cardiac monitor and pulse oximeter.
- ❑ Order appropriate labs, X-rays, and an ECG.
- ❑ Insert a NG tube and a Foley catheter.

19.4 History:

- ❑ Allergies: None.
- ❑ Medications: None.
- ❑ PMH: Fractured right femur with rod placement 10 years ago.
- ❑ Last meal: 10 hours ago.
- ❑ Family: Wife present to answer questions, family history non-contributory.
- ❑ Records: None.
- ❑ Immune: Up to date.
- ❑ Narcotics: Wife denies drug use.
- ❑ Doctor: No family physician.
- ❑ Social history: Drinks one beer per week, no tobacco use.

19.5 Secondary Survey:

- ❑ General: Patient is intubated in mild respiratory discomfort but he responds to commands.
- ❑ Skin: Warm, dry mucous membranes, no rash or petechiae.
- ❑ HEENT: Normal.
- ❑ Neck: Slight crepitance to palpation.
- ❑ Chest: Atraumatic, no palpable crepitance.
- ❑ Lungs: Diminished breath sounds on the left. Hamman's "crunch" present.
- ❑ Heart: Rapid rate, regular rhythm, no murmur.
- ❑ Abdomen: Mild epigastric tenderness present. Bowel sounds are normal, no masses, no organomegaly, no rebound or guarding.
- ❑ Rectal: Normal, heme negative.
- ❑ Back: Normal.
- ❑ Extremities: Normal.
- ❑ Neuro: No focal deficits, normal DTRs, patient obeys commands.

19.6 Laboratory:

- ❑ CBC: WBC 22, Hgb 13.5, Hct 42, Plt 150,000.
- ❑ Differential: Polys 80, Bands 5, Lymphs 10, Eos 1, Mono 3.
- ❑ Chemistry: Na 135, K 4.0, Cl 101, CO_2 18.
- ❑ BUN/Cr: 12/1.2.
- ❑ Glucose: 110.
- ❑ Ca/Mg: Normal.
- ❑ LFTs: Normal.
- ❑ Amylase/Lipase: Normal.
- ❑ PT/PTT: Normal.
- ❑ Cardiac enzymes: Pending.
- ❑ ABG: pH 7.29, pO_2 85, pCO_2 42, HCO_3 16 (before intubation, on room air).
- ❑ Blood cultures: Pending.
- ❑ U/A: Normal.

19.7 X-rays:

- ❑ CXR: Large left pleural effusion with a radiopaque substance present. A 30% pneumothorax present on the left side.
- ❑ Lateral neck: Air is present in the retropharyngeal space.
- ❑ Esophagram: Extravasation of the water-soluble agent is seen in the left pleural space.
- ❑ CT chest: Not available.

19.8 Special Tests:

- ❑ ECG: Sinus tachycardia with non-specific ST and T wave changes in the anterior leads.

19.9 Critical Actions:

- ❑ Initiate cardiac workup.
- ❑ Identify the esophageal rupture and obtain an esophagram.
- ❑ Start IV fluid resuscitation.
- ❑ Administer broad spectrum antibiotic coverage (include anaerobic coverage).
- ❑ Consult a thoracic or general surgeon immediately.
- ❑ Insert a chest tube.

19.10 Pearls:

❑❑ What is the most common area of rupture in the esophagus?

Left side of the distal portion, which is a physiologically weakened area.

❑❑ What is the role of esophagoscopy?

This is performed if a perforation is suspected but cannot be confirmed by contrast studies, if there is upper gastrointestinal bleeding associated with a partial-thickness laceration, or if the patient is unconscious and a contrast study cannot be performed.

❑❑ Why is early surgical repair important?

If surgical repair is done in less than 24 hours, the mortality rate is 5%. However, if repair is delayed, the mortality reaches 75%.

CASE 20 (Kawasaki's Disease)

Examiner

The patient's mother states that her child has had a fever and a poor appetite for the past 6 days. Today he broke out in a rash and his eyes started to drain. However, he has not vomited or does not have diarrhea, and his fever can be controlled by Tylenol.

The candidate should recognize this disease, know the diagnostic criteria, and understand and start the appropriate therapy. This patient requires admission, but be resistant to this until the potential complications are explained to the parent by the candidate.

20.1 Introduction:

A 3 year old male is brought in by his parents with a complaint of rash and fever.

Vital Signs are: BP 98/60, P 122, R 26, T 103.6 °F, Wt 15 kg.

20.2 Primary Survey:

- ❑ General: WN/WD male, sitting with parents, appears uncomfortable but in no distress.
- ❑ Airway: Intact.
- ❑ Breathing: Tachypnea, lungs clear.
- ❑ Circulation: Rash present, normal capillary refill, pulses strong and regular.
- ❑ Disability: Intact.
- ❑ Exposure: Child undressed except for underwear, no bruising, abrasions, or lacerations. Diffuse rash present.
- ❑ Finger: Intact.

20.3 Management:

- ❑ Patient is stable, proceed to the history and secondary survey.
- ❑ Laboratory and X-rays may be ordered now (not mandatory).

20.4 History:

- ❑ Allergies: None.
- ❑ Medications: Acetaminophen every 4 hours for past 2 days.
- ❑ PMH: No significant illnesses or injuries. No surgeries.
- ❑ Last meal: 2 hours ago.
- ❑ Family: Non-contributory.
- ❑ Records: None.
- ❑ Immune: Up to date.
- ❑ Doctor: The patient's pediatrician is on staff at your hospital.
- ❑ Social history: The patient lives with parents and three brothers, all have been well. No smoking within the household, no pets, and recent carpet cleaning.

20.5 Secondary Survey:

- ❑ General: Nontoxic but ill appearing child.
- ❑ Skin: The rash is a raised painful, deep red, plaque-like eruption present on the trunk, extremities (palms and soles), and perineum. No petechia or purpura
- ❑ HEENT: Normocephalic/atraumatic, PERRLA, EOM-I, fundi normal, conjunctiva injected. Throat is red, mucous membranes are moist, strawberry tongue present.
- ❑ Neck: 3 large (2.0 cm) anterior cervical nodes present. No meningeal signs.
- ❑ Lungs: Normal.

- ❑ Heart: Tachycardia with a regular rhythm, no murmur or rub.
- ❑ Abdomen: Normal.
- ❑ Perineum/GU: Desquamation of the perineum present.
- ❑ Rectal: Deferred.
- ❑ Back: Rash as described above.
- ❑ Extremities: Rash as described above with involvement of the palms of the hands and sole of the feet.
- ❑ Neuro: Normal.

20.6 Laboratory:

- ❑ CBC: WBC 20, Hgb 12, Hct 35, Plt 450,000.
- ❑ Differential: Polys 80, Bands 15, Lymphs 5, Eos 1, Mono 0.
- ❑ Chemistry: Na 140, K 4.5, Cl 98, CO_2 26.
- ❑ BUN/Cr: 10/1.0.
- ❑ Glucose: 95.
- ❑ Ca/Mg: Normal.
- ❑ LFTs: Normal.
- ❑ Amylase/Lipase: Normal.
- ❑ PT/PTT: Normal.
- ❑ Cardiac enzymes: Pending.
- ❑ Sed rate: 52.
- ❑ Blood cultures: Pending.
- ❑ U/A: Normal.

20.7 X-rays:

- ❑ CXR: Normal.

20.8 Special Tests:

- ❑ ECG: Sinus tachycardia.
- ❑ Echocardiogram: Normal.

20.9 Critical Actions:

- ☒ Start IV gamma globulin infusion at 2 g/kg over 10 hours. (May reference a book.)
- ☒ Administer aspirin, 80-100 mg/kg/day.
- ☒ Obtain CBC, Plt, and blood culture.
- ❑ Determine LFTs.
- ❑ Order an ECG. → ✓ for cardiac effects assoc c̄ Kawasacki's (usually farther down line)
- ☒ Admit.

20.10 Pearls:

❑❑ **Why should infusion of gamma globulin be started immediately**?

Early infusion of gamma globulin decreases the incidence of coronary artery aneurysms and promotes resolution of established aneurysms.

❑❑ **What are the diagnostic criteria for Kawasaki syndrome?**

Fever for at least 5 days along with the presence of 4 out of the following five conditions:

1) Bilateral conjunctivitis.
2) Polymorphous rash.
3) Cervical adenopathy.
4) Extremity changes.
5) Oral mucosa involvement.

❑❑ **What is the purpose of aspirin therapy?**

Aspirin may reduce the tendency toward thrombosis and associated coronary artery disease.

CASE 21 (Guillain-Barré)

Examiner

The patient states that she was feeling well until about 2 days ago when she felt a numbness to both hands which progressed up both arms, followed by both feet and legs. She awoke today unable to get out of bed and walk. She has had no recent illnesses, no fever, chills, night sweats, blurred or double vision, and no cough or difficulty swallowing. In addition, she has not traveled recently and has no know tick exposure.

This is a difficult case and obtaining an exact diagnosis is not required. The candidate should acquire an in depth history and physical exam, and should be able to develop a detailed differential diagnosis.

21.1 Introduction:

A 52 year old female is brought in from the car in a wheelchair with a complaint of weakness numbness in the arms and legs.

Vital Signs are: BP 138/60, P 60, R 21, T 99.6 °F.

21.2 Primary Survey:

- ❑ General: WN/WD female, looks younger than stated age, is in no apparent distress.
- ❑ Airway: Intact.
- ❑ Breathing: Tachypnea, lungs clear.
- ❑ Circulation: Normal.
- ❑ Disability: GCS 15, PERRLA.
- ❑ Exposure: No medic alert tags, no rash, bruising, or abrasions.

- ❑ Finger: Rectal deferred to secondary survey.

21.3 Management:

- ❑ No acute treatment is required at this time, may proceed to the history and secondary survey.
- ❑ Consider starting an IV of LR or 0.9 NS now.
- ❑ Consider placing on a pulse oximeter and cardiac monitor.

21.4 History:

- ❑ Allergies: None.
- ❑ Medications: None.
- ❑ PMH: No past illnesses or injuries. No past surgeries.
- ❑ Last meal: 3 hours ago.
- ❑ Family: Non-contributory.
- ❑ Records: None.
- ❑ Immune: Last tetanus shot 15 years ago.
- ❑ Narcotics: Denies illicit drug use.
- ❑ Doctor: No family physician.
- ❑ Social history: No alcohol or tobacco use. Lives with husband and 2 adolescent children all of which have been well.

21.5 Secondary Survey:

- ❑ General: Pleasant 52 year old female in no acute distress.
- ❑ Skin: No rash, no ticks.
- ❑ HEENT: Normal.
- ❑ Neck: Normal, no meningeal signs.
- ❑ Chest: Breast exam normal, no mass.
- ❑ Lungs: Clear and equal breath sounds.
- ❑ Heart: Normal.
- ❑ Abdomen: Bladder is distended and painful to palpation. Otherwise, the exam is normal.
- ❑ Pelvic: Normal.
- ❑ Rectal: Poor tone, stool in vault, heme negative.
- ❑ Back: Normal.
- ❑ Extremities: Normal.
- ❑ Neuro: Alert and oriented times 3. CN II-XII intact. Patellar and Achilles reflexes absent bilaterally with bicep and tricep reflexes 1/4 and symmetric. The patient has diminished hand grip strength and she is unable to dorsiflex and plantarflex against resistance. All proximal muscle groups are strong and equal. She is unable to distinguish sharp vs dull discrimination to the lower extremities. Toes are down-going and finger-to-nose test is normal. Unable to assess gait due to her inability to walk.

21.6 Laboratory:

- ❑ CBC: WBC 8, Hgb 12, Hct 35.2, Plt 250,000.
- ❑ Differential: Polys 58, Bands 3, Lymphs 35, Eos 1, Mono 3.
- ❑ Chemistry: Na 140, K 3.5, Cl 99, CO_2 24.
- ❑ BUN/Cr: 10/1.0.

- ❑ Glucose: 106.
- ❑ Ca/Mg: Normal.
- ❑ LFTs: Normal.
- ❑ Amylase/Lipase: Normal.
- ❑ PT/PTT: Normal.
- ❑ Cardiac enzymes: Pending.
- ❑ ABG: Normal.
- ❑ Sedimentation rate: Normal.
- ❑ Blood cultures: Pending.
- ❑ U/A: Normal.

21.7 X-rays:

- ❑ CXR: Normal.
- ❑ CT head: Normal.

21.8 Special Tests:

- ❑ Pulse oximeter: 99%.
- ❑ ECG: Normal.
- ❑ Lumbar puncture: Color clear, WBC 1, RBC 2, Protein 65, Glucose 52, Gram's stain is negative. Bacterial antigens negative.
- ❑ Pulm function tests: Pending.

21.9 Critical Actions:

- ☑ Complete a neurologic exam.
- ☑ Complete and detailed history, including questioning for tick exposure.
- ☑ Perform a lumbar puncture.
- ☑ Consult neurology.
- ☑ Admit.
- ☑ Obtain a CT of head.

21.10 Pearls:

❑❑ Discuss the pathophysiology of myasthenia gravis.

Myasthenia gravis is the most common disorder of the neuromuscular junction. It is an autoimmune disorder directed against the acetylcholine receptors. It reduces the number of available receptors thereby impairing neuromuscular transmission.

❑❑ Describe tick paralysis and its treatment.

A reversible, rapidly progressive ascending paralysis beginning at the extremities and trunk and moving up to involve the bulbar musculature. Treatment involves finding the tick, removing it, and providing supportive care with resolution of symptoms noted in 24 to 48 hours.

CASE 22 (DKA and Cellulitis)

Examiner

The patient states that he noticed swelling and increasing pain to his left leg over the past 3 days. He also complained of fever, chills, anorexia, night sweats, and polyuria. He denies nausea, vomiting, or diarrhea. The patient "scratched" his leg five days ago while he was working in his garden.

This is a sick patient who requires surgical intervention but needs stabilization first. He needs fluids, antibiotics, and correction of metabolic abnormalities.

22.1 Introduction:

A 51 year old male presents with left lower leg swelling.

Vital Signs are: BP 130/80, P 130, R 28, T 102.4 °F.

22.2 Primary Survey:

- ❑ General: Obese male who appears toxic. He is hyperalert and sweating.
- ❑ Airway: Intact.
- ❑ Breathing: Tachypneic, bilateral breath sounds present.
- ❑ Circulation: Capillary refill is diminished.
- ❑ Disability: Normal.
- ❑ Exposure: No gross findings.
- ❑ Finger: Deferred to secondary survey.

22.3 Management:

- ❑ Start IV of NS or LR with a bolus of 500 cc given.
- ❑ Place the patient on a cardiac monitor and pulse oximeter.
- ❑ Obtain quick glucose.
- ❑ Order appropriate labs and X-rays.
- ❑ Call family members.

22.4 History:

- ❑ Allergies: None.
- ❑ Medications: Insulin, 45 units NPH/21 units regular in the A.M. Procardia, XL 60 mg q day. Xanax, 0.25 mg prn.
- ❑ PMH: IDDM, HTN, and hyperlipidemia.
- ❑ Last meal: 24 hours ago.
- ❑ Family: Family history of stroke, HTN, and heart disease.
- ❑ Records: Medical records department is unable to find his records.
- ❑ Immune: Up to date.
- ❑ Narcotics: No illicit drug use.
- ❑ Doctor: His doctor is out of town.
- ❑ Social history: Married with three children. He does not drink or smoke.

22.5 Secondary Survey:

- General: Patient appears uncomfortable and continues to be diaphoretic and anxious.
- Skin: Pale, moist, no rash.
- HEENT: Normal.
- Neck: Normal.
- Chest: Normal.
- Lungs: Tachypneic, clear to auscultation bilateral.
- Heart: Tachycardia, no murmur or extra sounds.
- Abdomen: Soft, decreased bowel sounds; mild to moderate tenderness in the suprapubic region.
- Perineum/GU: Circumcised penis, non-tender testicles.
- Rectal: Normal rectal, normal prostate, heme negative stool.
- Back: Normal.
- Extremities: Left lower leg is large, swollen, with purulent drainage from an open wound. Crepitance is felt.
- Neuro: Normal.

22.6 Laboratory:

- CBC: WBC 25, Hgb 16, Hct 53, Plt 225,000.
- Differential: Polys 35, Bands 27, Lymphs 25, Eos 4, Mono 1.
- Chemistry: Na 148, K 4.8, Cl 108, CO_2 10.
- Anion gap: 30.
- BUN/Cr: 36/1.7.
- Glucose: 730.
- Ca/Mg: 11/1.4.
- LFTs: Normal.
- Amylase/Lipase: Normal.
- PT/PTT: 17/41.
- Cardiac enzymes: Normal.
- ABG: pH 7.15, pO_2 93, pCO_2 29, HCO_3 12.
- Blood cultures: Pending.
- Serum acetone: Moderate.
- U/A: Glucose 4+, Ketone 3+, Protein 250, Nitrite Negative, Leukocyte negative, RBC 1, WBC 6.

22.7 X-rays:

- CXR: Normal.
- Left leg: Gas present in the tissue. No foreign body, no fracture.

22.8 Special Tests:

- ECG: Sinus tachycardia, otherwise normal.

22.9 Critical Actions:

- Start IV fluid rehydration.

❑ Place on monitor, pulse oximeter, and O_2.
❑ Perform a quick glucose test.
❑ Determine ABG.
❑ Order appropriate labs.
❑ Administer insulin with or without a bolus.
❑ Order an ECG.
❑ Obtain an X-ray to identify free air in the left leg.
❑ Start appropriate antibiotics in the ED.
❑ Obtain intensive care consult.
❑ Admit to the ICU for stabilization prior to surgery.
❑ Stat orthopedic consult.

22.10 Pearls:

❑❑ What is the initial treatment for DKA?

IV fluids. Glucose-induced diuresis produces deficits averaging 5 L. Replace fluids with 0.9% normal saline at 1 L/hour for the first 2 to 3 hours.

❑❑ What are the precipitating factors leading to DKA?

Noncompliance with medications, infection, myocardial infarction, CVA, trauma, pregnancy, pancreatitis, or emotional stress.

CASE 23 (Triple)

Patient #1 (Hyperosmolar Coma and Pancreatitis)

Examiner

According to the EMTs, the staff at the nursing home where the patient lives noticed a decreased appetite, altered level of consciousness, and increasing lethargy.

This patient is in need of rapid diagnosis, (fingerstick glucose > 700), and fluid resuscitation. After a 500 cc bolus of NS, the patient will stabilize. The abdominal pain will persist and IV pain medication is appropriate once the diagnosis is made.

23.1 Introduction: (Patient #1)

A 70 year old female presents, via ambulance, from a nursing home, with a complaint of altered level of consciousness.

Vital Signs are: BP 80/40, P 130, R 30, T 100.2 °F.

23.2 Primary Survey:

- General: Chronically ill-appearing female with rapid respirations and tachycardic. Moans to painful stimuli.
- Airway: Intact.
- Breathing: Fine bibasilar crackles.
- Circulation: Poor turgor, delayed capillary refill.
- Disability: PERRLA, incomprehensible sounds, eyes open to pain.
- Exposure: No medic alert tags.

23.3 Management:

- Perform a quick bedside glucose test.
- Start IV bolus of NS (500 cc).
- Place on cardiac monitor, pulse oximeter, and O_2.
- Order appropriate labs and X-rays.

23.4 History:

- Allergies: None.
- Medications: Zaroxolyn, 5 mg po q day. Glyburide, 2.5 mg po q day. Colace, q day. Zantac, 150 mg po bid. Procardia XL, 60 mg po q day.
- PMH: Dementia, NIDDM, HTN, chronic gastritis.
- Last meal: 3 hours ago.
- Family: Unknown.
- Records: None.
- Immune: Unknown.
- EMTs: Present for questioning.
- Doctor: Private physician available for admission and information.
- Social history: Unknown.

23.5 Secondary Survey:

- General: If a fluid bolus is given the patient appears more awake.
- Skin: Dry mucosa, poor turgor, no rash.
- HEENT: Bilateral cataracts, cracked dry lips.
- Neck: Normal.
- Chest: Normal.
- Lungs: Bilateral fine crackles.
- Heart: Tachycardia, 3/6 systolic ejection murmur.
- Abdomen: Firm, bowel sounds present, tenderness over the epigastric region. No organomegaly, negative Cullin's, negative Grey-Turner's.
- Perineum/GU: Normal.
- Rectal: Heme negative.
- Back: Normal.
- Extremities: Normal.
- Neuro: Patient responds with incomprehensible sounds, and localizes to painful stimuli. DTRs normal, no focal deficits. Toes down going.

The nurse interrupts stating another pediatric patient who is very uncomfortable is waiting to be examined. Patient #1 is stable enough for the candidate to completely evaluate patients #2 and #3.

Patient #2 (Septic arthritis)

Examiner

The mother states that her child fell in the driveway 4 days ago sustaining an abrasion to the left knee. Yesterday his knee began to swell and today he started to vomit.

This is a straight forward case of a child with septic arthritis. Allow the candidate to complete the case before patient #3 arrives.

23.1 Introduction: (Patient #2)

Four year old male presents with a limp. He is accompanied by both parents.

Vital Signs are: BP 100/50, P 120, R 20, T 101.2 °F.

23.2 Primary Survey:

- ❑ General: WN/WD 4 year old male uncomfortable, but non-toxic appearing.
- ❑ Airway: Intact.
- ❑ Breathing: Normal.
- ❑ Circulation: Normal.
- ❑ Disability: Normal.
- ❑ Exposure: Swelling to the left knee.
- ❑ Finger: Deferred.

23.3 Management:

- ❑ Start IV.
- ❑ Administer bolus of 400 cc NS (20 mL/kg).
- ❑ Order appropriate labs and X-rays.

23.4 History:

- ❑ Allergies: None.
- ❑ Medications: None.
- ❑ PMH: No significant illnesses or injuries. No past surgeries.
- ❑ Last meal: 2 hours ago.
- ❑ Family: Noncontributory.
- ❑ Records: None.
- ❑ Immune: Up to date.
- ❑ Doctor: Family doctor is available for information regarding the patient's past history.
- ❑ Social history: The patient lives with both natural parents and 3 older siblings. No indication of physical abuse.

23.5 Secondary Survey:

- [ ] General: Alert and happy with no signs of distress.
- [ ] Skin: Warm, dry, no rash or petechiae. Moist mucous membranes.
- [ ] HEENT: Normal.
- [ ] Neck: Normal.
- [ ] Chest: Normal.
- [ ] Lungs: Normal.
- [ ] Heart: Normal.
- [ ] Abdomen: Normal.
- [ ] Perineum/GU: Normal.
- [ ] Rectal: Deferred.
- [ ] Back: Normal.
- [ ] Extremities: Warm, swollen, and red left knee. Decreased range of motion, cries when you attempt to examine it. Pulses are present distal to the knee. No other joints are involved.
- [ ] Neuro: Normal.

23.6 Laboratory:

- [ ] CBC: WBC 19, Hgb 15, Hct 46, Plt 450,000.
- [ ] Differential: Poly 80, Bands 25, Lymphs 15, Eos 1, Mono 3.
- [ ] Chemistry: Na 140, K 4.5, Cl 109, CO_2 22.
- [ ] BUN/Cr: 16/1.0.
- [ ] Glucose: 80.
- [ ] Ca/Mg: Normal.
- [ ] LFTs: Normal.
- [ ] Amylase/Lipase: Normal.
- [ ] PT/PTT: Normal.
- [ ] Sed rate: 88.
- [ ] Blood cultures: Pending.
- [ ] U/A: Normal.

23.7 X-rays:

- [ ] CXR: Normal.
- [ ] Left knee: No air, no fracture or periosteal reaction. Significant soft tissue swelling is present.

23.8 Special Tests:

- [ ] Joint fluid: WBC 75,000, Glc 30, Poly 80%, Turbid, Gram stain pending.

23.9 Critical Actions:

- [x] Start IV line.
- [x] Order appropriate labs.
- [x] Admit.
- [x] Start antibiotics in the ED. → Tx of septic arthritis 3mo - 14y
- [x] Arthrocentesis.

- vancomycin } until cxs return
- ceftriaxone }

'most common cause - Staph

Patient #3 (β-blocker OD)

Examiner

The patient, according to her sister, has been feeling depressed for the past year since her husband died. The family thought she was doing better because she seemed more "content" recently. She currently sold her house and moved in with her sister. She is otherwise in very good health and has no major complaints.

The patient has taken an intentional overdose of a β-blocker. This information should be hidden from the candidate until late in the case when her sister brings in the empty bottle and reveals that she has been depressed lately. The patient will be unable to provide any information until treated with glucagon.

23.1 Introduction: (Patient #3)

A 55 year old female is brought by the family who states she is tired and keeps vomiting.

Vital Signs are: BP 80/P, P 50, R 20, T 98.8 °F.

23.2 Primary Survey:

- ❑ General: WN/WD female who looks younger than stated age presents confused, disoriented, and lethargic.
- ❑ Airway: Intact.
- ❑ Breathing: Normal.
- ❑ Circulation: Delayed capillary refill, pulse regular but slow.
- ❑ Disability: PERRLA, opens eyes spontaneously, obeys verbal commands, disoriented but converses.
- ❑ Exposure: Medic alert tags indicated she has hypertension.
- ❑ Finger: Heme negative stools.

23.3 Management:

- ❑ Start IV fluids with a 250 cc bolus of NS. May repeat.
- ❑ Place on O_2, pulse oximeter, and cardiac monitor.
- ❑ Order appropriate labs, X-rays, and an ECG.
- ❑ Interview the family members and have sister bring all pill bottles.
- ❑ Candidate may administer atropine and dopamine when the pressure doesn't respond to fluids (this will also not work).
- ❑ Perform stat bedside glucose check.
- ❑ Administer Narcan.

23.4 History:

- ❑ Allergies: Unknown.
- ❑ Medications: Unknown.
- ❑ PMH: HTN, no previous suicide attempts.
- ❑ Last meal: Unknown.
- ❑ Family: Family present for questioning.
- ❑ Records: None.

- ❑ Immune: Unknown.
- ❑ Narcotics: No history of illicit drug use according to the family.
- ❑ Doctor: Family doctor is available if needed.
- ❑ Social history: No tobacco use, employed as a lawyer in an accounting firm.

23.5 Secondary Survey:

- ❑ General: Confused, but responds to commands.
- ❑ Skin: Normal.
- ❑ HEENT: Normal.
- ❑ Neck: Normal.
- ❑ Chest: Normal.
- ❑ Lungs: Normal.
- ❑ Heart: Bradycardia without a murmur or extra sounds.
- ❑ Abdomen: Normal.
- ❑ Perineum/GU: Normal.
- ❑ Rectal: Heme negative.
- ❑ Back: Normal.
- ❑ Extremities: Normal.
- ❑ Neuro: Normal.

Examiner

The sister of the patient brings back an empty bottle of Propranolol which was refilled 3 days ago. There are 60 pills missing. No other medications were noted but a suicide note was found. The candidate should immediately be treated with glucagon, 3-10 mg IV every, 15-20 minutes until improvement is seen. If glucagon is given, the patient will get better and become more responsive.

23.6 Laboratory:

- ❑ CBC: WBC 11, Hgb 12.2, Hct 39, Plt 255,000.
- ❑ Chemistry: Na 144, K 4.4, Cl 115, CO_2 23.
- ❑ BUN/Cr: 12/1.0.
- ❑ Glucose: 105.
- ❑ Ca/Mg: Normal.
- ❑ LFTs: Normal.
- ❑ Amylase/Lipase: Normal.
- ❑ PT/PTT: Normal.
- ❑ Cardiac enzymes: Normal.
- ❑ ABG: pH 7.43, pO_2 98, pCO_2 40, HCO_3 21, (room air).
- ❑ Blood cultures: Pending.
- ❑ Salicylate: Negative.
- ❑ Acetaminophen: Negative.
- ❑ β-HCG: Negative.
- ❑ Anion gap: 6.
- ❑ Osmolality: 290.
- ❑ Osmo gap: 10.

- ❑ ETOH: Negative.
- ❑ U/A: Normal.
- ❑ Urine drug screen: Negative.

23.7 X-rays:

- ❑ CXR: Normal.
- ❑ CT head: Normal.

23.8 Special Tests:

- ❑ ECG: Sinus bradycardia without ectopy or heart block.
- ❑ Pulse oximeter: 100% on room air.
- ❑ Cardiac monitor: Sinus bradycardia.

23.9 Critical Actions:

- ❑ Start IV fluids, O_2, and cardiac monitor.
- ❑ Obtain a history of depression and overdose with propranolol.
- ❑ Treat the low BP and altered level of consciousness with fluids and appropriate medications (glucose, Narcan, atropine, and possibly dopamine).
- ❑ Administer glucagon after determining a β-blocker is involved.
- ❑ Check salicylate, acetaminophen, urine drug screen, serum ETOH.
- ❑ Admit to the ICU.
- ❑ Place the patient on suicide precautions.
- ❑ Obtain a psychiatric consult.

Patient #1

23.6 Laboratory:

- ❑ CBC: WBC 18, Hgb 15.5, Hct 54, Plt 400,000.
- ❑ Differential: Polys 60, Bands 27, Lymphs. 11, Eos 2, Mono 0.
- ❑ Chemistry: Na 150, K 5.6, Cl 120, CO_2 22.
- ❑ BUN/Cr: 48/2.7.
- ❑ Glucose: 1205.
- ❑ Ca/Mg: 11.0/1.5.
- ❑ Phosphorus: 2.2.
- ❑ LFTs: Normal.
- ❑ Amylase/Lipase: 360/2102.
- ❑ PT/PTT: Normal.
- ❑ Cardiac enzymes: Normal.
- ❑ ABG: pH 7.35, pO_2 85, pCO_2 46, HCO_3 22.
- ❑ Serum ketones: Negative.
- ❑ Blood cultures: Pending.
- ❑ U/A: Protein 300, Glucose 3+, Ketone negative, WBC 0, RBC 0.

23.7 X-rays:

- ❑ CXR: Normal.
- ❑ Abdominal series: Sentinel loop with calcifications in the area of the pancreas. No free air.

23.8 Special Tests:

- ❑ Cardiac monitor: Sinus tachycardia.
- ❑ Pulse oximeter: 94% on room air.

23.9 Critical Actions:

- ❑ Start IV, O_2, and place on monitor.
- ❑ Administer fluid bolus.
- ❑ Check bedside glucose.
- ❑ Order appropriate labs.
- ❑ Relieve patient's pain.

23.10 Pearls: (Patient #1)

❑❑ What predisposing factors precipitate hyperosmolar, hyperglycemic, nonketotic coma?

Chronic renal insufficiency, pneumonia, gram-negative sepsis, myocardial infarction, pancreatitis, GI bleeding, and medication (thiazide diuretics, phenytoin, propranolol, cimetidine, and corticosteroids).

❑❑ What are the indications for insulin in HHNC?

Severe acidosis, hyperkalemia, or renal failure.

Pearls: (Patient #2)

❑❑ What are the bacterial etiologies of septic arthritis in children and adolescents?

Staphylococcus aureus and Group B *Streptococcus* are the most common pathogens in the first 2 months of life. From 3 months to 3 years, *Haemophilus influenzae* type B and *S. aureus* are the most common. *H. influenzae* has decreased since advent of the HIB vaccine. After 3 years of age, *S. aureus* predominates until adolescence, when *Neisseria gonorrhea* becomes a frequent cause.

❑❑ How does septic arthritis occur?

Seeding of a joint with bacteria occurs either by hematogenous spread, direct inoculation, or spread from an adjacent site of infection. Hematogenous dissemination is secondary to the spread of colonized invasive organisms that breach mucosal defenses, resulting in bacteremia.

Pearls: (Patient #3)

❑❑ Why is glucagon useful in the treatment of β-blocker overdose?

IV glucagon enhances myocardial contractility, heart rate, and AV conduction by stimulating the production of intracellular cyclic AMP.

❑❑ **What are the potential ECG abnormalities seen in a β-blocker overdose?**

Sinus bradycardia, first-degree block, widening of the QRS complex, peaked T waves, and ST changes.

❑❑ **What clinical presentation may be seen with β-blocker poisoning?**

Bradyrhythmias, hypotension, conduction abnormalities, CHF (more likely in those with heart disease),bronchospasm (especially in those with history of bronchospasm), seizures, altered mental status, and hypoglycemia.

CASE 24 (Alcoholic Ketoacidosis, Pubic Lice)

Examiner

According to a neighbor, the patient drinks alcohol. However, he told her last night that he stopped drinking due to abdominal pain. The neighbor checked on him this morning and he still had pain and nausea had developed. After work today, the patient was complaining of pain and vomiting. She then forced the patient to come to the ED.

This patient will refuse to cooperate and will be combative. His neighbor gives an accurate history. He will require sedation and IV rehydration will normalize his vital signs and mental status.

24.1 Introduction:

A 70 year old male is brought by ambulance screaming obscenities.

Vitals Signs: BP 140/75, P 114, R 34, T 99.6 °F.

24.2 Primary Survey:

- ❑ General: Unkept, unshaven obese male holding his abdomen and smelling of alcohol with 10,000 lice all screaming "Please save our host!".
- ❑ Airway: Intact.
- ❑ Breathing: Tachypneic.
- ❑ Circulation: Rapid thready pulse.
- ❑ Disability: Normal.
- ❑ Exposure: No medic alert tags.
- ❑ Finger: Trace positive blood in stool.

24.3 Management:

- ❑ Start IV of NS with a 500 cc bolus.
- ❑ Perform bedside glucose check (35 mg/dL).
- ❑ Place on cardiac monitor, pulse oximeter, and O_2.
- ❑ Sedate to calm the patient.
- ❑ Order appropriate labs, CXR, head CT, and ECG.
- ❑ Administer thiamine, 100 mg IM or IV.

24.4 History:

- ❑ Allergies: None.
- ❑ Medications: None.
- ❑ PMH: His neighbor is unsure of his past medical problems. She does not remember whether he had his gallbladder or appendix removed.
- ❑ Last meal: 2 days ago.
- ❑ Family: Unknown.
- ❑ Records: None.
- ❑ Immune: Unknown.
- ❑ EMTs: They are present to comment on his appearance.
- ❑ Narcotics: No illicit drug use.
- ❑ Doctor: None.
- ❑ Social history: Retired lawyer. Divorced four times. Smokes 2 packs of cigarettes per day and drinks about one-fifth of bourbon daily.

24.5 Secondary Survey:

- ❑ General: As above. If given a fluid bolus and glucose, he will be more awake and alert.
- ❑ Skin: Multiple old well-healed scars and bruises of varying age. Pruritic rash, located in genital region.
- ❑ HEENT: Left frontal ecchymosis, beefy red tongue, dental caries, PERRLA, EOM-I. Fundi normal.
- ❑ Neck: Normal.
- ❑ Chest: Tenderness to palpation along left ribs, old ecchymosis present.
- ❑ Lungs: Tachypnea, diffuse rhonchi.
- ❑ Heart: Tachycardia. No murmur, rub, or gallop.
- ❑ Abdomen: Tenderness to the epigastric region without guarding.
- ❑ Perineum/GU: Atrophic testicles.
- ❑ Rectal: Trace guaiac positive stools, normal prostate.
- ❑ Back: Normal.
- ❑ Extremities: No clubbing, wasted musculature present, no edema.
- ❑ Neuro: Resting tremor is present, otherwise normal.

24.6 Laboratory:

- ❑ CBC: WBC 4.4, Hgb 12.3, Hct 34.7, Plt 145,000.
- ❑ Differential: Polys 77, Bands 2, Lymphs 18, Eos 2, Mono 5.
- ❑ Chemistry: Na 146, K 5.2, Cl 108, CO_2 9.
- ❑ BUN/Cr: 28/1.1.
- ❑ Glucose: 35.
- ❑ Ca/Mg: 8.4/1.6.
- ❑ Phosphorus: 2.8.
- ❑ LFTs: Normal.
- ❑ Amylase/Lipase: 350/200.
- ❑ PT/PTT: 13/38.
- ❑ Cardiac enzymes: Normal.
- ❑ ABG: pH 7.15, pO_2 94, pCO_2 .27, HCO_3 10.
- ❑ Blood cultures: Pending.

- ❑ Anion gap: 29.
- ❑ Osmolality: 370.
- ❑ Serum acetone: Moderate.
- ❑ ETOH: 205.
- ❑ U/A: Normal.

24.7 <u>X-rays</u>:

- ❑ CXR: No pneumothorax or infiltrate.
- ❑ CT head: Diffuse cortical atrophy.

24.8 <u>Special Tests</u>:

- ❑ ECG: Sinus tachycardia.
- ❑ Wood's Lamp: Fluoresce nits.
- ❑ Microscopic: *P. pubis.*

24.9 <u>Critical Actions</u>:

- ❑ Start IV with fluid bolus and O_2. Place on monitor and pulse oximeter.
- ❑ Perform bedside glucose test with correction of low sugar.
- ❑ Order appropriate labs, X-rays, and ECG.
- ❑ Determine ABG.
- ❑ Add thiamine, vitamins, and magnesium to IV.
- ❑ Order head CT.
- ❑ Sedate accordingly.
- ❑ Admit to a monitored bed.
- ❑ Administer topical 1% Permethrin, or 0.5% Malathion, or Lindane.

24.10 <u>Pearls</u>:

❑❑ Why would a patient with alcoholic ketoacidosis be negative for ketone bodies?

There are three types of ketone bodies; acetone and the two acids, β-hydroxybutyrate (βHB) and acetoacetate (AcAc). The nitroprusside reaction, commonly used to detect ketones, may give a false negative because only AcAc and acetone cause a positive reaction and βHB is the dominant ketone in AKA.

❑❑ What is the classic historical presentation for a patient with AKA?

The patient is a chronic alcoholic with poor caloric intake, vomiting, anorexia, abdominal pain, and a recent termination of binge drinking. Patients often present 24-48 hours after last alcohol use.

Case 25 (Heat Stroke, Rhabdomyolysis)

Examiner

A neighbor of the patient called the EMTs because the patient has not left her apartment for four days and does not answer the door or phone. The neighbor does not know anything else about the history of the patient.

This is a simple, straight-forward case of hyperthermia requiring rapid immediate cooling and rhabdomyolysis. If cooling is performed, the patient will respond by becoming more responsive and the neurologic findings will disappear. Only state the temperature when asked a second time by the candidate. Have the candidate describe their cooling technique of choice, in detail.

25.1 Introduction:

A 70 year old female arrives, via ambulance, with an altered level of consciousness.

Vital Signs are: BP 90/P, P 120, R 36.

25.2 Primary Survey:

- ❑ General: Obtunded female, speaking incomprehensible words.
- ❑ Airway: Intact.
- ❑ Breathing: Lungs clear, tachypneic.
- ❑ Circulation: Rapid thready pulse, delayed capillary refill.
- ❑ Disability: PERRL. Opens eyes to verbal command, localizes pain, incomprehensible words.
- ❑ Exposure: No medic alert tags.
- ❑ Finger: Negative.

25.3 Management:

- ❑ Determine rectal temperature (106.5 ^{o}F) with continuous rectal temperature probe.
- ❑ Start IV of NS at 250 mL/hour.
- ❑ Place on cardiac monitor, pulse oximeter, and O_2.
- ❑ Insert Foley catheter - rose colored urine.
- ❑ Order appropriate labs.
- ❑ Begin rapid cooling.
- ❑ Administer thiamine, glucose, Narcan.
- ❑ Candidate may elect to administer sodium bicarbonate if rhabdomyolysis is recognized.

25.4 History:

- ❑ Allergies: Unknown.
- ❑ Medications: Unknown.
- ❑ PMH: Unknown.
- ❑ Last meal: Unknown.
- ❑ Family: Unknown.
- ❑ Records: None.

- ❑ Immune: Unknown.
- ❑ EMTs: They noted the apartment was hot, the windows were closed, and the patient was lying on the bed asleep. No pill bottles or alcohol were present in the house.
- ❑ Narcotics: Unknown.
- ❑ Doctor: The internist on call is available.
- ❑ Social history: Unknown.

25.5 <u>Secondary Survey</u>:

- ❑ General: Patient is more awake and gives some history if appropriate cooling measures and fluids are given.
- ❑ Skin: Hot, dry, pale.
- ❑ HEENT: Dry, parched mouth otherwise, normal.
- ❑ Neck: Normal.
- ❑ Chest: Normal.
- ❑ Lungs: Tachypneic.
- ❑ Heart: Tachycardia without murmur.
- ❑ Abdomen: Normal.
- ❑ Perineum/GU: Normal.
- ❑ Rectal: Heme negative.
- ❑ Back: Normal.
- ❑ Extremities: Normal.
- ❑ Neuro: Cranial nerves intact. DTRs hyperactive and equal. Toes upgoing bilateral. Unable to assess cerebellar function.

25.6 <u>Laboratory</u>:

- ❑ CBC: WBC 22, Hgb 14, Hct 41, Plt 200,000.
- ❑ Chemistry: Na 145, K 4.5, Cl 110, CO_2 24.
- ❑ BUN/Cr: 40/1.7.
- ❑ Glucose: 80.
- ❑ Ca/Mg: Normal.
- ❑ LFTs: SGOT 45, GGT 80, Alk Phosp 110.
- ❑ Amylase/Lipase: Normal.
- ❑ PT/PTT: 13/25.
- ❑ Cardiac enzymes: CPK 1110 (122,600), CKMB 2%.
- ❑ ABG: pH 7.40, pO_2 92, pCO_2 40, HCO_3 23.
- ❑ Blood cultures: Pending.
- ❑ U/A: ø WBC, ø RBC.
- ❑ Urine dip: Positive for blood and protein.
- ❑ Urine myoglobin: Negative.

25.7 <u>X-rays</u>:

- ❑ CXR: Normal.
- ❑ CT head: Normal.

25.8 Special Tests:

- ❑ ECG: Sinus tachycardia without abnormalities.
- ❑ Pulse oximeter: 93% on room air.
- ❑ Cardiac monitor: Sinus tachycardia without ectopy.

25.9 Critical Actions:

- ❑ Recognize hyperthermia and begin rapid cooling.
- ❑ Recognize rhabdomyolysis and initiate treatment with volume resuscitation.
- ❑ Place on O_2 and monitor cardiac responses.
- ❑ Insert Foley catheter.
- ❑ Order CBC, chemistry profile, LFTs, coagulation studies, U/A, urine myoglobin, and ECG.
- ❑ Admit to ICU.

25.10 Pearls:

❑❑ **What is the etiology and treatment for myoglobinuria?**

The cause is rhabdomyolysis, and the treatment is IV hydration, osmotic diuretics, and alkalinization of the urine.

❑❑ **Which medications can cause hyperthermia?**

Neuroleptic agents, anticholinergics, salicylate toxicity, PCP, amphetamine, cocaine, and lithium.

CASE 26 (Hypothermia)

Examiner

This patient presents with an altered level of consciousness due to hypothermia. The candidate should use a rectal probe because standard thermometers monitor only down to a temperature of 95 °F. Implementing a coma protocol is required. If the candidate aggressively warms the patient, he will become more responsive. If not, he will go into VF and will remain in VF until he is warmed.

26.1 Introduction:

A 45 year old homeless male presents, via ambulance, unconscious.

Vital Signs are: BP 90/P, P 50, R 10.

26.2 Primary Survey:

- ❑ General: Give the temperature as 95 °F unless the candidate asks for a rectal probe. The probe will read 80 °F. The patient is a poorly nourished male who is unresponsive to painful stimuli with a poor respiratory effort.
- ❑ Airway: Intact.

- ❑ Breathing: Decreased respiratory rate.
- ❑ Circulation: Capillary refill 4 seconds.
- ❑ Disability: Pupils dilated and nonreactive.
- ❑ Exposure: No medic alert tags, no gross abnormalities. A bottle of whiskey is in his pocket.
- ❑ Finger: Heme negative.

26.3 Management:

- ❑ Intubate with c-spine precaution.
- ❑ Start two large bore IVs. Infuse 250 mL bolus of warm saline and continue warm saline.
- ❑ Apply an external warming device.
- ❑ Insert a NG tube and a Foley catheter. Remove all clothing.
- ❑ Place on cardiac monitor and pulse oximeter.
- ❑ Order appropriate labs, X-rays, and an ECG.
- ❑ Administer thiamine, Narcan, glucose IV.
- ❑ Active core rewarming.

26.4 History:

- ❑ Allergies: Unknown.
- ❑ Medications: Unknown.
- ❑ PMH: Unknown.
- ❑ Last meal: Unknown.
- ❑ Family: None.
- ❑ Records: None.
- ❑ Immune: Unknown.
- ❑ EMTs: The patient was found behind a building unconscious, wet, cold without signs of trauma.
- ❑ Narcotics: Unknown.
- ❑ Doctor: Unknown.
- ❑ Social history: Unavailable.

26.5 Secondary Survey:

- ❑ General: No change from the primary survey.
- ❑ Skin: Cold, moist, clammy, poor turgor., old healed scars
- ❑ HEENT: Normocephalic and atraumatic head. Pupils dilated, non-reactive; Fundi normal.
- ❑ Neck: Supple, no JVD, no nodes.
- ❑ Chest: Atraumatic. No palpable crepitance.
- ❑ Lungs: Clear.
- ❑ Heart: Bradycardic without a murmur.
- ❑ Abdomen: Soft, bowel sounds decreased. No mass, no organomegaly.
- ❑ Perineum/GU: Normal.
- ❑ Rectal: Normal.
- ❑ Back: Normal.
- ❑ Extremities: Diminished pulses, abrasions to the left forearm.
- ❑ Neuro: No eye opening, incomprehensible sounds, and flexion withdraw reaction to pain. Toes equivocal. DTRs +1/+4 and symmetric.

26.6 Laboratory:

- CBC: WBC 7.5, Hgb 18, Hct 59, Plt 35,000.
- Differential: Polys 70, Bands 3, Lymphs 20, Eos 1, Mono 3.
- Chemistry: Na 140, K 4.5, Cl 106, CO_2 24.
- BUN/Cr: 28/1.6.
- Glucose: 130.
- Ca/Mg: Normal.
- LFTs: Normal.
- Amylase/Lipase: 300/650.
- PT/PTT: 17/45.
- Cardiac enzymes: Normal.
- ETOH: 355.
- ABG: pH 7.16, pO_2 90, pCO_2 50, HCO_3 24.
- Blood cultures: Pending.
- Urine drug: Negative.
- U/A: Negative.

26.7 X-rays:

- C-spine: Normal.
- CXR: Normal.
- Pelvis: Normal.
- CT head: Normal.
- Left forearm: Normal.

26.8 Special Tests:

- Cardiac monitor: Sinus bradycardia.
- Pulse oximeter: 86% on room air initially.
- ECG: Sinus bradycardia with Osborne J waves.

26.9 Critical Actions:

- Intubate with c-spine precautions.
- Obtain an accurate core temperature.
- Perform active rewarming.
- Insert a NG tube and a Foley catheter.
- Place on cardiac monitor.
- Administer tetanus, 0.5 cc IM.
- Administer thiamine, Narcan, glucose.
- Obtain CT of the head.
- Admit to the ICU.

26.10 Pearls:

❑❑ What constitutes active rewarming?

Techniques that warm the core of the body directly. Such techniques include heated IV fluids, peritoneal lavage, gastrointestinal and bladder irrigation, heated inhalation, thoracostomy tube irrigation and extracorporeal rewarming.

❑❑ What are the indications for active rewarming?

When the temperature is below 90 °F, cardiovascular instability, neurologic, or endocrinologic insufficiency.

CASE 27 (Epiglottitis)

Examiner

Child presents, via EMS, with suspected epiglottitis. The child has a cough, sore throat, and a fever throughout the day, which has quickly worsened.

The physician should allow mother to ride in ambulance and remain with child in ED despite the nurse's desire to remove the parent. Paramedics should not be told to intubate the patient.

On arrival, evidence of epiglottitis is easily discovered. Physician should avoid any intervention, despite nurse's, lab tech's, and respiratory therapist's attempts to perform tests.

Physician should have crash cart available while arranging for OR, calling anesthesiology, and having ENT enroute as quickly as possible.

Once initial stabilization is achieved, the emergency physician should be asked to see a patient with an ankle injury that is demanding immediate attention. The emergency physician should ask the nurse to obtain X-rays but they should not leave the patient's bedside. If they do, the patient requires immediate crash intubation and results in the patient's death. The role of ED physician should be close observation without active intervention until the appropriate consultants are immediately available.

27.1 Introduction:

A 4 year old child presents, via EMS, with a sore throat, drooling, and difficulty in breathing. Mother says the child has had a fever at home.

Vital Signs are: BP N/A, P 120, R 30, T N/A.

Nurse should be instructed to take P and RR, avoid BP and T.

27.2 Primary Survey:

- ❑ General: Toxic appearing child is sitting propped up on his hands with his head forward and his tongue out.
- ❑ Airway: Avoid examination of airway. If airway is examined the child immediately goes into respiratory distress, intubation is impossible, and the child dies.
- ❑ Breathing: Child is moving air. Stridor. Lungs clear and equal.
- ❑ Circulation: Distal pulse intact, rate of 120.
- ❑ Disability: Alert, moving all extremities.

- ❑ Exposure: Avoid.
- ❑ Finger: Avoid.

27.3 Management:

- ❑ Ensure that a pediatric crash cart is located at bedside.
- ❑ Place an immediate call to anesthesiology.
- ❑ Call ENT in from home.
- ❑ Allow parent to remain with child.

27.4 History:

- ❑ Allergies: None.
- ❑ Medications: None.
- ❑ PMH: None.
- ❑ Last meal: 8 hours ago.
- ❑ Events: Child has had a cough, sore throat, and fever today, which has quickly became worsened.
- ❑ Family: None.
- ❑ Records: None.
- ❑ Immune: Child is Hispanic and his family is visiting the US. The child has not received the Haemophilus b vaccine.
- ❑ EMTs: Avoid treatment enroute.
- ❑ Narcotics: None.
- ❑ Doctor: Pages to Dr. Pediatrician, Dr. Anesthesiologist, and Dr. ENT.
- ❑ Social history: None.

27.5 Secondary Survey:

- ❑ General: Toxic 4 year old in moderate respiratory distress. Distress increases if any active intervention occurs.
- ❑ Skin: Warm and dry.
- ❑ HEENT: Drooling.
- ❑ Neck: Avoid.
- ❑ Chest: Tachypnea.
- ❑ Lungs: Clear.
- ❑ Heart: Regular and tachy.
- ❑ Abdomen: Avoid.
- ❑ Rectal: Avoid.
- ❑ Back: No gross abnormality.
- ❑ Extremities: No gross abnormality.
- ❑ Neuro: Toxic. Moving all extremities.

27.6 Laboratory:

- ❑ Avoid lab draws.
- ❑ Pulse oximeter may be obtained: 96%.

27.8 X-rays:

- ❑ CXR: Avoid.
- ❑ Soft tissue neck: Avoid.

27.9 Critical Actions:

- ❑ Ensure that intubation equipment is readily available, including needle cricothyrotomy prep.
- ❑ Page anesthesiology and ENT quickly.
- ❑ Prepare OR for patient.
- ❑ Avoid unnecessary interventions (blood draws, monitors, and radiographs).
- ❑ Allow patient to remain with parent.
- ❑ Avoid leaving patient's bedside.
- ❑ Treat family members with rifampin.

27.10 Pearls:

❑❑ What is the most common cause of epiglottitis in children? In adults?

Children: *Haemophilus influenzae type B*. Adults: *Haemophilus influenzae type B* and Group A *Streptococcus*.

❑❑ If *Haemophilus influenzae* is isolated, what should be done for family members and close contacts?

Close contacts and family members under 4 should be treated with rifampin.

CASE 28 (Crotalidae Envenomation)

Examiner

Patient is intoxicated. With difficulty, physician learns that the patient was bitten in the buttocks when he sat on a snake while he and his friends were "whooping it up" by the campfire. He has had increasing pain and swelling of the buttock since the event occurred one hour ago. He also feels light-headed.

The patient has a high envenomation bite and eventually requires antivenom.

28.1 Introduction:

A 24 year old male, very intoxicated, complaining of pain in the butt.

Vital Signs are: BP 80/60, P 128, R 20, T 99 °F.

28.2 Primary Survey:

- ❑ General: Intoxicated, very wild, poor historian, complaining of severe pain.
- ❑ Airway: Intact.

- ❑ Breathing: Regular.
- ❑ Circulation: Tachy.
- ❑ Disability: None.
- ❑ Exposure: Buttock swelling and 2 clear puncture wounds.
- ❑ Finger: Normal rectal tone, guaiac negative.

28.3 Management:

- ❑ Start IV, O_2, and place on monitor.
- ❑ Orders labs.
- ❑ Fluid challenge.

28.4 History:

- ❑ Allergies: None.
- ❑ Medications: None.
- ❑ PMH: Previous rattlesnake bite.
- ❑ Last meal: Had several beers in the last few hours.
- ❑ Family: None.
- ❑ Records: None.
- ❑ Immune: None.
- ❑ EMTs: None.
- ❑ Doctor: Consult private MD for ICU admission.
- ❑ Social history: History of excessive alcohol use.

28.5 Secondary Survey:

- ❑ VS: Minimal response to fluid challenge.
- ❑ General: Vomiting, complaining of pain.
- ❑ Skin: Two fang marks on buttock, extensive soft tissue swelling, and edema.
- ❑ HEENT: Numbness and tingling to mouth and tongue.
- ❑ Neck: Normal.
- ❑ Chest: Normal.
- ❑ Lungs: Normal.
- ❑ Heart: Tachycardia.
- ❑ Abdomen: Mild non-focal tenderness.
- ❑ Rectal: Normal.
- ❑ Back: Normal.
- ❑ Extremities: Normal.
- ❑ Neuro: Decreased motor strength, muscle fasciculations, somnolent.

28. 6 Laboratory:

- ❑ CBC: WBC 12, Hgb 11, Hct 33, Plt 200.
- ❑ Chemistry: Na 135, K 4.8, Cl 110, CO_2 24.
- ❑ BUN/Cr: 18/1.2.
- ❑ Glucose: 130.
- ❑ Ca/Mg: Normal.

- ❑ LFTs: Normal.
- ❑ Amylase/Lipase: Normal.
- ❑ PT/PTT: 16/30.
- ❑ U/A: +++ Glucose, protein, and blood.
- ❑ ETOH: 146.
- ❑ Type and Cross: Pending.
- ❑ Drug screen: Negative.

28.7 X-rays:

- ❑ CXR: Normal.

28.8 Critical Actions:

- ❑ Determine Td status.
- ❑ Relieve pain with narcotics or Tylenol.
- ❑ Determine if patient has history of horse serum allergy prior to treatment.
- ❑ Determine systemic symptoms and administer appropriate drugs: First skin test, if negative, start 5 vials of antivenin in 250 mL normal saline IV fluid, one vial every 15 minutes.
- ❑ Avoid NSAIDs and ASA which may increase bleeding.
- ❑ Admit to ICU.

28.9 Pearls:

❑❑ What percentage of rattle snake bites are dry bites?

25%.

❑❑ What signs and symptoms suggest the need for antivenom?

Systemic symptoms such as tachycardia, hypo/hypertension, muscle fasciculations, and change in mental status.

❑❑ How much antivenom is typically required?

Up to 30 vials may be required for severe envenomations.

CASE 29 (Multiple Blunt Trauma)

Examiner

This patient has hit a parked car. She was found passed out behind the wheel of the car with no seatbelt. There is extensive damage to the front end of the vehicle.

This is the trauma case from hell. The patient has a C-5 step-off fracture, a left-pneumothorax, is pregnant with the uterus placing pressure on the vena cava until she is rolled. The patient also has a bladder rupture, an abruption, a pelvic fracture, and a dislocated open fracture of the left-ankle.

The patient was involved in a high-speed head on collision into a parked car. The reason for the accident was severe hypoglycemia and opiate-induced somnolence.

The examiner should be careful not to give anything away. The physician must remember to roll the patient 30 degrees to the left or the vital signs will continue to drop. The fetus also is in distress until the patient is rolled. In addition, the patient only responds to pain until both dextrose and Narcan are given.

The physician must consult several specialists, including the trauma surgeon, urologist, obstetrician, and orthopedic surgeon. However, all of these individuals are out on the golf course with a dead cell phone and can't be reached until all of the patient's problems are diagnosed and treated.

A 24 year old female crashes her car into another parked car. Backboard, but no c-spine precautions.

Vital Signs are: BP 90/60, P 128, R 30, T 97.6 °F.

29.2 Primary Survey:

- ❑ General: Non-responsive female.
- ❑ Airway: No gag.
- ❑ Breathing: Tachypnea. No breath sounds on the left.
- ❑ Circulation: 4 second capillary refill.
- ❑ Disability: Does not respond to painful stimuli. Pupils reactive.
- ❑ Exposure: No medic alert tags. Trachea deviated to the right. Left ankle is deformed. Patient is obviously pregnant but this information is only provided if the candidate asks or examines the abdomen.
- ❑ Finger: Rectal tone intact, no blood. Blood in vaginal vault os closed.

29.3 Management:

- ❑ Restrain with cervical collar.
- ❑ Intubate by using in-line immobilization.
- ❑ Insert left chest tube. Obtain 200 cc of blood.
- ❑ Start large bore IVs, 1-2 L wide open. Place on O_2 and monitor.
- ❑ Insert a NG tube but do not insert a Foley catheter due to blood.
- ❑ Order trauma labs.
- ❑ Administer dextrose, Narcan, and thiamine.
- ❑ Evaluate Csp, CXR, and pelvis.
- ❑ Relocate ankle, apply traction, and order X-rays.
- ❑ Administer antibiotics for open fracture.
- ❑ Roll patient on the left side by placing a blanket roll under the right side of the backboard.

29.4 History:

- ❑ Allergies: Unknown.
- ❑ Medications: Unknown.
- ❑ PMH: Unknown.
- ❑ Last meal: Unknown.
- ❑ Events: Hit a parked car. Found passed out behind the wheel of the car. No seatbelt. Extensive damage to front end of vehicle.
- ❑ Family: Unknown.

- ❑ Records: Unknown.
- ❑ Immune: Unknown.
- ❑ EMTs: Extensive vehicle damage.
- ❑ Narcotics: Search reveals empty bottle of Tylenol #3 (20 tabs).
- ❑ Doctor: Dr. Wow on pill bottle. If called, answering service says the dentist is not in until tomorrow morning.
- ❑ Social history: Unknown.

29.5 Secondary Survey:

- ❑ General: Non-responsive unless given Narcan and dextrose.
- ❑ Skin: Multiple tattoos.
- ❑ HEENT: Normal.
- ❑ Neck: Palpable step-off at C-5.
- ❑ Chest: Palpable crepitance on the left.
- ❑ Lungs: Breath sounds equal with tube placement.
- ❑ Heart: Tachy.
- ❑ Abdomen: BS +. Soft. Pelvic mass present. If specifically asked, palpably enlarged uterus, 6 months.
- ❑ Perineum/GU: Blood in vaginal vault and around urethra.
- ❑ Rectal: Guaiac negative.
- ❑ Back: Normal.
- ❑ Extremities: Dislocated left ankle, open fracture, pulseless until relocated.
- ❑ Neuro: Minimal response to painful stimuli while moving all extremities. The patient wakes up and fights tube if given Narcan and glucose.

29.6 Laboratory:

- ❑ CBC: WBC 18, Hgb 11, Hct 33, Plt 400.
- ❑ Chemistry: Na 135, K 4.0, Cl 110, CO_2 24.
- ❑ BUN/Cr: 18/1.2.
- ❑ Glucose: 20; 150 if given glucose.
- ❑ LFTs: Normal.
- ❑ Amylase/Lipase: Normal.
- ❑ PT/PTT: Normal.
- ❑ ABG: pH 7.4, pO_2 95, pCO_2 24, HCO_3 20.
- ❑ U/A: Large blood.
- ❑ Urine pregnancy test: Positive.
- ❑ Drug Screen: Opiates.

29.7 X-rays:

- ❑ CXR: ET, good placement. No pneumo after tube. Left pulmonary contusion.
- ❑ Csp: Step off at C-5-6.
- ❑ Pelvis: Left pubic rami fracture. Fetus.
- ❑ Urethrogram: Bladder extravasation.
- ❑ L Ankle: Trimalleolar fracture.

29.8 Special Tests:

- ❑ US Pelvis: Placenta abruption.
- ❑ Fetal monitor: Shows distress until mother put in left lateral position.
- ❑ CT: Down.
- ❑ ECG: Normal sinus rhythm, tachycardia.
- ❑ Lavage: Should be avoided as patient will go to OR with ruptured bladder. If performed without open technique, amniotic fluid present on tap.

29.9 Critical Actions:

- ☑ Place a cervical collar on the patient.
- ☑ Intubate by using in-line immobilization.
- ☑ Insert left chest tube.
- ☑ Use large bore IVs, 1-2 L wide open. Start O_2 and monitor.
- ☑ Insert a NG tube. Hold off on a Foley due to blood.
- ☑ Order trauma labs. Obtain blood, even though it is not needed.
- ❑ Administer dextrose, Narcan, and thiamine.
- ☑ Relocate ankle, apply traction, and order X-rays.
- ☑ Administer antibiotics for open fracture.
- ☑ Roll patient on left side.
- ☑ Obtain fetal evaluation, i.e., ultrasound and fetal monitor.
- ❑ Avoid peritoneal lavage or CT.
- ☑ Consult trauma, ortho, Ob/Gyn, and urology.
- ❑ Diagnosis: C-spine Fx, pneumo, bladder rupture, pelvic Fx, and fracture and dislocated ankle.

29.10 Pearls:

❑❑ What percentage of patients with bladder rupture have hematuria?

94%.

❑❑ Does a bladder rupture typically cause peritonitis?

No.

❑❑ What are common risk factors for bladder rupture?

Full bladder at the time of the trauma and prior pelvic or bladder surgery.

CASE 30 (Asthma)

Examiner

A patient with history of asthma is brought in by paramedics. Enroute she receives several treatments. The paramedics indicate that shortly before arrival the patient became significantly worse. All attempts at medical therapy fail, such as subcutaneous and IV epinephrine, Solu-Medrol, magnesium, and inhalers.

Intubation does not help. The patient is very tight and breath sounds cannot be distinguished. The only X-ray technician in the hospital is in the ICU at a code.

The patient has a pneumothorax that can only be diagnosed by performing a needle thoracostomy. The physician must needle both sides to find the pneumothorax. Following needling the chest, it is critical that a chest tube is placed in both sides as a pneumothorax has been created by the act of needling both chests.

30.1 Introduction:

A 28 year old female with history of asthma arrives, via paramedics, in acute respiratory distress.

Vital Signs are: BP 160/80, P 130, R 34, T 98.6 °F.

30.2 Primary Survey:

- ❑ General: Acute distress, unable to speak.
- ❑ Airway: No gag.
- ❑ Breathing: No breath sounds.
- ❑ Circulation: 3s capillary refill.

30.3 Management:

- ❑ Intubate.
- ❑ Administer β-agonists.
- ❑ Administer epinephrine.
- ❑ Administer Solu-Medrol.
- ❑ Administer magnesium.
- ❑ Consider Heliox.
- ❑ Start IV, O_2, and place on monitor.
- ❑ Order labs and ABGs.
- ❑ CXR ordered but is not available.
- ❑ Needle L or R chest (no response).
- ❑ Needle other chest (rush of air).
- ❑ Place chest tube bilaterally.

30.4 History:

- ❑ Allergies: None.
- ❑ Medications: Proventil inhaler, prednisone, Cipro, and theophylline.
- ❑ PMH: N/A.
- ❑ Last meal: N/A.
- ❑ Events: Family says patient ran out of inhalers and steroids 2 days ago and today she became much worse.
- ❑ Family: None.
- ❑ Records: None.
- ❑ Immune: N/A.
- ❑ EMT: Gave two breathing treatments when she suddenly became much worse.
- ❑ Narcotics: None.
- ❑ Doctor: Available for admission.

- ❑ Social history: None.

30.5 Secondary Survey:

- ❑ General: Acute distress.
- ❑ Skin: Warm.
- ❑ HEENT: Normal.
- ❑ Neck: Retractions.
- ❑ Chest: Retractions and tachypnea.
- ❑ Lungs: No breath sounds until chest tube placement and then diffuse wheezes.
- ❑ Heart: Normal.
- ❑ Abdomen: Normal.
- ❑ Pelvic: Deferred.
- ❑ Rectal: Deferred.
- ❑ Back: Normal.
- ❑ Extremities: Normal.
- ❑ Neuro: Obtunded.

30.6 Laboratory:

- ❑ CBC: WBC 15, Hgb 12, Hct 36.
- ❑ Chemistry: Normal.
- ❑ BUN/Cr: Normal.
- ❑ Glucose: Normal.
- ❑ ABG: pH 7.3, pO_2 70, pCO_2 20, HCO_3 22.
- ❑ U/A: + Bacteria and WBCs.
- ❑ Theophylline: 24.

30.7 X-rays:

- ❑ CXR: Bilateral chest tubes, ETT in place.

30.8 Critical Actions:

- ❑ Intubate.
- ❑ Administer β-agonists.
- ❑ Administer epinephrine.
- ❑ Administer Solu-Medrol.
- ❑ Start IV, O_2, and place on monitor.
- ❑ Assess CXR and check tube placement.
- ❑ Needle L and R chest.
- ❑ Place chest tube on both sides after bilateral needle thoracostomies.
- ❑ Admit to ICU.

30.9 Pearls:

❑❑ **What risk factors increase the mortality from asthma?**

Greater than 3 ED visits/year or greater than 2 hospitalizations/year, nocturnal symptoms, previous ICU admissions, previous mechanical ventilation, steroid dependence, and history of syncope with asthma.

❑❑ **Which common drugs slow theophylline clearance and result in increased theophylline levels?**

Erythromycin and ciprofloxacin.

CASE 31 Triple (Intussusception and dehydration, TTP, and Glaucoma)

Patient #1 (Intussusception and dehydration)

Examiner

Patient presents with triage note of vomiting, fever, and diarrhea. Child has been very tearful; however, just prior to the physician's exam the child has sustained a miraculous recovery. The mother is in the process of bundling up the child to take him home when the physician walks into the room. The mother says that she is tired of waiting and wants to take the patient home. Only with reluctance is the physician able to persuade the mother to stay for a complete history and physical. At this time, red tinged stool becomes apparent which mother attributed to beats. The child suddenly starts to cry and grabs at his stomach. Tests are ordered, including a barium enema.

The case is interrupted by Cases 2 and 3. Eventually the patient comes back from X-ray with a diagnosis of intussusception and is admitted for observation following the procedure.

31.1 Introduction: (Patient #1)

An 8 month old with intermittent crying, impossible to console, and multiple episodes of vomiting for 12 hours.

Vital Signs are: BP N/A, P 130, R 28, T 100.2 °F, Wt 30 kg.

31.2 Primary Survey:

- ❑ General: Fussy child, crying in mother's arms. Listless.
- ❑ Airway: Intact.
- ❑ Breathing: Normal.
- ❑ Circulation: Normal.
- ❑ Disability: None.
- ❑ Exposure: Normal.
- ❑ Finger: Guaiac positive stool and current jelly stool.

31.3 Management:

- ❑ Order appropriate lab work-up for toxic child.
- ❑ Start NS Fluid bolus at 20 cc/kg.
- ❑ Order abdominal X-rays, CXR, and BE.

31.4 History:

- ❑ Allergies: None.
- ❑ Medications: Amoxicillin for otitis.
- ❑ PMH: Recent diagnosis of otitis in right ear 4 days ago.
- ❑ Last meal: Milk, 8 hours ago.
- ❑ Events: Intermittent intense crying. Child flexes legs, lasts 5-20 minutes. Red mucous stool if asked.
- ❑ Family: None.
- ❑ Records: Normal birth.
- ❑ Immune: Up to date.
- ❑ EMTs: Via private vehicle.
- ❑ Narcotics: None.
- ❑ Doctor: Dr. Stork.
- ❑ Social history: None.

31.5 Secondary Survey:

- ❑ General: Lethargic, irritable, and listless.
- ❑ Skin: Decreased turgor.
- ❑ HEENT: Mucous membranes dry.
- ❑ Neck: Supple.
- ❑ Chest: Normal.
- ❑ Lungs: Clear.
- ❑ Heart: Regular.
- ❑ Abdomen: Distended and swollen, oblong mass RLQ.
- ❑ Perineum/GU: Normal.
- ❑ Rectal: Guaiac positive, current jelly stool.
- ❑ Back: Normal.
- ❑ Extremities: Normal.
- ❑ Neuro: Listless.

At this point the nurse asks you to see a patient that is having a stroke.

Patient #2 (TTP)

Examiner

Patient has had two episodes of slurred speech and tingling in the right arm, hand, and face, i.e., one episode yesterday lasting one hour and one today which has lasted over one hour but is improving.

The patient has a physical exam consistent with a CVA; however, the CT comes back negative and the patient's symptoms resolve while in the scanner. The managed care physician thinks the patient is having a TIA and wants to send her home for an outpatient work-up. This should be resisted by the physician. The diagnosis is verified by checking the platelet count, which is very low. The candidate may actually be given a second chance at the diagnosis as the private physician may ask if any of the labs are abnormal.

31.1 Introduction: (Patient #2)

A 40 year old female presents with slurred speech and tingling in the right face, arm, and hand.

Vital Signs are: BP 126/90, P 96, R 20, T 98.6 °F.

31.2 Primary Survey:

- ❑ General: Normal.
- ❑ Airway: Normal.
- ❑ Breathing: Normal.
- ❑ Circulation: Normal.
- ❑ Disability: Slurred speech.
- ❑ Exposure: Normal.
- ❑ Finger: Normal.

31.3 Management:

- ❑ Order CT scan.
- ❑ Order labs and ECG.

31.4 History:

- ❑ Allergies: None.
- ❑ Medications: Doans Pills.
- ❑ PMH: Bladder infections.
- ❑ Last meal: 4 hours ago.
- ❑ Family: DM and cancer.
- ❑ Records: None.
- ❑ Immune: Up to date.
- ❑ EMTs: None.
- ❑ Narcotics: None.
- ❑ Doctor: Dr. Manage Care.
- ❑ Social history: Non-smoker, non-drinker.

31.5 Secondary Survey:

- ❑ General: Alert, no distress.
- ❑ Skin: Normal.
- ❑ HEENT: Normal.
- ❑ Neck: Normal.
- ❑ Chest: Normal.

- ❑ Lungs: Normal.
- ❑ Heart: Normal.
- ❑ Abdomen: Normal.
- ❑ Perineum/GU: Normal.
- ❑ Rectal: Normal.
- ❑ Back: Normal.
- ❑ Extremities: Normal.
- ❑ Neuro: Slurred speech, minimal decreased sensation right arm compared to left, otherwise normal exam.

At this point the nurse asks you to see a third patient that is experiencing severe eye pain.

Patient #3 (Glaucoma)

Examiner

The patient has severe eye pain and does not speak English, which increases the difficulty of acquiring a history. The pain began shortly after attending a movie with her daughter and grandchild.

The diagnosis may be obtained by taking a history from the English speaking daughter and from the clinical exam.

31.1 Introduction: (Patient 3)

A 52 year old Eskimo female is in severe distress complaining of left eye pain, nausea, and vomiting.

Vital Signs are: BP 160/90, P 105, R 22, T 98.6 °F.

31.2 Primary Survey:

- ❑ General: Severe distress.
- ❑ Airway: Normal.
- ❑ Breathing: Normal.
- ❑ Circulation: Normal.
- ❑ Disability: None.
- ❑ Exposure: Normal.
- ❑ Finger: Normal.

31.3 Management:

- ❑ None at this time.

31.4 History:

- ❑ Allergies: Sulfa causes severe anaphylaxis.
- ❑ Medications: None.
- ❑ PMH: Asthma.
- ❑ Last meal: None.

- ❑ Events: Severe eye pain began shortly after attending a movie with her daughter and grandchild.
- ❑ Family: None.
- ❑ Records: None.
- ❑ Immune: Up to date.
- ❑ EMTs: None.
- ❑ Narcotics: None.
- ❑ Doctor: None.
- ❑ Social history: Non-smoker, non-drinker.

31.5 Secondary Survey:

- ❑ General: Acute pain.
- ❑ Skin: Normal.
- ❑ HEENT: Diffuse injection with watery discharge. Vision is markedly blurred in the left eye. Cornea is hazy. Pupils are mid-dilated with little reaction to light. Anterior chamber is shallow. Intraocular pressure is 80 mm Hg (less than 20 mm Hg is normal).
- ❑ Neck: Normal.
- ❑ Chest: Normal.
- ❑ Lungs: Rare wheeze.
- ❑ Heart: Normal.
- ❑ Abdomen: Normal.
- ❑ Perineum/GU: Normal.
- ❑ Rectal: Normal.
- ❑ Back: Normal.
- ❑ Extremities: Normal.
- ❑ Neuro: Normal.

31.6 Laboratory:

- ❑ Not indicated.

31.7 X-rays:

- ❑ CXR: Not indicated.

31.8 Special Tests:

- ❑ ECG: Not indicated.

31.9 Critical Actions:

- ❑ Consult ophthalmology.
- ❑ Evaluate anterior angle depth.
- ❑ Evaluate intraocular pressure.
- ❑ Avoid β-blockers such as timolol maleate due to asthma.
- ❑ Start pilocarpine hydrochloride 1%, one drop every 30 minutes until the pupil constricts, followed by one drop every 6 hours.
- ❑ Administer prednisolone acetate 1%, one drop every 30 minutes to 1 hour until surgery.
- ❑ Avoid acetazolamide as the patient is allergic to sulfa drugs and cross reactivity may occur.
- ❑ Administer mannitol, 20% 1-2 g/kg IV over 30-60 minutes, or glycerin 75%, 1 to 1.5 g/kg po, or Isosorbide, 45% 1.5 g/kg po (only one of these three agents should be given).

Patient # 1

31.6 Laboratory:

- CBC: WBC 18,000, Hgb 14, Hct 42, Plt 385.
- Differential: Pending.
- Chemistry: Na 132, K 4.2, Cl 98, CO_2 10.
- BUN/Cr: 30/1.0.
- Glucose: 130.
- Ca/Mg: Pending.
- LFTs: Pending.
- Amylase/Lipase: Pending.
- PT/PTT: Pending.
- Blood cultures: Pending.
- U/A: Spec G 1.036, 2 + ketones. Otherwise normal.

31.7 X-rays:

- CXR: Normal.
- Abdominal: Decreased bowel gas and fecal material in right colon. Small bowel distention and air-fluid levels. Oblong area of colon outlined by gas.
- BE: Diagnostic for intussusception.

31.8 Special Tests:

- ECG: None.

31.9 Critical Actions:

- Start IV fluid bolus of 20 cc/kg of NS.
- Obtain a surgical consult.
- Order abdominal X-ray.
- Order BE.
- Admit for observation.
- Start antibiotics for potential perforation, i.e., ampicillin, 100-200 mg/kg, or clindamycin, 30-40 mg/kg, or gentamicin, 5.0-7.5 mg/kg.

Patient #2

31.6 Laboratory:

- CBC: WBC 13, Hgb 9.5, Hct 30, Plt 13.
- Differential: Segs 55%, Lymphs 38%, Monos 5%, Eosins 1%.
- Chemistry: Na 140, K 3.8, Cl 105, CO_2 28.
- BUN/Cr: 15/1.0.
- Glucose: 120.
- Ca/Mg: Pending.
- LFTs: Pending.
- Amylase/Lipase: Pending.

- ❑ PT/PTT: 12/28.
- ❑ Cardiac enzymes: Not indicated.
- ❑ ABG: Not indicated.
- ❑ Blood cultures: Not indicated.
- ❑ U/A: Normal.

31.7 X-rays:

- ❑ CXR: Normal.

31.8 Special Tests:

- ❑ ECG: NSR.
- ❑ CT Head: Normal.

31.9 Critical Actions:

- ❑ Do not allow the patient to go home.
- ❑ Consult Dr. Managed Care.
- ❑ Consult neurology.
- ❑ Consult hematology - "I will be down to take care of the patient".

31.10 Pearls: (Patients 1-3)

❑❑ What are the common complications of intussusception?

Perforation, peritonitis, shock, sepsis, and re-intussusception.

❑❑ When do you expect to see current jelly stools?

Within 12-24 hours, mucus or blood may be found per rectum.

❑❑ For whom should β-blockers be avoided?

In patients with asthma, heart-block, or heart failure.

❑❑ What is the differential of an acutely painful red eye?

Keratitis, iritis, ulcer, erosion, foreign body, conjunctivitis, glaucoma, and trauma.

CASE 32 (Myxedema Coma, Pneumonia, Hyponatremia)

Examiner

Patient has pneumonia which has made her chronic hypothyroid state significantly worse. In the last few days, she has had a fever, chills, and a productive cough. For the last several weeks, she has noticed increased episodes of constipation, fatigue, muscle cramps, and a sensation of always being cold. She has also been gaining weight and has been "slowing down" lately. She now presents in acute distress but does not require intubation.

32.1 Introduction:

A 62 year old female in mild respiratory distress.

Vital Signs are: BP 90/60, P 60, R 14, T 96 °F.

32.2 Primary Survey:

- General: Late middle aged female in moderate respiratory distress. Patient is coughing.
- Airway: Gag.
- Breathing: Crackles at left base, rare rhonchi.
- Circulation: 3s capillary refill.
- Disability: None.
- Exposure: No gross abnormality.
- Finger: Deferred.

32.3 Management:

- Start IV, O_2, and place on monitor.
- Order CXR.
- Order CBC, Chem, and U/A.
- Obtain blood, urine, and sputum cultures.

32.3 History:

- Allergies: None.
- Medications: None.
- PMH: Appendicitis, T &A.
- Last meal: Light breakfast earlier today.
- Family: Non-contributory.
- Records: N/A.
- Immune: Normal.
- EMTs: No further information.
- Narcotics: None.
- Doctor: Dr. Family.
- Social history: Drinks alcohol socially.

32.4 Secondary Survey:

- General: Mild lethargy.
- Skin: Dry yellow skin, course hair, diffuse non-pitting edema.
- HEENT: Large tongue, puffy eyes and face, loss of lateral part of eyebrows.
- Neck: Normal.
- Chest: No retractions.
- Lungs: Crackles at left base.
- Heart: Regular and slow.

- ❑ Abdomen: Slight abdominal distention, bowel sound low pitched.
- ❑ Perineum/GU: Normal.
- ❑ Rectal: Normal.
- ❑ Back: Normal.
- ❑ Extremities: Puffy hands and legs.
- ❑ Neuro: Slow DTRs, ataxia, and paresthesias.

32.5 Laboratory:

- ❑ CBC: WBC 16, Hgb 11, Hct 39, Plt 350.
- ❑ Differential: Elevated bands.
- ❑ Chemistry: Na 121, K 5.2, Cl 102, CO_2 25.
- ❑ BUN/Cr: 18/1.4.
- ❑ Glucose: 60.
- ❑ Ca/Mg: Normal.
- ❑ LFTs: Mild elevation SGOT, LDH.
- ❑ Amylase/Lipase: Pending.
- ❑ PT/PTT: Pending.
- ❑ Cardiac enzymes: Pending.
- ❑ ABG: pH 7.36, pO_2 77, pCO_2 26, HCO_3 24.
- ❑ Blood cultures: Pending.
- ❑ U/A: Normal.
- ❑ T4, TSH: Pending.

32.6 X-rays:

- ❑ CXR: Cardiomegaly, LLL pneumonia.
- ❑ Abd series: Mild ileus.

32.7 Special Tests:

- ❑ ECG: Bradycardia, low voltage, prolonged PR and inverted T waves.

32.8 Critical Actions:

- ☑ Administer IV 0.9 NS to correct hyponatremia, O_2, and place on monitor.
- ☑ Administer hydrocortisone, 300 mg.
- ☑ Administer glucose.
- ☑ Administer L-thyroxine, 400-500 μg slow IV, or triiodothyroxine, 12.5-25 μg q 6-8 hours (dose should be decreased in the presence of cardiac ischemia).
- ☑ Admit to ICU.
- ☑ Obtain endocrine or IM consult.
- ❑ Obtain blood, urine, and sputum cultures.
- ☑ Start antibiotics for treatment of pneumonia.

32.9 Pearls:

❑❑ **When should the L-thyroxine dose be decreased?**

When cardiac ischemia is present.

❑❑ **What lab abnormalities available in the ED are expected in severe hypothyroidism?**

Anemia, elevated cholesterol, LDH, AST, CPK, and hyponatremia.

CASE 33 (Thyroid Storm, CHF)

Examiner

The patient presents in moderate CHF with atrial fibrillation. This evening the daughter found her mother breathing with difficulty. According to the daughter, the patient has had intermittent episodes of palpitations and gradually increasing SOB. For the last week, she has been having diarrhea, nausea, and vomiting with crampy abdominal pain. She has also noticed that her mother is more nervous than usual, has lost a lot of weight, and has been complaining of being warm all the time.

A thorough history and physical reveals that the patient is suffering from severe hyperthyroidism. The patient's CHF is relieved by standard therapy and she does not require intubation. The daughter and eventually the patient is able to describe symptoms of CHF and progressive hyperthyroidism.

33.1 Introduction:

A 52 year old female presents SOB, sitting up, and in respiratory distress.

Vital Signs are: BP 140/70, P 130, R 28, T 103 °F.

33.2 Primary Survey:

- ❑ General: Obvious respiratory distress, diaphoretic, cool, and clammy.
- ❑ Airway: Gag.
- ❑ Breathing: Diffuse crackles at bases, respiratory retractions.
- ❑ Circulation: 3s capillary refill.
- ❑ Disability: Able to make very brief gasping statements "I", "can't", "breath".
- ❑ Exposure: No gross abnormalities.
- ❑ Finger: Deferred.

33.3 Management:

- ❑ Start IV, O_2, and place on monitor, O_2 Sat.
- ❑ Order labs, CBC, Chem, U/A, CXR, and ECG.
- ❑ Administer Lasix.
- ❑ Administer nitroglycerin.

33.4 History:

- ❑ Allergies: None.
- ❑ Medications: None.
- ❑ PMH: N/A.
- ❑ Last meal: N/A.
- ❑ Family: None.
- ❑ Records: None.
- ❑ Immune: None.
- ❑ EMTs: None.
- ❑ Narcotics: None.
- ❑ Doctor: Dr. Medicine is available to admit the patient.
- ❑ Social history: Rarely consumes alcohol and is a non-smoker.

33.5 Secondary Survey:

- ❑ General: Middle aged female in moderate respiratory distress.
- ❑ Skin: Warm and moist, hair is fine and silky if asked.
- ❑ HEENT: Exophthalmos, inflamed conjunctiva.
- ❑ Neck: Enlarged thyroid with bruit over the gland.
- ❑ Chest: Respiratory retractions.
- ❑ Lungs: Diffuse crackles.
- ❑ Heart: Tachy and irregular.
- ❑ Abdomen: Soft, BS +, No focal tenderness.
- ❑ Perineum/GU: Normal.
- ❑ Rectal: Heme negative.
- ❑ Back: Normal.
- ❑ Extremities: Normal.
- ❑ Neuro: Brisk return phase of DTRs, symmetrical decreased muscle strength, slight tremor.

33.6 Laboratory:

- ❑ CBC: WBC 15, Hgb 12, Hct 36, Plt 400.
- ❑ Differential: Pending.
- ❑ Chemistry: Na 140, K 4.4, Cl 102, CO_2 29.
- ❑ BUN/Cr: 11/1.2.
- ❑ Glucose: 180.
- ❑ Ca/Mg: Normal.
- ❑ LFTs: Normal.
- ❑ Amylase/Lipase: Pending.
- ❑ PT/PTT: Pending.
- ❑ Cardiac enzymes: Normal.
- ❑ ABG: pH 7.38, pO_2 76, pCO_2 30, HCO_3 22.
- ❑ Blood cultures: Pending.
- ❑ U/A: Normal.
- ❑ T4, TSH, T3U: Pending.

33.7 X-rays:

- ❑ CXR: CHF.

33.8 Special Tests:

- ❑ ECG: Atrial fibrillation.

33.9 Critical Actions:

- ❑ Start IV, O_2, and place on monitor.
- ❑ Administer Tylenol and cover with cooling blanket.
- ❑ Administer Lasix.
- ❑ Administer nitroglycerin.
- ❑ Administer methimazole, 90-120 mg po, or PTU, 900-1200 mg po.
- ❑ Administer Digitalis, 0.25-0.5 mg.
- ❑ Avoid Propranolol.
- ❑ One hour after PTU or methimazole, give sodium iodide, 1 g IV over 8-12 hours, or Lugol solution, 30 drops per day or lithium carbonate, 300-450 mg po tid.
- ❑ Administer hydrocortisone, 300 mg IV.
- ❑ Consult endocrinology or internal medicine.
- ❑ Admit to ICU.

33.10 Pearls:

❑❑ What is the mortality rate of thyroid storm?

10%-20%.

❑❑ What are the most common causes?

Infection, trauma, vascular accident, diabetes, and nonthyroidal surgery.

❑❑ What are the common diagnostic criteria?

T > 100 °F, tachycardia, peripheral manifestations, and CNS, CV, and GI dysfunction.

CASE 34 (Pyloric Stenosis)

Examiner

Hispanic child, with parent that does not speak English, is brought to the ED. Physician must find an interpreter. Child has classic history of progressive symptoms over 3-4 weeks and blood-tinged vomitus. However, because mother speaks little English, all she initially describes is that her baby is yellow.

34.1 Introduction:

Five week old Hispanic male presents with mother who speaks very little English.

Vital Signs are: BP N/A, P 100, R 26, T 100.1 °F, Wt 5 kg.

34.2 Primary Survey:

- ❑ General: Awake, hungry, mildly lethargic.
- ❑ Airway: Intact.
- ❑ Breathing: Normal.
- ❑ Circulation: Normal.
- ❑ Disability: Normal.
- ❑ Exposure: Normal.
- ❑ Finger: Normal.

34.3 History:

- ❑ Allergies: None.
- ❑ Medications: None.
- ❑ PMH: None.
- ❑ Last meal: 2 hours ago.
- ❑ Events: In the past few days the child has become more yellow. For the last 2-3 weeks the child has been vomiting, but recently with increasing frequency. Today the mother noticed the vomit is blood tinged.
- ❑ Family: Normal.
- ❑ Records: None.
- ❑ Immune: Up to date.
- ❑ EMTs: None.
- ❑ Narcotics: None.
- ❑ Doctor: None.
- ❑ Social history: None.

34.4 Secondary Survey:

- ❑ General: 5 week old child, who is on the bottle, is mildly lethargic.
- ❑ Skin: Jaundiced.
- ❑ HEENT: Normal.
- ❑ Neck: Normal
- ❑ Chest: Normal.
- ❑ Lungs: Clear.
- ❑ Heart: Normal.
- ❑ Abdomen: Palpable mass just below the liver edge and just lateral to the rectus abdominal muscle.
- ❑ Perineum/GU: Normal.
- ❑ Rectal: Guaiac negative.
- ❑ Back: Normal.
- ❑ Extremities: Normal.
- ❑ Neuro: Normal.

34.5 Laboratory:

- ❑ CBC: WBC 16, Hgb 14 , Hct 42, Plt 400.
- ❑ Differential: Pending.
- ❑ Chemistry: Na 136, K 3.2, Cl 96, CO_2 35.

- ❑ BUN/Cr: 28/1.2.
- ❑ Glucose: 130.
- ❑ Ca/Mg: Pending.
- ❑ LFTs: Pending.
- ❑ Amylase/Lipase: Not indicated.
- ❑ PT/PTT: Pending.
- ❑ Cardiac enzymes: Not indicated.
- ❑ ABG: Not indicated.
- ❑ Blood cultures: Pending.
- ❑ U/A: Pending.

34.6 X-rays:

- ❑ CXR: Normal.

34.7 Special Tests:

- ❑ Abdomen films: Gastric dilation.
- ❑ Ultrasound: Pyloric stenosis.
- ❑ BE: String sign (Elongated pyloric canal).

34.8 Critical Actions:

- ❑ Administer 0.9 NS at 20 mL/kg over 30-60 minutes.
- ❑ Insert NG tube at low-intermittent suction.
- ❑ Obtain surgery consult.
- ❑ US or BE.

34.9 Pearls:

❑❑ What is the cause of pyloric stenosis?

Hypertrophy and hyperplasia of the circular antral and pyloric musculature results in gastric outlet obstruction.

❑❑ Which type of chemical imbalance is expected in pyloric stenosis?

Hypochloremic metabolic alkalosis is due to large losses of hydrochloric acid through vomiting.

CASE 35 (Ethylene Glycol)

Examiner

A seven year old male presents to the ED with slurred speech and lethargy. The patient is unable to provide answers to questions. Reluctantly, the nine year old brother provides information that they were playing in an old barn and the younger child consumed an unknown quantity of liquid three hours ago. The police or paramedics are sent to the barn and find ethylene glycol. Otherwise, diagnosis is made by finding crystals in the urine.

35.1 Introduction:

A 7 year old male presents to the ED very lethargic.

Vital Signs are: BP 90/60, P 90, R 20, T 100.5 °F.

35.2 Primary Survey:

- ❑ General: Slurred speech and very lethargic.
- ❑ Airway: + Gag.
- ❑ Breathing: = Breath sounds.
- ❑ Circulation: 3s capillary refill.
- ❑ Disability: Responds to verbal stimuli with confused unclear response.
- ❑ Exposure: No gross abnormalities.
- ❑ Finger: NG tube, Foley catheter.

35.3 Critical Event:

- ❑ Child has a tonic-clonic seizure.

35.4 Management:

- ❑ Start IV, O_2, and place on monitor.
- ❑ Administer diazepam, phenytoin, or phenobarbital.

35.5 History:

- ❑ Allergies: Unknown.
- ❑ Medications: Unknown.
- ❑ PMH: Unknown
- ❑ Last meal: Four hours ago.
- ❑ Family: Unknown.
- ❑ Records: Unavailable.
- ❑ Immune: Unknown.
- ❑ EMTs: Police or paramedics sent to site and find ethylene glycol.
- ❑ Narcotics: None.
- ❑ Doctor: Dr. Peds.
- ❑ Social history: Parents could not be located. Children were discovered by the police and brought into the ED by paramedics.

35.6 Secondary Survey:

- ❑ General: Appears intoxicated but no odor of ETOH. If asked, a faint, sweet, aromatic odor is detected on the child's breath.
- ❑ Skin: Dry.
- ❑ HEENT: Nystagmus, vertical and horizontal.
- ❑ Neck: Supple.
- ❑ Chest: Normal.
- ❑ Lungs: Normal.

- ❑ Heart: Regular, Tachy.
- ❑ Abdomen: Soft, BS +.
- ❑ Perineum/GU: Normal.
- ❑ Rectal: Normal.
- ❑ Back: Normal.
- ❑ Extremities: Normal.
- ❑ Neuro: Responds to pain. Moves all extremities. Very lethargic.

35.7 Laboratory:

- ❑ CBC: WBC 14.0, Hgb 13.0, Hct 39.0.
- ❑ Chemistry: Na 140, K 5.0, Cl 90, CO_2 10.
- ❑ BUN/Cr: 9/1.0.
- ❑ Glucose: 180.
- ❑ Ca: 6.
- ❑ O_2 sat: 95%
- ❑ ABG: pH 7.05, pO_2 110, pCO_2 20, HCO_3 12.
- ❑ U/A: Protein 3+, Blood 2+, Calcium oxalate crystal 1+.
- ❑ Wood's lamp: Fluorescence of urine.
- ❑ Amylase: 140.
- ❑ Measured serum osm: 350.
- ❑ Calculated serum osm: 303.

  [2(Na + K) + Glu/18 + BUN/3]

  [2(140 + 5) + 180/18 + 9/3] = 303

- ❑ Tox screen: Pending.
- ❑ Anion Gap: 40 (Normal 10-12) [Na - (Cl + HCO_3)].

35.8 X-rays:

- ❑ CXR: Normal.

35.9 Special Tests:

- ❑ ECG: Normal.
- ❑ Ethylene glycol: 55 mg/dL.

35.10 Critical Actions:

- ☑ Access ABCs.
- ☑ Administer IV bicarbonate in small increments.
- ☑ Treat hypocalcemia with IV calcium chloride or gluconate, 1-7 mEq for children, 7-14 mEq for adults.
- ☑ Treat seizures with diazepam, phenytoin or barbiturates.
- ☑ Give ethanol if serum EG is greater than 20 mg/dL or acidemia. Goal is a serum ethanol concentration of 100 mg/dL. Load 10 mL/kg of 10% ethanol with glucose to avoid hypoglycemia. Maintenance infusion as 1.5 mL/kg/hour.

- ❑ Administer pyridoxine and thiamine as they are precursors to cofactors in the degradation of EG.
- ❑ Admit to ICU.
- ❑ Consider giving fomepizole (Antizol) 15 mgl/kg followed by doses of 10 mg/kg q 12 hours for 4 doses, then 15 mg/kg every 12 hours until EG levels have been reduced below 20 mg/dL.

35.11 Pearls:

❑❑ Explain the competitive metabolism of ethylene glycol and ethanol.

EG is metabolized to glycoaldehyde by alcohol dehydrogenase. Alcohol dehydrogenase has a much higher affinity for ethanol than for EG. When both alcohols are present, ethanol is metabolized. Thus, ethanol inhibits the metabolism of EG.

❑❑ What is the significance of calcium oxalate crystals in EG ingestion?

EG results in the accumulation of glycolic acid resulting in decreased bicarbonate levels, acidotic symptoms, renal tubular damage, interstitial edema, and increased mortality. Glycolic acid metabolism results in the production of oxalic acid which precipitates as calcium oxalate crystals.

❑❑ What is the lethal dose of EG?

0.1 mL/kg may produce toxic levels, even a mouthful could be hazardous. Less than 60 mL has resulted in death.

❑❑ What late findings can be expected?

Hypertension, tachycardia, dysrhythmias, and pulmonary edema develop 12-36 hours after ingestion.

❑❑ Describe the appearance and frequency of calcium oxalate crystals.

Needle-shaped crystals are present in the urine in 30% to 50% of ingestions.

CASE 36 (Rotator Cuff Strain, Drug Seeking, Anemia)

Examiner

This patient presents with a complaint of acute pain in the right shoulder from an old injury. On first blush, the patient appears to be a drug seeker. However, a careful physical exam must be performed by the candidate to reveal the patient also has severe anemia. The patient is an evasive historian and does not provide this information nor does she reveal the signs and symptoms of her anemia unless specifically asked. She concentrates on her shoulder pain and requests a large dose of Demerol. Furthermore, she denies shortness of breath, headaches, black stools, or vomiting blood.

After the pain shot, the patient wants to leave. At this point the labs return and the diagnosis of severe anemia is made. The patient says she does not want to stay in the hospital and, for religious reasons, she does not want a transfusion.

The candidate should call the private managed care physician who wants to send her home, i.e., he will see her in his office in the morning. The candidate should indicate that this is not safe and convince the private physician to admit the patient for a work-up. The private physician will eventually agree to the admission.

The patient continues to refuse admission until the candidate asks the husband to come in from the waiting room. With his help the patient agrees to stay in the hospital.

If the candidate should send the patient home, an AMA form should be completed; however, she returns to the ED immediately, vomiting blood and then dies.

36.1 Introduction:

A 37 year old female with complaint of severe right shoulder pain.

Vital Signs are: BP 100/80, P 104, R 24, T 99.1 °F.

36.2 Primary Survey:

- ❑ General: Cachectic white female appearing much older than her stated age.
- ❑ Airway: Intact.
- ❑ Breathing: Shallow. Crackles at the right base which clear when the patient is asked to cough.
- ❑ Circulation: 4s capillary refill.
- ❑ Disability: None.
- ❑ Exposure: Normal.
- ❑ Finger: Guaiac negative.

36.3 History:

- ❑ Allergies: Penicillin.
- ❑ Medications: Toradol and Vicodin.
- ❑ PMH: On disability for rotator cuff tear for the past ten months. She has had two operations that have not helped relieve her shoulder pain. Also, she has a history of anemia and her uterus has been removed.
- ❑ Last meal: 4 hours ago.
- ❑ Family: Husband is in the waiting room.
- ❑ Records: Rotator cuff repair.
- ❑ Immune: Up to date.
- ❑ EMTs: None.
- ❑ Narcotics: Out of meds.
- ❑ Doctor: Dr. Bone and Dr. Medicine.
- ❑ Social history: Smokes 2 packs per day.

36.4 Secondary Survey:

- ❑ General: Cachectic white female.
- ❑ Skin: Pale.
- ❑ HEENT: Inner lids pale.
- ❑ Neck: Supple.
- ❑ Chest: Normal.
- ❑ Lungs: Crackles at right base which clear with cough.
- ❑ Heart: RRR with no murmur.

- ❑ Abdomen: Soft.
- ❑ Perineum/GU: Normal.
- ❑ Rectal: Guaiac negative.
- ❑ Back: Normal.
- ❑ Extremities: Severe pain with all attempts at evaluating right shoulder.
- ❑ Neuro: Motor strength is decreased but equal, otherwise normal exam.

36.5 Management:

- ❑ Order pain shot for the patient.
- ❑ Order labs and possibly a CXR.

36.6 Laboratory:

- ❑ CBC: WBC 12, Hgb 4.4, Hct 14.6, Plt 590.
- ❑ MCV: 57.
- ❑ Differential: Pending.
- ❑ Chemistry: Na 134, K 4.0, Cl 104, CO_2 24.
- ❑ BUN/Cr: 10/1.0.
- ❑ Glucose: 120.
- ❑ Ca/Mg: Normal.
- ❑ LFTs: Normal.
- ❑ Amylase/Lipase: Normal.
- ❑ PT/PTT: Normal.
- ❑ Cardiac enzymes: Normal.
- ❑ Saturation: 98% on room air.
- ❑ Blood cultures: Not indicated.
- ❑ U/A: Normal.

36.7 X-rays:

- ❑ CXR: Cardiomegaly.

36.8 Special Tests:

- ❑ ECG: NSR.

36.9 Critical Actions:

- ❑ Convince MD to admit.
- ❑ Convince patient to admit.
- ❑ Relieve patient's pain.

36.10 Pearls:

❑❑ When should a patient with chronic anemia be admitted?

Most textbooks generally recommend admission and transfusion for hemoglobins below 9. Patients with sickle cell and renal failure may be allowed to carry slightly lower counts.

❑❑ **What is the most common cause of microcytic anemia?**

Iron deficiency often caused by chronic blood loss.

CASE 37 (Black Widow Spider Bite)

Examiner

The patient is a 8 year old child who is bitten by a black widow spider. The child is not able to provide much of a history other than he was playing in a wood shed. The patient is brought in by the grandmother who was watching the child. According to his grandmother, he came into the house with a complaint of increasing abdominal pains/cramps as well as pain in the neck, back, and legs. The child is also experiencing nausea, headache, and priapism.

37.1 Introduction:

An 8 year old child presents with a complaint of abdominal pain.

Vital Signs are: BP 150/110, P 110, R 24, T 99.0 °F.

37.2 Primary Survey:

- ❑ General: Moderate distress.
- ❑ Airway: Intact.
- ❑ Breathing: Normal.
- ❑ Circulation: Normal.
- ❑ Disability: None.
- ❑ Exposure: If specifically asked, the child has a circular area of pallor surrounded by a ring of erythema located on his upper back.
- ❑ Finger: Guaiac negative.

37.3 Management:

- ❑ Candidate may order initial screening labs at this time.

37.4 History:

- ❑ Allergies: None.
- ❑ Medications: None.
- ❑ PMH: None.
- ❑ Last meal: 5 hours ago.
- ❑ Events: Child has been playing in the wood shed all day. He came into the house with a complaint of increasing abdominal pains/cramps as well as pain in the neck, back, and legs. The child is also experiencing nausea, headache, and priapism.
- ❑ Family: None.
- ❑ Records: None.
- ❑ Immune: Td up to date.

- ❑ EMTs: None.
- ❑ Narcotics: None.
- ❑ Doctor: No family doctor, child is visiting grandmother, parents are traveling in Europe.
- ❑ Social history: None.

37.5 Secondary Survey:

- ❑ General: Child in moderate distress, moving intermittently but unable to find a comfortable position.
- ❑ Skin: Circular area of pallor surrounded by a ring of erythema located on the upper back. Two small puncture wounds in center of lesion.
- ❑ HEENT: Periorbital ecchymosis.
- ❑ Neck: Supple.
- ❑ Chest: Normal.
- ❑ Lungs: Clear.
- ❑ Heart: RRR.
- ❑ Abdomen: BS +, tender abdomen with rigid abdominal muscles. Guarding with no rebound.
- ❑ Perineum/GU: Child has an erect penis.
- ❑ Rectal: Guaiac negative, non-tender.
- ❑ Back: Normal.
- ❑ Extremities: Normal.
- ❑ Neuro: Normal.

37.6 Laboratory:

- ❑ CBC: WBC 12, Hgb 14, Hct 44, Plt 300.
- ❑ Differential: Pending.
- ❑ Chemistry: Na 140, K 4.0, Cl 105, CO_2 24.
- ❑ BUN/Cr: 10/1.0.
- ❑ Glucose: 125.
- ❑ Ca/Mg: Normal.
- ❑ LFTs: Normal.
- ❑ Amylase/Lipase: Normal.
- ❑ PT/PTT: Normal.
- ❑ Blood cultures: Pending.
- ❑ U/A: Normal.

37.7 X-rays:

- ❑ CXR: Normal.
- ❑ Abdomen: Normal.

37.8 Special Tests:

- ❑ ECG: Not indicated.

37.9 Critical Actions:

- ❑ Treat patient with grandmother's approval.

- ❑ Recognize lesion as black widow spider bite.
- ❑ Treat patient's pain.
- ❑ Provide muscle relaxation and amnesia with lorazepam.
- ❑ Recognize severe hypertension as indication for antivenin.
- ❑ Check skin for antivenin sensitivity before administering this medication. Dose is generally one vial of antivenin regardless of patients weight. Physician may check with Poison Center for dose or read package insert.

37.10 Pearls:

❑❑ What is the role of calcium in the treatment of black widow spider bites?

There is not scientific evidence that calcium is effective, there are only anecdotal reports of its benefit.

❑❑ When is antivenin indicated for a black widow spider bite?

Severe pain or dangerous hypertension.

CASE 38 (Eclampsia, Aspiration)

Examiner

A two days post-partum female presents due to eclampsia. Physician must follow appropriate seizure treatment and diagnose aspiration.

38.1 Introduction:

A 38 year old female presents seizing.

Vital Signs are: BP 160/110, P 110, R 24, T 101 °F.

38.2 Primary Survey:

- ❑ General: Seizing female.
- ❑ Airway: Gag intact.
- ❑ Breathing: Spontaneous.
- ❑ Circulation: 3s capillary refill.
- ❑ Disability: Seizing.
- ❑ Exposure: No gross deformity.
- ❑ Finger: Pending.

38.3 History:

- ❑ Allergies: None.
- ❑ Medications: Vitamins.
- ❑ PMH: G2P2.

- ❑ Last meal: Two hours prior to seizure.
- ❑ Family: Normal.
- ❑ Records: Not available.
- ❑ Immune: Up to date.
- ❑ EMTs: No further information.
- ❑ Narcotics: None.
- ❑ Doctor: Dr. Ob.
- ❑ Social history: None.

38.4 Secondary Survey:

- ❑ General: Seizing.
- ❑ Skin: Normal.
- ❑ HEENT: Normal.
- ❑ Neck: Normal.
- ❑ Chest: Normal.
- ❑ Lungs: Crackles at right base.
- ❑ Heart: Regular.
- ❑ Abdomen: Soft, BS positive.
- ❑ Perineum/GU: Dark discharge per vagina.
- ❑ Rectal: Normal.
- ❑ Back: Normal.
- ❑ Extremities: 3+ edema.
- ❑ Neuro: Seizing, hyperactive DTRs, and ankle clonus present.

38.5 Management:

- ❑ Administer 2-4 g magnesium sulfate as a 20% solution IV over 5-10 minutes, followed by 1-3 g per hour.
- ❑ Administer lorazepam, 1-2 mg/minute, or diazepam, 5 mg/minute.
- ❑ Consult Ob attending.
- ❑ Start IV, O_2, and place on monitor.
- ❑ Check gag.

38.6 Laboratory:

- ❑ CBC: WBC 14, Hgb 13, Hct 39, Plt 400.
- ❑ Differential: Pending.
- ❑ Chemistry: Pending.
- ❑ BUN/Cr: Pending.
- ❑ Glucose: 140 by glucometer.
- ❑ Ca/Mg: Pending.
- ❑ LFTs: Pending.
- ❑ Amylase/Lipase: Pending.
- ❑ PT/PTT: Not indicated.
- ❑ Cardiac enzymes: Pending.
- ❑ Pulse oximeter: 95%.
- ❑ ABG: pH 7.42, pO_2 84, pCO_2 35, HCO_3 40.

- ❑ Blood cultures: Pending.
- ❑ U/A: Pending.

38.7 X-rays:

- ❑ CXR: Segmental RLL infiltrate.

38.8 Special Tests:

- ❑ ECG: N/A.

38.9 Critical Actions:

- ❑ Administer 2-4 g magnesium sulfate as a 20% solution IV over 5-10 minutes, followed by 1-3 g per hour.
- ❑ Administer lorazepam, 1-2 mg/minute, or diazepam, 5 mg/minute.
- ❑ Consult Ob attending.
- ❑ Start IV, O_2, and place on monitor.
- ❑ Check gag.
- ❑ Admit to ICU.
- ❑ Recognize probable aspiration, ~~hold antibiotics pending culture.~~

38.10 Pearls:

❑❑ What physical finding is most predictive of impending eclampsia?

Ankle Clonus.

❑❑ How do you evaluate the patient for Mg toxicity?

Loss of patellar reflex occurs at 7-10 mEq/L and respiratory depression occurs at 12 mEq/L.

❑❑ What is the antidote for Mg toxicity?

10% Calcium gluconate, 10-20 mL.

❑❑ When should antibiotics be started in aspiration pneumonia?

When clinical evidence of infection occurs.

CASE 39 (Calcium Channel Blocker Poisoning)

Examiner

The patient is a middle aged male with a history of depression. He called EMS after swallowing a "nearly full bottle" of sustained release diltiazem with a large quantity of alcohol. On arrival, the paramedics noted that the patient vomited once and was coughing. However, no pill fragments were seen in the emesis. Paramedics reported an empty fifth of vodka, several beer cans, and an empty bottle of diltiazem. A suicide note was at the scene. No other medications were found. There was no evidence of trauma.

The physician should treat the patient for a toxic ingestion and altered mental status while protecting the airway before gastric lavage.

39.1 Introduction:

A 50 year old male is brought to the ED smelling strongly of alcohol, with emesis on clothing, and responding to sternal rub.

Vital Signs are: BP 90/60, P 76, R 12, T 97 °F.

39.2 Primary Survey:

- ❑ General: Disheveled male, decreased responsiveness.
- ❑ Airway: Patent after chin lift to clear tongue.
- ❑ Breathing: Inspiratory crackles at bases.
- ❑ Circulation: 2+ capillary refill, pulses symmetric.
- ❑ Disability: PERRLA, pupils mid-range, strong smells of ethanol, responds slowly to noxious stimuli for brief period.
- ❑ Exposure: No evidence of trauma, no track marks, no scars.
- ❑ Finger: Normal rectal tone, guaiac negative.

39.3 Management:

- ❑ Intubate patient and place on pulse oximeter.
- ❑ Establish large bore IV. Obtain stat glucose, electrolytes, renal and liver function tests, PT/PTT, osm, Mg, and Ca. Start bolus with NS 500 mL IV.
- ❑ Place on cardiac monitor and evaluate rhythm. Order ECG.
- ❑ Administer D_{50}, thiamine, and Narcan.
- ❑ Insert 36-40 French OG tube. Lavage with 150-200 mL boluses of normal saline until aspirate is clear.
- ❑ Administer activated charcoal, 1 g/kg, and cathartic. Consider whole bowel irrigation.
- ❑ Administer calcium chloride or calcium gluconate for hypotension or bradyrhythmias.
- ❑ Consider glucagon, atropine, isoproterenol, epinephrine, amrinone, dopamine, norepinephrine, pacemaker, or intra-aortic balloon pump as indicated by patient condition.

39.4 History:

- ❑ Allergies: Unknown.
- ❑ Medications: Diltiazem, others unknown.
- ❑ PMH: Hypertension.
- ❑ Last meal: Recent alcohol.
- ❑ Family: Unknown.
- ❑ Records: None.
- ❑ Immune: Unknown.
- ❑ EMTs: Less responsive enroute to the ED. Initial BP 120/80, P 90, stated wife left him yesterday. Suicide note was at scene.
- ❑ Narcotics: Empty fifth of vodka, empty cans of beer at scene.
- ❑ Doctor: Name on pill bottle.

- Social history: Married, unknown history of previous drugs or alcohol abuse, smokes cigarettes.

39.5 Secondary Survey:

- General: Intubated male, no obvious injuries.
- Skin: Warm, moist, no skin lesions.
- HEENT: Anicteric, oropharynx-normal moisture, TMs-normal.
- Neck: No deformity, no JVD, supple.
- Chest: Chest wall symmetric, no injury.
- Lungs: Inspiratory crackles at bases.
- Heart: Regular rhythm, no rub or gallop.
- Abdomen: Normal.
- Perineum/genital: Normal.
- Rectal: Normal tone, guaiac negative.
- Extremities: Normal.
- Neuro: Responds to noxious stimuli, PERRLA, moving all four extremities, DTRs intact and symmetric.

39.6 Laboratory:

- CBC: WBC 11, Hgb 13, Hct 39, Plt 230.
- Chemistry: Na 140, K 4.0, Cl 110, CO_2 22.
- BUN/Cr: 14/1.0.
- Glucose: 140.
- Ca/Mg: 10/2.0.
- LFTs: Normal.
- Amylase/Lipase: Normal.
- PT/PTT: Normal.
- Cardiac enzymes: Normal.
- ABG: pH 7.40, pO_2 150, pCO_2 30, HCO_3 22, (post-intubation).
- U/A: Normal.

39.7 X-rays:

- CXR: Mild failure, borderline increased heart size, ETT in good position.

39.8 Special Tests:

- ECG: NSR with first degree heart block.

39.10 Critical Actions:

- Access ABCs, intubate to provide patent and protected airway.
- Treat hypotension with IV fluids. Consider glucagon, isoproterenol, epinephrine, amrinone, norepinephrine, dopamine, and intra-aortic balloon pump if refractory.
- Administer calcium chloride or gluconate for hypotension and bradyrhythmias.
- Administer dextrose, Narcan, and thiamine.
- Gastric lavage with administration of charcoal and cathartic. Consider whole bowel irrigation.
- Arrange ICU admission.

39.11 Pearls:

❑❑ **How do calcium channel blockers exert their therapeutic effect?**

They interfere with calcium entry into the myocardial tissue and the vascular smooth muscle resulting in decreased conduction through the A-V node, decreased S-A node discharge, vasodilation, and decreased cardiac contractility.

❑❑ **Do all the calcium channel blockers have the same effect on the heart and vascular smooth muscle?**

No. The different classes of calcium channel blockers vary in their effects on conduction, contractility, and vasodilation.

❑❑ **Which calcium channel blocker is associated with hyperglycemia?**

Verapamil may inhibit the release of insulin. Administering calcium can decrease this effect.

CASE 40 (Disc Battery Ingestion)

Examiner

A child is brought in by his parents who report he swallowed a disc battery one hour ago. The child is crying but has no drooling and has taken his bottle without difficulty since the ingestion. There is no evidence of aspiration of the battery.

The physician should assess for aspiration, location of the battery, whether the battery appears intact, and for any evidence of abdominal obstruction.

40.1 Introduction:

A 2 year old child is brought to the ED by his parents who report that he swallowed a disc battery from a calculator one hour ago.

Vital Signs are: P 100, R 22, T 98.6 °F.

40.2 Primary Survey:

- ❑ General: Well developed, well nourished child in no respiratory distress and is consolable by parents.
- ❑ Airway: Patent, normal cry.
- ❑ Breathing: Clear, symmetric breath sounds, no use of accessory muscles.
- ❑ Circulation: 2+ capillary refill.
- ❑ Disability: Alert, responds appropriately to parents.
- ❑ Exposure: No evidence of any injury.
- ❑ Finger: Deferred.

40.3 Management:

- ❑ Order CXR (include view of the neck) and KUB.
- ❑ Allow parents to remain with child.
- ❑ Keep patient NPO while X-ray is pending.

40.4 History:

- ❑ Allergies: None.
- ❑ Medications: None.
- ❑ PMH: None.
- ❑ Last meal: Had bottle enroute to hospital..
- ❑ Family: Noncontributory.
- ❑ Records: None.
- ❑ Immune: Up to date.
- ❑ Narcotics: No other ingestion.
- ❑ Doctor: Consult with PMD regarding disposition after work-up.
- ❑ Social history: Lives with parents.

40.5 Secondary Survey:

- ❑ General: Healthy appearing, active child.
- ❑ Skin: Normal.
- ❑ HEENT: Oropharynx clear, pink, moist, no drooling.
- ❑ Neck: No stridor, supple.
- ❑ Chest: No use of accessory muscles.
- ❑ Lungs: Clear, equal breath sounds.
- ❑ Heart: RRR, no murmurs.
- ❑ Abdomen: Normal bowel sounds, no tenderness, no distention, no masses, no organomegaly.
- ❑ Perineum/GU: Normal.
- ❑ Rectal: Deferred.
- ❑ Back: Normal.
- ❑ Extremities: Normal.
- ❑ Neuro: Active, alert, normal exam.

40.6 Laboratory:

- ❑ None indicated.

40.7 X-rays:

- ❑ CXR: Normal X-ray, no foreign bodies, normal lung fields.
- ❑ Abdomen X-ray: Opaque disc detected in the stomach. Object appears intact. Remainder of abdomen is normal.

40.8 Special Tests:

- ❑ None indicated.

40.9 Critical Actions:

- ❑ Obtain accurate history of type and time of ingestion as well as history of any vomiting or respiratory distress.
- ❑ Avoid inducing vomiting.
- ❑ Obtain X-ray to determine the position of the battery and if the battery appears intact
- ❑ Explain follow-up to parents, i.e., observe for abdominal pain, distention, vomiting, strain stool to look for battery passage, and repeat X-ray to follow passage through GI tract. Consult with PMD to arrange follow-up X-ray.

40.10 Pearls:

❑❑ **Name the materials contained in disc batteries.**

Disc, or button, batteries may contain salts of metals, including zinc, cadmium, mercury, silver, nickel, and lithium as well as concentrated alkaline media, usually potassium or sodium hydroxide.

❑❑ **What are the potential complications of disc battery ingestion?**

Complications include obstruction, aspiration, heavy metal absorption, and perforation. Lodged batteries may lead to pressure necrosis, liquefaction, necrosis if leakage of contents occurs, or electrical injury through conduction to tissues. Most batteries pass uneventfully in two to three days.

❑❑ **Name possible interventions for a battery lodged in the esophagus.**

Glucagon, nitrates, or benzodiazepines may be useful in relaxing esophageal tone, allowing the battery to pass into the stomach.

CASE 41 (Cyanide Poisoning)

Examiner

A laboratory worker is brought to the ED after suddenly collapsing while at lunch. Colleagues know of no ingestion or medical conditions.

The physician is presented with a comatose patient who is bradycardic and is breathing agonally. He does not have a palpable blood pressure. The physician must secure the ABCs, administer dextrose, Narcan, and thiamine, and obtain appropriate laboratory data/studies in an attempt to discover the etiology of the patient's moribund state.

While working on the patient, a medical student, who worked in a laboratory, recognizes the aroma of bitter almonds associated with cyanide. Patient improves after treatment. The physician then initiates specific treatment for cyanide poisoning and arranges for ICU admission. Further questioning of the patient's colleagues reveals that the he had appeared depressed recently. They report he had access to numerous chemicals, including cyanide.

41.1 Introduction:

Vitals Signs are: BP non-palpable, P 58, R 8, T 98.0 °F.

41.2 Primary Survey:

- ❑ General: Comatose male with no evidence of trauma.
- ❑ Airway: Patent.
- ❑ Breathing: Agonal respirations, pulse oximetry 95% on room air.
- ❑ Circulation: Unable to obtain blood pressure, weak carotid pulse, delayed capillary refill.
- ❑ Disability: Pupils are equal and reactive, no response to deep pain.
- ❑ Exposure: Blisters in oropharynx, no other injury or lesions.
- ❑ Finger: Normal rectal tone, guaiac negative.

41.3 Management:

- ❑ Intubate patient and start O_2. Obtain ECG.
- ❑ Initiate fluid resuscitation via large bore IVs. Order laboratory work for blood count, electrolytes, glucose, renal function, toxicology, lactate, and blood gas analysis.
- ❑ Administer dextrose, Narcan, thiamine.

A medical student who is working in the adjacent area reports he smells a bitter almond odor, associated with cyanide, emanating from the comatose patient. Management now includes:

- ❑ Administer sodium nitrite, 300 mg, followed by sodium thiosulfate, 12.5 g, contained in the Lilly Cyanide Antidote Kit.
- ❑ Lavage patient and administer charcoal.
- ❑ Arrange admission to the ICU.

41.4 History:

- ❑ Allergies: Unknown.
- ❑ Medications: Unknown.
- ❑ PMH: None.
- ❑ Last meal: Ate recently.
- ❑ Events: Colleagues report that patient has appeared depressed recently and collapsed suddenly at lunch, while sitting in chair. They report he had access to numerous chemicals, including cyanide.
- ❑ Family: Unknown.
- ❑ Records: None.
- ❑ Immune: Unknown.
- ❑ EMTs: Confirm above history, no vomiting, no trauma.
- ❑ Narcotics: No known drug ingestion.
- ❑ Doctor: Unknown.
- ❑ Social history: No regular alcohol or cigarette use. Recently overlooked for promotion.

41.5 Secondary Survey:

- ❑ General: Comatose male, no cyanosis.
- ❑ Skin: Slightly cool, no track marks.
- ❑ HEENT: No evidence of trauma. Eyes are clear, retinal vessels appear cherry red. Blistering of oropharynx is evident.
- ❑ Neck: No step-off, supple, no stridor prior to intubation.

- ❑ Chest: No crepitus.
- ❑ Lungs: Clear, equal breath sounds bilaterally.
- ❑ Heart: RRR, bradycardic, no murmurs.
- ❑ Abdomen: Normal bowel sounds, non-distended, no masses.
- ❑ Perineum/GU: Normal male.
- ❑ Rectal: Normal tone, guaiac negative.
- ❑ Back: Normal.
- ❑ Extremities: Normal.
- ❑ Neuro: Comatose, pupils equal and reactive.

41.6 Laboratory:

- ❑ CBC: WBC 10.0, Hgb 14, Hct 40, Plt 232.
- ❑ Differential: Normal.
- ❑ Chemistry: Na 140, K 4.2, Cl 104, CO_2 8.
- ❑ BUN/Cr: 12/1.0.
- ❑ Glucose: 86.
- ❑ Ca/Mg: Normal.
- ❑ LFTs: Normal.
- ❑ Amylase/Lipase: Normal.
- ❑ PT/PTT: Normal.
- ❑ Cardiac enzymes: Normal.
- ❑ ABG: pH 7.11, pO_2 90, pCO_2 28, HCO_3 12.
- ❑ U/A: Normal.
- ❑ Lactate: 5.0.

41.7 X-rays:

- ❑ CXR: Clear lung fields, normal heart size.

41.8 Special Tests:

- ❑ ECG: Sinus bradycardia.

41.9 Critical Actions:

- ❑ Support ABCs, intubate the patient, and start O_2.
- ❑ Administer dextrose, Narcan, and thiamine.
- ❑ Administer antidote for cyanide poisoning.
- ❑ Lavage and administer charcoal.
- ❑ Admit to ICU with psychiatric evaluation when patient awakens.

41.10 Pearls:

❑❑ How does cyanide exert its effect?

Cyanide combines with the enzyme cytochrome oxidase. Binding with cytochrome oxidase disrupts the final step in mitochondrial oxidative phosphorylation preventing oxygen utilization and aerobic metabolism.

The body, therefore, cannot utilize oxygen and anaerobic metabolism ensues.

❑❑ **How does the antidote work?**

Nitrites induce formation of methemoglobin which avidly binds to cyanide. The cyanide is removed from the cytochrome oxidase thereby allowing oxidative phosphorylation to resume. Sodium thiosulfate acts as a sulfur donor to the body's rhodanese enzyme which transfers sulfur to cyanide converting it to thiocyanate. Thiocyanate is then renally excreted.

❑❑ **What are some sources of cyanide?**

Cyanide is widespread in various industries, including electroplating, fumigation, precious metal refining, photography, and chemical production. It is also found in acetonitrile, a solvent used as an artificial nail remover. Cyanide may also be released when various materials are burned, including silk, wool, synthetic rubber, polyurethane, and nitrocellulose.

CASE 42 (Isopropanol Poisoning)

Examiner

A patient is brought to the ED appearing severely intoxicated. On initial arrival of the paramedics, he complained of abdominal pain. There is no history of trauma. He had no visual complaints, but is hypotensive. The patient was found wandering in the street. There is no other history.

The physician should stabilize the patient's blood pressure, assess for etiology of altered mental status, and evaluate for abdominal pain.

The Paramedics subsequently report finding an empty bottle of rubbing alcohol at the site.

42.1 Introduction:

A disheveled, intoxicated male is brought to the ED after paramedics were called when he was found wandering in the street. There is no evidence of trauma.

Vital Signs are: BP 86/58, P 104, R 14, T 98.0 °F, O_2 sat = 95%.

42.2 Primary Survey:

- ❑ General: Disheveled, intoxicated male, faint odor of acetone.
- ❑ Airway: Patent.
- ❑ Breathing: Essentially clear, equal breath sounds.
- ❑ Circulation: Symmetric pulses, 2+ capillary refill, 86/58.
- ❑ Disability: Rouses with noxious stimuli, pupils equal and reactive.
- ❑ Exposure: No evidence of trauma.
- ❑ Finger: Normal rectal tone, guaiac + tan stool.

42.3 Management:

- ❑ Assess ABCs, bolus with IV fluid to treat hypotension.

- ❑ Obtain laboratory work for electrolytes, glucose, renal and hepatic function, CBC, coagulation studies, amylase, lipase, toxicology screen, ethanol level, osmolality, arterial blood gases, isopropanol level and urinalysis, hold type and screen.
- ❑ Administer dextrose, thiamine, and Narcan.
- ❑ Assess gag, insert airway as needed.
- ❑ Insert a NG tube to assess for upper GI bleeding.

42.4 History:

- ❑ Allergies: Unknown.
- ❑ Medications: Unknown.
- ❑ PMH: Unknown.
- ❑ Last meal: Unknown, probable recent alcohol ingestion.
- ❑ Family: None.
- ❑ Records: None.
- ❑ Immune: Unknown.
- ❑ EMTs: Paramedics find, when going through his belongings, an empty bottle of rubbing alcohol.
- ❑ Narcotics: Intoxicated, no response to Narcan.
- ❑ Doctor: None.
- ❑ Social history: Probably homeless, not known to ED staff.

42.5 Secondary Survey:

- ❑ General: Poor hygiene, intoxicated, BP increased with IVF.
- ❑ Skin: No track marks, ruddy.
- ❑ HEENT: No evidence of trauma, anicteric, oropharynx-slightly dry, poor dentition, normal nose, ears.
- ❑ Neck: No deformity, moving head freely on arrival, no meningismus, no nodes, no stridor, no JVD.
- ❑ Chest: No deformity or crepitus, gynecomastia.
- ❑ Lungs: Essentially clear, equal breath sounds.
- ❑ Heart: RRR, no murmurs, rubs, or gallops.
- ❑ Abdomen: Normal bowel sounds, tenderness to deep palpation in left upper quadrant, no peritoneal signs, no masses or organomegaly, non-distended
- ❑ Perineum/genital: Normal male.
- ❑ Rectal: As above.
- ❑ Back: No deformity.
- ❑ Extremities: No deformity, tobacco stains on fingers.
- ❑ Neuro: PERRLA, rouses to noxious stimuli, intoxicated, face symmetric, + gag, tongue midline, face symmetric, moves all extremities, DTRs are symmetric, toes are downgoing bilaterally.

42.6 Laboratory:

- ❑ CBC: WBC 10, Hgb 10, Hct 30, Plt 150.
- ❑ Differential: Normal.
- ❑ Chemistry: Na 140, K 3.8, Cl 105, CO_2 22.
- ❑ BUN/Cr: 10/1.0.
- ❑ Glucose: 60.
- ❑ Ca/Mg: 10/1.1.

- LFTs: LDH 290, AST 80, ALT 55, GGT 75, Alk Phos 40, Bili 1.3.
- Amylase/Lipase: 120/15.
- PT/PTT: 13/33.
- ABG: pH 7.4, pO_2 90, pCO_2 40, HCO_3 22.
- Osmolality: 360, osmol gap = 74.
- ETOH: 5 mg/dL.
- U/A: + ketones, - glucose.
- Isopropanol: Still pending.
- Toxicology: Negative.

42.7 X-rays:

- CXR: No acute infiltrate.

42.8 Special Tests:

- ECG: Normal sinus rhythm, normal intervals, no acute changes.
- NG aspirate: No blood or coffee ground material.

42.9 Critical Actions:

- Stabilize ABCs.
- Administer dextrose, Narcan, thiamine.
- Assess for cause of hypotension/altered mental status/abdominal pain. Eliminate possibility of acute GI bleed.
- Provide supportive care for isopropanol ingestion. Consider hemodialysis if patient has persistent hypotension or coma, or if isopropanol level is greater than 400 mg/dL.
- Admit to hospital; ICU if severe symptoms persist.

42.10 Pearls:

❑❑ What are the findings that may be associated with isopropanol intoxication?

CNS depression, prolonged intoxication, abdominal pain, hemorrhagic gastritis, hypotension secondary to peripheral vasodilatation, odor of acetone or rubbing alcohol, mild or no acidosis, ketonuria, ketonemia, elevated osmol gap, normal to low glucose.

❑❑ What is the major pathway for isopropanol metabolism?

It is metabolized by alcohol dehydrogenase to acetone in the liver.

CASE 43 (Triple)

Patient #1 (Subarachnoid Hemorrhage)

Examiner

This patient presents with a 3 day history of a severe headache that is partially relieved by acetaminophen with codeine. She is nauseated, photophobic, and has an abnormal mental status and positive funduscopic findings.

This patient is stable but the candidate should perform a complete exam, order a CT scan, and perform an LP once the CT comes back as negative. Since the patient remains stable throughout the case, Critical actions involve diagnosing a SAH by LP and instituting appropriate supportive therapy.

43.1 Introduction:

A 45 year old female presents with a complaint of headache

Vital Signs are: BP 198/120, P 88, R 18, T 100.1°F

43.2 Primary Survey:

- ❑ General: WN/WD female in moderate discomfort, sitting still with sun glasses on. She is in no respiratory distress.
- ❑ Airway: Intact
- ❑ Breathing: Intact
- ❑ Circulation: Intact
- ❑ Disability: GCS 15, PERRLA
- ❑ Exposure: No medic alert tags
- ❑ Finger: Deferred to secondary exam

43.3 Management:

- ❑ Start an IV, place on a monitor and pulse oximeter
- ❑ You may order appropriate diagnostic studies now or after the history and secondary survey.

43.4 History:

- ❑ Allergies: None
- ❑ Medications: None
- ❑ PMH: Migraine headaches controlled by acetaminophen and ibuprofen
- ❑ Last meal: 6 hours ago
- ❑ Events: 3 days ago she experienced and explosive headache lasting 1 hour with vomiting and photophobia. The intensity decreased but the headache remained. No complaint of fever, chills, or vomiting now. This headache is worse than her usual migraines. No history of trauma.
- ❑ Family : Non-contributory
- ❑ Records: None
- ❑ Immune: Up to date

- ❑ EMTs: Non-contributory
- ❑ Narcotics: No illicit drug use
- ❑ Doctor: No doctor
- ❑ Social history: Patient is sexually active. No alcohol or tobacco use.

43.5 <u>Secondary Survey:</u>

- ❑ General: Continues to complain of a headache, with VS unchanged.
- ❑ Skin: Normal
- ❑ HEENT: Small round hemorrhages seen near the optic nerve.
- ❑ Neck: Mild nuchal rigidity
- ❑ Chest: Normal
- ❑ Lungs: Normal
- ❑ Heart: Normal
- ❑ Abdomen: Normal
- ❑ Perineum/genital: Normal
- ❑ Rectal: Normal
- ❑ Back: Normal
- ❑ Extremities: Normal
- ❑ Neuro: Alert to person, place, but not time. CN II - XII intact, bilateral Babinskis present.

43.6 <u>Management:</u>

- ❑ Appropriate labs and x-rays can be ordered now.
- ❑ Allow candidate to send the patient to CT scan.
- ❑ You may treat the headache.

While the patient is in CT scan, the nurse tells you that another patient is in room #2.

Patient #2 (Human Bite)

Examiner

This patient presents with a human bite to the second metacarpal-phalangeal joint of the right hand. Do not tell the candidate it was a result of hitting someone's tooth, unless specifically asked. This patient requires admission but is resistant, have the candidate talk him in to it. He can be completely worked up and dispositioned without interruption. If the candidate takes too long, have the third patient arrive.

43.1 <u>Introduction</u>: (Patient #2)

A 21 year old male presents with a cut to his right hand.

Vital Signs are: BP 126/72, P 88, R 16, T 100.8° F

43.2 Primary Survey:

- General: Pleasant 21 year old right-handed male sitting upright on the cart, asking for his hand to be "fixed" so he can go.
- Airway: Intact
- Breathing: Normal
- Circulation: Normal
- Disability: Normal

43.3 History:

- Allergies: Penicillin.
- Medications: None.
- PMH: No significant illnesses or injuries. No past surgeries.
- Last meal: 1 hour ago
- Events: Patient states he was at a bar, had a "few too many drinks," and cut his hand. Only after specifically asking him how he did it, does he say that he punched someone in the mouth.
- Family: Older brother is in the waiting area
- Records: None
- Immune: Up to date
- Narcotics: No illicit drug use
- Doctor: None
- Social history: Smokes 2 packs per day, drinks 1 case of beer per week.

43.4 Secondary Survey:

- General: No change in vital signs
- Skin: Normal
- HEENT: Normal
- Neck: Normal
- Chest: Normal
- Lungs: Normal
- Heart: Normal
- Abdomen: Normal
- Perineum/genital: Normal
- Rectal: Deferred
- Back: Normal
- Extremities: A full-thickness laceration over the second MP joint with extension into the joint is present. There is normal sensation, motor function, and capillary refill to that digit. Red streaks are present and moderate swelling to the dorsum of the hand is noted.
- Neuro: Normal

43.5 Laboratory:

- CBC: WBC 19, Hgb 12.5, Hct 37.5, Plt 240,000
- Differential: Polys 80, Bands 38, Lymphs 15, Eos 2, Mono 3.
- Chemistries : Na 138, K 4.0, Cl 109, CO2 32.
- BUN/Cr: 10/0.9.

- ❑ Glucose: 90.
- ❑ PT/PTT: Normal.
- ❑ Blood cultures: Pending.
- ❑ Wound Culture: Pending.
- ❑ U/A: Normal.
- ❑ Drug screen: Negative.
- ❑ ETOH: 80.

43.6 X-Rays:

- ❑ Right hand: No fracture or foreign body.

43.7 Management:

- ❑ IV.
- ❑ Irrigate wound.
- ❑ Start antibiotics.
- ❑ Consult a hand surgeon.
- ❑ Convince patient to be admitted.

The nurse informs you the patient in room 3 is not breathing well.

Patient #3 (Anaphylactic Shock)

Examiner

This patient was stung by a bee and is in acute respiratory distress. Regardless of the treatment rendered, the patient deteriorates requiring airway management and pressor support. The candidate will be unable to intubate, thereby requiring a cricothyrotomy. Once the airway is established and appropriate therapy is given, the patient will stabilize. A family member arrives after the primary survey and initial management.

43.1 Introduction:

A 32 year old male presents via ambulance in respiratory distress with a rash.

Vital Signs are: BP 80/P, P 124, R 40, T 98.8° F.

43.2 Primary Survey:

- ❑ General: 32 year old male in acute respiratory distress.
- ❑ Airway: Significant oral angioedema, patient continually grabs his throat, drooling.
- ❑ Breathing: Diminished breath sounds in both bases with wheezing in the upper fields.
- ❑ Circulation: Capillary refill is delayed, peripheral pulses are weak.
- ❑ Disability: GCS 15, PERRLA
- ❑ Exposure: Medic-alert tag indicates allergic to bee stings.
- ❑ Finger: Deferred

43.3 Management:

- ❑ IV.
- ❑ Monitor.
- ❑ Albuterol 2.5 mg per nebulizer.
- ❑ Epinephrine 0.3 mL (1:1000) subcutaneously x 3, 15 minutes apart.
- ❑ 1 liter bolus of .9% NS.
- ❑ Solumedrol 125 mg IV.
- ❑ Benadryl 50 mg IV.
- ❑ H2 blocker IV.
- ❑ Tetanus prophylaxis.

43.4 Primary Survey (recheck)

- ❑ Patient is still in respiratory distress, requires rapid sequence intubation. Endotracheal intubation is unsuccessful, requiring a cricothyrotomy. Have the candidate describe the procedure.

43.5 History:

The patient is unable to give a history, the EMTs are gone, but the patient's wife is in the waiting room.

- ❑ Allergies: Bee stings (last bee sting caused a mild case of wheezing and a rash), and Sulfa.

- ❑ Medications: None.
- ❑ PMH: No illnesses or injuries. No surgeries.
- ❑ Last meal: Unknown.
- ❑ Events: Wife states per husband was working in the garden when she heard him call too her. When she arrived he was lying on the ground, unable to speak, in respiratory distress.
- ❑ Family: Non-contributory.
- ❑ Records: None.
- ❑ Immune: Last tetanus 15 years ago.
- ❑ EMTs: Gone.
- ❑ Narcotics: None.
- ❑ Doctor: None.
- ❑ Social history: No alcohol or tobacco use.

43.6 Secondary Survey:

- ❑ General: Patient is paralyzed, being ventilated on 100% FiO2.
- ❑ Skin: Raised wheels, diffuse distribution.
- ❑ HEENT: Clear rhinorrhea, eye lid edema, chemosis, tongue and uvular swelling.
- ❑ Neck: Urticaria.
- ❑ Chest: Urticaria.
- ❑ Lungs: Wheezing present but louder than before.
- ❑ Heart: Rapid rate, no murmur
- ❑ Abdomen: Normal.
- ❑ Perineum/genital: Normal.
- ❑ Rectal: Normal.

- ❑ Back: Urticaria
- ❑ Extremities: After fluid bolus capillary refill is < 2 seconds, pulses equal and stronger.
- ❑ Neuro: Patient paralyzed.

43.7 Laboratory:

- ❑ CBC: WBC 21, Hgb 15, Hct 45, Plt 300,000.
- ❑ Differential: Polys 65, Bands 8, Lymphs 10, Eos 20, Mono 5.
- ❑ Chemistries: Na 138, K 4.5, Cl 112, CO2 24.
- ❑ BUN/Cr: 9/1.0.
- ❑ Glucose: 138.
- ❑ Ca/Mg: Normal.
- ❑ LFTs: Normal.
- ❑ Amylase/Lipase: Normal.
- ❑ PT/PTT: Normal.
- ❑ Cardiac enzymes: Normal.
- ❑ ABG: pH 7.45, pO2 360, pCO2 27, HCO3 25.
- ❑ U/A: Normal.

43.8 X-Rays:

- ❑ CXR: No pulmonary edema, cric tube in place.

43.9 Special Tests:

- ❑ ECG: Sinus tachycardia.

43.10 Management:

- ❑ The patient's vital signs stabilize, Contact the ICU physician on call for admission.

Patient #1 returns from the CT scan with the headache still present and vital signs and neurologic status unchanged.

Patient #1

43.1 Laboratory:

- ❑ CBC: WBC 12, Hgb 13.2, Hct 39.6, Plt 185,000
- ❑ Chemistries: Na 125, K 3.8, Cl 108, CO2 24
- ❑ BUN/Cr: 15/1.0
- ❑ Glucose: 140
- ❑ Ca/Mg: Normal
- ❑ LFTs: Normal
- ❑ Amylase/Lipase: Normal
- ❑ PT/PTT: Normal
- ❑ Cardiac enzymes: Normal
- ❑ ABG: pH 7.48, pO2 98, pCO2 27, HCO3 23, (room air)
- ❑ Blood cultures: Pending

- ❑ U/A: Normal
- ❑ Drug screen: Negative
- ❑ ETOH: Negative

43.2 X-Rays:

- ❑ CXR: Normal
- ❑ CT head: Normal

43.3 Special Tests:

- ❑ ECG: Non-specific ST-T wave abnormalities
- ❑ Spinal Tap: Opening pressure 200, Protein 600, glucose normal, RBCs 100,000, WBCs 500, Appearance xanthochromia, Gram's stain negative, Latex pending.

43.4 Management:

- ❑ Call a neurosurgeon.
- ❑ Call the radiologist to set up cerebral angiography.
- ❑ Elevate the head of the bed to 30°.
- ❑ Start Nitroprusside to lower the diastolic below 100 mm Hg.
- ❑ Give phenytoin (15 - 20 mg/kg loading dose), for seizure prophylaxis.
- ❑ Use antiemetic if vomiting continues.
- ❑ Start nimodipine to decrease the risk of cerebral vasospasm.
- ❑ Call a Neurosurgeon.
- ❑ Admit to the ICU.
- ❑ Perform LP when CT is negative.
- ❑ Institute head injury precautions.
- ❑ Decrease the diastolic blood pressure below 100 mm Hg.

43.5 Pearls (Patient #1)

❑❑ When does xanthochromia first appear in the cerebral spinal fluid?

4 to 6 hours after the initial hemorrhage.

❑❑ What is the cause of hyponatremia seen in some patients with a subarachnoid hemorrhage?

Inappropriate secretion of antidiuretic hormone or excessive release of natriuretic peptides.

❑❑ What are the CNS complications commonly seen in patients surviving an initial subarachnoid hemorrhage?

Rebleeding, vasospasm, and acute hydrocephalus.

Patient #2 (Human Bite)

43.1 Critical Actions:

- ❑ Admit.
- ❑ Consult a hand surgeon.
- ❑ Start IV antibiotics.
- ❑ Do not suture the wound.
- ❑ Irrigate wound.

43.2 Pearls (Patient #2)

❑❑ What are the indications for admission in a patient with a human bite?

Lymphangitis, adenopathy, symptoms of systemic infection, suspected joint, tendon, or bone infection, and patients that are immunocompromised or have vascular insufficiency.

❑❑ What are the most common bacteria found in infected human bite wounds?

Staphylococcus aureus and streptococcus species.

Patient #3 (Anaphylactic Shock)

43.1 Critical Actions:

- ❑ Epinephrine.
- ❑ Early airway when the epi doesn't work.
- ❑ Describe how to perform a cricothyrotomy.
- ❑ Steroids.
- ❑ Fluid bolus to correct hypotension.
- ❑ ICU admission.
- ❑ Tetanus prophylaxis

43.2 Pearls (Patient #3)

❑❑ What is the most common cause of life-threatening anaphylaxis?

Penicillin.

❑❑ What is the most common cause of death from anaphylaxis?

Laryngeal edema resulting in upper airway obstruction.

CASE 44 (Mesenteric Ischemia)

Examiner

This is a difficult case but the patient has many risk factors for mesenteric ischemia/occlusion. Have the candidate call and talk with the radiologist and the surgeon. The radiologist will be resistant to performing an abdominal angiogram unless the candidate presents the risk factors, lab findings and ECG indicating the potential for this disorder. The surgeon will accept the consult without complaint. Continue to point out how much pain the patient has despite the paucity of physical findings.

44.1 Introduction:

An 80 year old male presents via ambulance from a retirement home, with a complaint of abdominal pain.

Vital signs are: BP 100/70, P 92, (irregular only if asked), R 26, T 100.6°F.

44.2 Primary Survey:

- ❑ General: Slender, cachectic appearing male, pale, diaphoretic, sitting upright holding his abdomen, in severe pain.
- ❑ Airway: Intact.
- ❑ Breathing: Normal.
- ❑ Circulation: Capillary refill > 2 seconds, weak peripheral pulses.
- ❑ Disability: Normal.
- ❑ Exposure: Medic alert tag stating "Heart disease."
- ❑ Finger: Deferred to secondary survey

44.3 Management:

- ❑ IV.
- ❑ O2.
- ❑ Pulse oximeter.
- ❑ Cardiac monitor.
- ❑ May order appropriate labs and x-rays now.

44.4 History:

- ❑ Allergies: None.
- ❑ Medications: Furosemide 40 mg bid.
  Digoxin 0.125 mg qd
  Glipizide 5 mg qd
  Nitroglycerine SL prn chest pain
  Aspirin 160 mg qd
  Mylanta 30 cc ac + hs
- ❑ PMH: Cardiac Angioplasty 1994
  Carotid endarterectomy 1995
  NIDDM
  S/P myocardial infarction 1990, 1994
- ❑ Last meal: 1 hour ago.

- ❑ Events: This 80 year old patient began complaining of pain shortly after eating breakfast. The pain is crampy, diffuse, nonradiating, and increasing in intensity. The patient complains of nausea, no vomiting, diarrhea, fever, chills, or urinary complaints. Last bowel movement was 10 hours ago and it was normal. A 20 pound weight loss has been noted over the past 4 months.
- ❑ Family: Father, mother, and brother all died from heart disease.
- ❑ Records: None.
- ❑ Immune: "Flu" shot this year.
- ❑ EMTs: Left department.
- ❑ Doctor: Dr. Internist.
- ❑ Social history: Retired accountant, smokes 1/2 pack per day for 40 years, quit 15 years ago. No alcohol use.

44.5 Secondary Survey:

- ❑ General: Patient appears very uncomfortable complaining of increasing pain.
- ❑ Skin: Pale, moist, no rash or petechiae.
- ❑ HEENT: Arcus senilis, EOM-I.
- ❑ Neck: Normal.
- ❑ Chest: Normal.
- ❑ Lungs: Normal.
- ❑ Heart: Irregular rhythm, loud III/VI systolic ejection murmur, laterally displaced PMI.
- ❑ Abdomen: Soft, mild diffuse tenderness to palpation. No rebound or guarding. Bowel sounds are present but diminished. No pulsatile mass or organomegaly.
- ❑ Perineum/genital: Normal.
- ❑ Rectal: Slightly enlarged, firm prostate, brown stool, hemoccult positive.
- ❑ Back: Normal.
- ❑ Extremities: Femoral pulses are strong but peripheral pulses are weak in the lower extremities. Pretibial edema, no calf tenderness, negative Homan's sign.
- ❑ Neuro: Intact.

44.6 Laboratory:

- ❑ CBC: WBC 14.2, Hgb 16.6, Hct 50, Plt 240,000.
- ❑ Differential: Polys 68, Bands 29, Lymphs 18,, Eos 1, Mono 0.
- ❑ Chemistries: Na 150, K 4.0, Cl 112, CO2 15.
- ❑ BUN/Cr: 60/2.5.
- ❑ Glucose: 201.
- ❑ Ca/Mg: 10/2.1.
- ❑ LFTs: Normal.
- ❑ Amylase/Lipase: 150/15.
- ❑ PT/PTT: 13.5/36.
- ❑ Cardiac enzymes: Normal.
- ❑ ABG: pH 7.10 pO2 94, pCO2 40, HCO3 13.
- ❑ Blood cultures: Pending.
- ❑ Digoxin: 1.7 (0.8 - 2.1).
- ❑ Phosphorus 7.0 (3 - 4.5).
- ❑ Type & Cross: Pending.
- ❑ U/A: Ketones 2+, all other values are negative.

44.7 X-Rays:

- ❑ CXR: Normal
- ❑ Abdominal series: Normal.

44.8 Special Tests:

- ❑ ECG: Atrial fibrillation
- ❑ Aortic and mesenteric angiography: Vasoconstriction in the superior mesenteric artery.
- ❑ CT abdomen: Negative.

44.9 Management:

- ❑ Consult interventional radiologist.
- ❑ Consult surgeon.
- ❑ 2 large bore IVs.
- ❑ Small doses of IV pain medication.
- ❑ Foley catheter for I & O measurements.
- ❑ Nasogastric tube.

44.10 Critical Actions:

- ❑ Pain medication.
- ❑ IV, O2, monitor.
- ❑ Recognize the diagnosis from the presence of all the risk factors.
- ❑ Consult a radiologist.
- ❑ Consult a surgeon.
- ❑ Obtain an angiogram
- ❑ Use normal saline and not vasopressors for resuscitation.

44.10 Pearls

❑❑ What are the risk factors for mesenteric ischemia?

Advanced age, advanced cardiovascular disease, history of thromboembolic events, concurrent medication with digoxin and a diuretic, and atrial fibrillation.

❑❑ What are the plain radiographic findings seen in mesenteric ischemia?

Thumb-printing of the intestinal mucosa, gas in the intestinal wall, gas in the portal venous system, and an ileus pattern. In the majority of cases, the films will be normal or have nonspecific findings.

❑❑ What is the gold standard test for diagnosing mesenteric ischemia/infarct?

Mesenteric angiography.

CASE 45 (Hemophilia C)

Examiner

A 12 year old female presents after a fall with acute pain to the right knee and severe swelling. She has a known history of hemophilia C. The case should demonstrate the candidate's ability to treat hemophilia as well as evaluate a severe knee injury and patellar dislocation.

45.1 Introduction:

A 12 year old female is brought to the ED by her mother with a complaint of severe right knee pain after she fell down the steps. The mother indicates the child has hemophilia C.

Vital signs are: BP 110/80, P 80, R 20, T 98.6 °F

45.2 Primary Survey:

- ❑ General impression: Child in severe pain with very swollen right knee.
- ❑ Airway: Normal.
- ❑ Breathing: Normal.
- ❑ Circulation: Normal.
- ❑ Disability: Normal.
- ❑ Exposure: No signs of trauma other than right knee, hemophilia medic alert tag.
- ❑ Finger: Not indicated.

45.3 Management:

- ❑ Start IV.
- ❒ Administer appropriate IV pain medicine (avoid a NSAID or aspirin)
- ❒ Order CBC, Factor XIII and XI levels, and von Willebrand factor level, PT, PTT, and Thrombin time.
- ❒ Order x-ray of both knees.
- ❒ Order ice packs to the right knee.
- ❒ Order Fresh Frozen Plasma 15-20 mL/kg IV loading dose.

45.4 History:

- ❑ Allergies: None.
- ❑ Medications: None.
- ❑ PMH: No significant illnesses or major injuries.
- ❑ Last meal: 2 hours ago.
- ❑ Family: Mother is present to answer questions. Family history is not applicable as child is adopted. The patient's hematologist is available for more information if needed.
- ❑ Records: None.
- ❑ Immune: Up to date.
- ❑ Doctor: Dr. Hematologist.

45.5 Secondary Survey:

- ❑ General: Awake and alert in severe pain.
- ❑ Skin: Normal.
- ❑ HEENT: Normal.
- ❑ Neck: Supple, no nodes.
- ❑ Chest: Normal.
- ❑ Lungs: Clear to auscultation.
- ❑ Heart: Normal.
- ❑ Abdomen: Normal.
- ❑ Perineum/GU: Normal.
- ❑ Rectal: Not indicated.
- ❑ Back: Normal.
- ❑ Extremities: Normal and equal pulses. Right knee severe swelling and pain with any attempt at movement.
- ❑ Neuro: Normal.

45.6 Laboratory:

- ❑ CBC: Normal.
- ❑ Chemistry: Normal.
- ❑ BUN/Cr: Normal.
- ❑ Glucose: Normal.
- ❑ PT Normal, PTT Moderately elevated, Thrombin Time Normal.
- ❑ U/A: Normal.
- ❑ Factor levels: Pending.

45.7 X-rays:

- ❑ Knee: Right patella dislocated.

45.8 Critical Actions:

- ❑ Appropriate early pain relief.
- ❑ Administer FFP.
- ❑ Relocate dislocated patella and immobilize knee.
- ❑ Consult hematologist and orthopedic surgeon.
- ❑ Admit for 23 observation and additional doses of FFP as needed.

45.9 Pearls:

❑❑ What concerns do you have with FFP administration?

Volume overloading, hypersensitivity reactions, and transmission of infection from plasma products.

❑❑ Why should you double check the current treatment recommendations before administering FFP?

In Europe Factor XI concentrates are available. Soon they should be available in the United States.

CASE 46 (Lithium Toxicity)

Examiner

A thirty-four year old female patient presents with nausea, vomiting, diarrhea, weakness, and confusion. She has a tremor and had a first time seizure witnessed by her husband. A detailed history taken from her husband will reveal that she has a history of manic-depression and takes lithium. He does not think that she is taking more than her usual dose. She is also taking tetracycline for her chronic acne and recently started taking Advil® for muscle cramps and pain from long distance running. The candidate should request a detailed neurologic examination which will reveal muscle fasciculations, choreoathetosis, hyperreflexia, clonus, and opisthotonos.

As part of the work-up, the candidate should order a lithium level, however, this test should be slow to return and the lab should call and indicate the lithium level will have to be sent to another institution due to equipment malfunction. The lab studies will reveal a low serum sodium and decreased anion gap. EKG will show depressed ST segments and T wave inversion. From the history of taking tetracycline and Advil® which increase lithium levels, long distance running which may cause dehydration and low sodium, and a neurologic exam, lab and EKG changes consistent with lithium toxicity, the student should be able to make the diagnose and began therapy.

46.1 Introduction:

A 34-year-old female presents from home complaining of nausea, vomiting, diarrhea, and weakness. Symptoms have gotten worse over the last three days.

Vital Signs are: BP 100/70, P 110, R 20, T 99.0 °F.

46.2 Primary Survey:

- ❑ General: The patient is a trim female actively vomiting. The patient is sitting on a commode and the room is odiferous. She is anxious, awake, pale, and in obvious discomfort. She is a very poor historian, however, her husband, with prompting, reports a history of confusion and a seizure and symptoms getting worse over the last three days. With further questioning, he provides a history or running a 10K race five days ago and taking Advil for a muscle pull. She also takes tetracycline for her acne.
- ❑ Airway: Intact.
- ❑ Breathing: Slightly increased rate.
- ❑ Circulation: Rapid pulse.
- ❑ Disability: Negative.
- ❑ Exposure: No obvious injuries.
- ❑ Finger: Normal rectal, heme negative.

46.3 Management:

- ❑ Determine that patient is at risk for lithium toxicity.
- ❑ Start IV with NS bolus.
- ❑ Place on O_2, pulse oximeter, and cardiac monitor.
- ❑ Perform frequent VS.
- ❑ Offer to change commode.

- ❑ Order screening labs, lithium level, ECG, and possibly head CT.

46.4 History:

- ❑ Allergies: None.
- ❑ Medications: Lithium, Advil®, and Tetracycline, dose taken is not known. The husband thinks she take her lithium several times a day and that "slow release" lithium was tried in the past and did not work.
- ❑ PMH: Well controlled manic-depression.
- ❑ Last meal: Yesterday evening.
- ❑ Family: Husband is present for information. Family doctor is available. Both of the patient's parents died from cancer in their 70's.
- ❑ Records: Available upon request.
- ❑ Immune: Up to date.
- ❑ Narcotics: No illicit drug use.
- ❑ Doctor: Consultants are available.
- ❑ Social history: No alcohol or tobacco use. Lives with his husband. Occupation is a psychologist.

46.5 Secondary Survey:

- ❑ General: Continues to be anxious, uncomfortable, vomiting, and had multiple episodes of diarrhea.
- ❑ Skin: Pale, dry.
- ❑ HEENT: Mucous membranes dry.
- ❑ Neck: Normal.
- ❑ Chest: Nontender.
- ❑ Lungs: Clear.
- ❑ Heart: Tachy and regular.
- ❑ Abdomen: Bowel sounds are normal and no pain to palpation is noted.
- ❑ Perineum/GU: Normal.
- ❑ Rectal: Normal.
- ❑ Back: No CVA tenderness.
- ❑ Extremity: Slow capillary refill, pulses are equal.
- ❑ Neuro: Severe tremor, muscle fasciculations and symmetrical weakness, choreoathetosis, hyperreflexia, clonus, and opisthotonos. Confusion.

46.6 Laboratory:

- ❑ CBC: Normal.
- ❑ Chemistry: Na 124, K 3.5, Cl 98, CO_2 20.
- ❑ BUN/Cr: 28/1.5.
- ❑ Glucose: Normal.
- ❑ Ca/Mg: Normal.
- ❑ LFTs: Normal.
- ❑ Amylase/Lipase: Normal.
- ❑ Cardiac Enzymes: Normal.
- ❑ U/A: Normal.
- ❑ Stool: Guic negative.
- ❑ Lithium: Comes back after full work-up and admit to ICU at a level of 4.4 mEq/L.

46.7 X-rays:

- ❑ Chest X-ray: Normal.
- ❑ CT Head: Normal.

46.8 Special Tests:

- ❑ ECG: Depressed ST segments and T wave inversion.

46.9 Critical Actions:

- ❑ Elicit a history from husband of taking lithium, Advil®, tetracycline.
- ❑ Give a normal saline bolus and repeat.
- ❑ O2 and Monitor.
- ❑ Admit to ICU.
- ❑ Arrange hemodialysis for probably chronic lithium toxicity.
- ❑ Consult renal and internal medicine physicians.
- ❑ Do not give activated charcoal as it is NOT effective in treating acute or chronic lithium ingestion and the patient has an altered level of consciousness.

46.10 Pearls:

❑❑ What electrolyte and EKG findings are associated with lithium toxicity?

Lithium toxicity is one of the few clinical entities that may be associated with a decrease in the anion gap. Both Na and K may be low. Chronic lithium toxicity is frequently associated with depressed ST segments and T wave inversion, in acute toxicity, complete heart block may occur.

❑❑ When should dialysis be used in lithium toxicity?

Guidelines for hemodialysis are controversial in patients with acute intoxication but it is generally recommended for high lithum levels despite minor symptoms. Change in mental status increases the need for hemodialysis. Consider dialysis in patients with chronic toxicity and serum lithium concentrations higher than 4 mEq/L and in unstable chronic patients with lithium levels higher than 2.5 mEq/L.

CASE 47 (Anthrax Infection)

Examiner

This case tests the candidate's ability to recognize Anthrax infection as well as activate reasonable exposure precautions. The patient is a psychotic microbiologist who arrives with respiratory distress, advanced active disease and initially no reported history of exposure. As the case develops, he has physical findings highly suggestive of anthrax and the substance is on his clothes. Shortly after the emergency physician questions the patient about possible exposure to something at work, the patient bolts from the treatment room and in the course of being tackled by security in the waiting room, dumps a plastic sac containing white powder into the air. He has exposed nine individuals in the waiting room, the triage nurse, the patient care nurse, two security officers, and the candidate.

After the incident, candidate must suspect the diagnosis, confront the patient, treat the patient, treat the exposure within the department, and contact the appropriate physicians, hazemat team and law enforcement agency to assist with management of the patient and exposure, and CDC.

47.1 Introduction:

A 44 year old male presents with fever, nonproductive cough, malaise, shortness of breath, and vomiting. Patient is very evasive but admits to symptoms getting worse over the last few days. Patient denies tobacco use or history of asthma. He says he is a microbiologist, knows what he has, and requests Cipro®.

Vital Signs are: BP 120/80, P 100, R 24, T 102.2° F

47.2 Primary Survey:

- ❑ General: 44 year old male, who appears in moderate respiratory distress.
- ❑ Airway: Intact.
- ❑ Breathing: Tachypneic with retractions.
- ❑ Circulation: Capillary refill 4 seconds.
- ❑ Disability: Pupils normal.
- ❑ Exposure: Patient has all his clothes on and did not put on the hospital gown provided.

47.3 Management:

- ❑ Initiate IV rehydration with NS.
- ❑ Order appropriate labs, including blood and urine cultures, and chest x-ray.
- ❑ Place on O_2, cardiac monitor, and pulse oximeter.

47.4 History:

- ❑ Allergies: None.
- ❑ Medications: None.
- ❑ PMH: None.
- ❑ Last meal: 24 hours ago.
- ❑ Family: None.
- ❑ Records: None.
- ❑ Immune: Up to date.
- ❑ Doctor: None.
- ❑ Social: Anxious, admits to being fired from job teaching microbiology at a local college.

47.5 Secondary Survey:

- ❑ General: Anxious and hyper alert.
- ❑ Skin: Normal.
- ❑ HEENT: Sclera nonicteric, PERRL, oral mucosa dry, pharynx normal, TMs normal.
- ❑ Neck: Supple, no meningeal signs.
- ❑ Chest: Nontender to palpation.
- ❑ Lungs: Crackles with basilar consolidation.
- ❑ Heart: Tachy, no murmur.

- ❑ Abdomen: Non-tender, no masses, no organomegaly.
- ❑ Perineum/GU: Normal.
- ❑ Rectal: Heme negative.
- ❑ Back: Normal.
- ❑ Extremities: Delayed capillary refill.
- ❑ Neuro: No focal deficits, normal DTRs.
- ❑ Lymphatic: Multiple sites of shoddy lymph nodes.

47.6 Laboratory:

- ❑ CBC: WBC 14, Hgb 14.1, Hct 43, Plt 225,000.
- ❑ Chemistry: Na 132, K 4.0, Cl 80, CO_2 13.
- ❑ BUN/Cr: 26/0.9.
- ❑ Glucose: 130.
- ❑ Ca/Mg: Normal.
- ❑ LFTs: Normal.
- ❑ PT/PTT: Normal.
- ❑ Pulse Ox: 91%.
- ❑ ABG: pH 7.27, pO_2 93, pCO_2 30, HCO_3 14.
- ❑ Cultures: Blood/urine/ pending.
- ❑ Gram Stain: Gram positive rods.
- ❑ U/A: RBC 0-2, WBC 0-2, Ketones 2+, Specific gravity 1.025.

47.7 X-rays:

- ❑ CXR: Wide mediastinum with paratracheal and hilar fullness and bibasilar pleural effusions.

47.8 Critical Actions:

- ❑ Start fluid bolus therapy with 0.9 NS or LR.
- ❑ Restrain patient or appropriate security in ED.
- ❑ Re-evaluation of VS following each bolus.
- ❑ Admit to ICU in isolation with security detail.
- ❑ Start IV ciprofloxin 400 mgs q12 hours.
- ❑ Consult infectious disease and internal medicine physicians.
- ❑ Call hazemat emergency and close down emergency department and waiting room for decontamination.
- ❑ All exposed should be hosed down and should scrub with soap and water.
- ❑ All exposed should be started on ciprofloxin 500 mg bid for 60 days.
- ❑ Call CDC to report high-probability exposure and obtain access to vaccine.
- ❑ Call local authorities.

47.9 Pearls:

❑❑ What is the key lab finding in patients with anthrax?

Gram positive rods.

❑❑ **What are the expected chest x-ray findings in inhalational anthrax?**

Prominent mediastinum with hilar adenopathy and pleural effusions.

CASE 48 (Acute Airway Obstruction, Cricothyroidotomy)

Examiner

An eleven-year old male presents acutely with impending airway obstruction. Paramedics indicate he was riding his bicycle and according to his sister, he apparently struck a small thin wire stretched across a bridge in the neck. Paramedics arrive in the ED and indicate they have attempted to intubate the patient but have been unable to do so with three attempts. O2 saturation has been dropping and on arrival is 91%. The paramedic screams they are having increasing difficulty bagging the patient as they wheel the patient into the trauma room.

When the candidate enters the room, the nurse says the patient is worse and the saturation has dropped to 85%. The patient has very course weak respirations. Any attempt at intubation fails. The candidate should perform a needle cricothyroidomy, appropriate x-rays, and ENT consultation. A cricothyroidotomy is not recommended in patients under 12 and should the candidate attempt this, the patient should develop severe hemorrhage, inability to access the airway, and the patient should expire.

48.1 Introduction:

A 11 year old male is brought to the ED by paramedics in severe respiratory distress. According to the paramedics, he sustained a neck injury from hitting a wire while riding his bicycle.

Vital Signs are: BP 90/60, P 130, R 30, T 98.6

48.2 Primary Survey:

- ❑ General: 11 year old in severe respiratory distress with stridor and shallow rapid respirations.
- ❑ Airway: Nearly impossible to bag.
- ❑ Breathing: Rapid.
- ❑ Circulation: Normal.
- ❑ Disability: Minimally responsive.
- ❑ Exposure: Large red mark in anterior neck, with extensive soft tissue swelling, and subcutaneous air. No C-collar has been placed on the patient.

48.3 Management:

- ❑ Ask the paramedics to maintain in-line traction and stabilize the neck.
- ❑ Attempt immediate intubation (which fails).
- ❑ Perform needle cricothyroidotomy (ask candidate to describe the procedure in detail).
- ❑ Place on 100% O_2 with intermittent jet insuflation and have assistant hold the catheter in place at all times.
- ❑ Cardiac monitor and pulse oximeter.
- ❑ Order portable C-spine and chest x-ray.

- ❑ Call anesthesiology and ENT on call for immediate surgery.

48.4 History:

- ❑ Allergies: Unknown.
- ❑ Medication: Unknown .
- ❑ PMH: Unknown.
- ❑ Last meal : 1 hour ago.
- ❑ Family: Unknown, cannot reach mother, eight year old sister is crying and cannot be calmed.
- ❑ Records: None.
- ❑ Immune: Unknown.
- ❑ Doctor: Dr. Pediatrician.
- ❑ Social: Unknown.

48.5 Secondary Survey:

- ❑ General: Improved after placement of needle cricothyroidotomy.
- ❑ Skin: Normal.
- ❑ HEENT: Normal.
- ❑ Neck: Red deep line across anterior neck with extensive soft tissue swelling.
- ❑ Chest: Normal.
- ❑ Lungs: Good breath sounds with insuflation.
- ❑ Heart: Normal.
- ❑ Abdomen: Normal.
- ❑ Perineum/GU: Normal.
- ❑ Rectal: Not indicated.
- ❑ Back: Normal.
- ❑ Extremities: Normal.
- ❑ Neuro: Normal.

48.6 Laboratory:

- ❑ CBC: Normal.
- ❑ Chemistry: Normal.
- ❑ BUN/Cr: Normal
- ❑ Glucose: Normal.
- ❑ PT/PTT: Normal.
- ❑ U/A: Normal.

48.7 X-rays:

- ❑ Neck: Extensive soft tissue swelling with fracture of hyoid bone.
- ❑ Chest: Chest x-ray normal.

48.8 Critical Actions:

- ❑ Attempt oral intubation.
- ❑ Perform needle cricothyroidotomy.

- ❑ C-spine precautions until cleared.
- ❑ Immediate consult of anesthesiology and ENT surgeons.
- ❑ Attempt to contact parents but send patient to OR even though parents cannot be reached.

48.9 Pearls:

❑❑ What is the minimum recommended age for surgical cricothyroidotomy?

12.

❑❑ What should always be continued until a surgical tracheostomy can be performed?

It is very important that a reliable operator continue to be present until another choice of airway is established, either tracheostomy or oro- or nasotracheal intubation.

REFERENCES

BOOKS:

Advanced Cardiac Life Support. Dallas: American Heart Association, 2001.

Advanced Trauma Life Support. Chicago: American College of Surgeons, 1997.

Anderson, J.E. Grant's Atlas of Anatomy (8th Ed.). Baltimore: Williams & Wilkins, 1983.

Bakerman, S. A B C'S of Interpretive Laboratory Data (2nd Ed.). Greenville: Interpretive Laboratory Data, Inc., 1984.

Berkow, R. The Merck Manual (17th Ed.). Rahway: Merck Sharp & Dohme Research Laboratories, 1999.

Bork, K. Diagnosis and Treatment of Common Skin Diseases (2nd Ed). Philadelphia: W.B. Saunders Company, 1999.

Dambro, M.R. Griffith's 5 Minute Clinical Consult. Williams and Wilkins, 1998.

DeGowin, E.L. Bedside Diagnostic Examination (7th Ed.). New York: Macmillan Publishing Co. Inc., 1999.

Fitzpatrick, T.B. Color Atlas and Synopsis of Clinical Dermatology (4th Ed.). New York: McGraw-Hill Publishing Company, 2000.

Harris, J.H. The Radiology of Emergency Medicine (4th Ed.). Baltimore: Lippincott, Williams and Wilkins, 2000.

Harrison, T.R. Principles of Internal Medicine (15th Ed.). New York: McGraw-Hill Book Company, 2001.

Harwood-Nuss, A. The Clinical Practice of Emergency Medicine (3rd Ed). Philadelphia: J.B. Lippincott Company, 2001.

Hoppenfeld, S. Physical Examination of the Spine and Extremities. Norwalk: Appleton-Century-Crofts, 1976.

Marriott, H.J.L. Practical Electrocardiography (10th Ed.). Baltimore: Lippincott, Williams and Wilkins, 2001.

Moore, K.L. Clinically Oriented Anatomy (4th Ed). Baltimore: Lippincott, Williams & Wilkins, 1999.

Perkins, E.S. An Atlas of Diseases of the Eye (3rd Ed.). London: Churchill Livingstone, 1986.

Physicians' Desk Reference. Oradell: Medical Economics Company Inc., 1999.

Plantz, SH. Emergency Medicine PreTest, Self-Assessment and Review, McGraw- Hill, 1990.

Plantz, S.H. & Adler, J.N. Emergency Medicine. Lippincott, Williams & Wilkins, 1998.

Plantz, S.H., Adler, J.N., et al., Emergency Medicine, eMedicine.com, Inc., 1999.

Plantz, S.H., Adler, J.N. & Collman, D. Emergency Medicine Pearls of Wisdom (6th Ed). Boston: Boston Medical Publishing, 1999.

Robbins, S.L. Pathologic Basis of Disease (6th Ed.). Philadelphia: W.B. Saunders Company, 1999.

Roberts. J.R. & Hedges, J.R. Clinical Procedures in Emergency Medicine (3rd Ed.). Philadelphia: W.B. Saunders Company, 1998

Rosen, P. Emergency Medicine Concepts and Clinical Practice (5th Ed.). St. Louis: Mosby , 2002.

Simon, R.R. Emergency Orthopedics The Extremities (3rd Ed.). Norwalk: Appleton & Lange, 1994.

Simon, R.R. Emergency Procedures and Techniques (3rd Ed.). Baltimore: Lippincott, Williams and Wilkins, 1999.

Slaby, F. Radiographic Anatomy. New York: John Wiley & Sons, 1990.

Squire, L.F. Fundamentals of Radiology (5th Ed.). Cambridge: Harvard University Press, 1997.

Stedman, T.L. Illustrated Stedman's Medical Dictionary (27th Ed.). Baltimore: Williams & Wilkins, 2000.

The Hand Examination and Diagnosis (2nd Ed.). London: Churchill Livingstone, 1983.

The Hand Primary Care of Common Problems (2nd Ed.). London: Churchill Livingstone, 1990.

Tintinalli, J.E. Emergency Medicine A Comprehensive Study Guide (5th Ed.). New York: McGraw-Hill, Inc., 1999.

Weinberg, S. Color Atlas of Pediatric Dermatology (2nd Ed.). New York: McGraw-Hill, 1990.

Weiner, H.L. Neurology for the House Officer (4th Ed.). Baltimore: Williams & Wilkins, 1989.

OTHER REVIEW BOOKS AVAILABLE FOR EXAM PREPARATION:

PHYSICIANS/PHYSICIAN ASSISTANTS:

PALS Pearls of Wisdom
Anesthesiology Pearls of Wisdom
Cardiology Pearls of Wisdom
Critical Care Pearls of Wisdom
Emergency Medicine Oral Pearls of Wisdom
Emergency Medicine Written Pearls of Wisdom
Family Practice Pearls of Wisdom
Gastroenterology Pearls of Wisdom
Internal Medicine Pearls of Wisdom
Neurology Pearls of Wisdom
Ob/Gyn Pearls of Wisdom
Ophthalmology Pearls of Wisdom
Otolaryngology Pearls of Wisdom
Pathology Pearls of Wisdom
Pediatrics Pearls of Wisdom
Emergency Pediatric Pearls of Wisdom
Podiatric Medicine Pearls of Wisdom
Psychiatry Pearls of Wisdom
Pulmonary Pearls of Wisdom
Sports Medicine Pearls of Wisdom
Surgery, General Pearls of Wisdom
Toxicology Pearls of Wisdom
Urology Pearls of Wisdom
Physician Assistant Pearls of Wisdom

NURSES/NURSE PRACTITIONERS:

Family Nurse Practitioner Pearls of Wisdom
Pediatric Nurse Practitioner Pearls of Wisdom
Critical Care Nursing Pearls of Wisdom
Emergency Nursing Pearls of Wisdom
Nursing NCLEX-RN Pearls of Wisdom
LPN Pearls of Wisdom

ALLIED HEALTH:

Medical Laboratory Technology Pearls of Wisdom
Pharmacy Pearls of Wisdom
The Poison Quiz Book Pearls of Wisdom
Paramedic Pearls of Wisdom
EMT- Intermediate Pearls of Wisdom
EMT- Basic Pearls of Wisdom

MEDICAL STUDENTS:

Internal Medicine Medical Student USMLE Parts II & III Pearls of Wisdom
Medical Student USMLE Parts II & III Pearls of Wisdom
Ob/Gyn Medical Student USMLE Parts II & III Pearls of Wisdom
Pathology Medical Student USMLE Part I Pearls of Wisdom
Pediatric Medical Student USMLE Parts II & III Pearls of Wisdom
General Surgery Medical Student USMLE Parts II & III Pearls of Wisdom
Anatomy Pearls of Wisdom
Medical Genetics Pearls of Wisdom
Microbiology Pearls of Wisdom
Pharmacology Pearls of Wisdom

BASIC SCIENCES:

MCAT Pearls of Wisdom
Chemistry, General Pearls of Wisdom
Organic Chemistry Pearls of Wisdom
Physics, General Pearls of Wisdom

- contraindications to thrombolytics
- Dosage of thrombolytics

- c̄ CP arrest in field:
  - ask for rhythm strip & direct resuscitation over radio